Introduction to
MEDICAL PRACTICE
MANAGEMENT

Deborah Montone and Michelle Lenzi

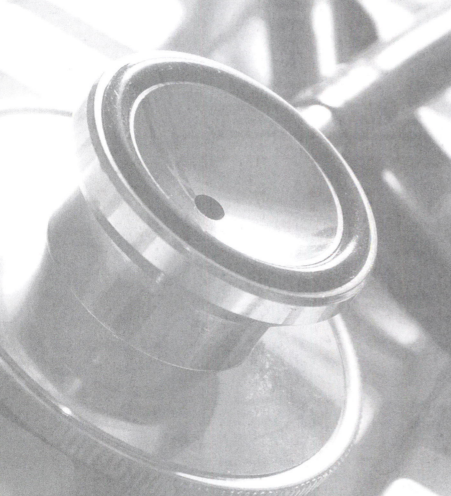

Introduction to
MEDICAL PRACTICE
MANAGEMENT

Deborah Montone and Michelle Lenzi

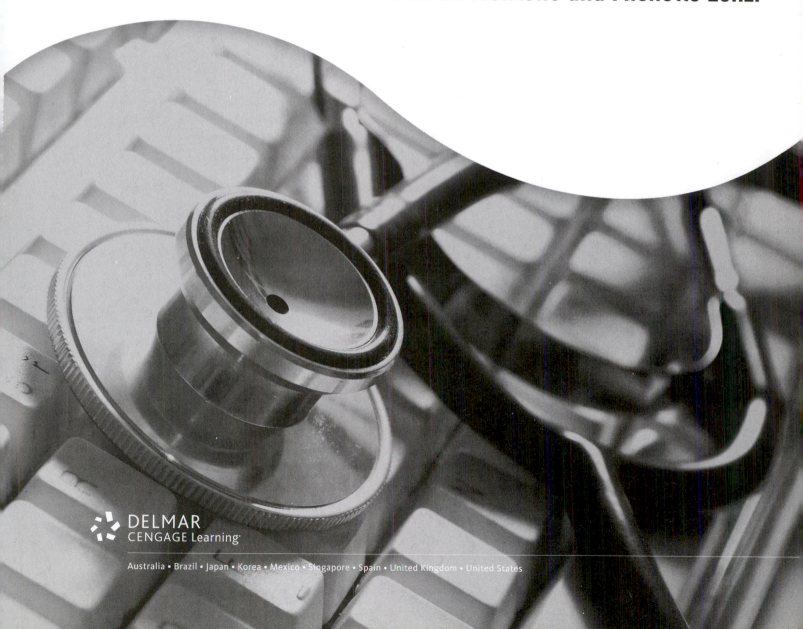

DELMAR
CENGAGE Learning·

Australia • Brazil • Japan • Korea • Mexico • Singapore • Spain • United Kingdom • United States

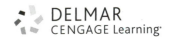
DELMAR
CENGAGE Learning·

Introduction to Medical Practice Management
Deborah Montone and Michelle Lenzi

Vice President, Careers & Computing: Dave Garza

Director of Learning Solutions: Matthew Kane

Executive Acquisitions Editor: Rhonda Dearborn

Managing Editor: Marah Bellegarde

Product Manager: Natalie Pashoukos

Editorial Assistant: Lauren Whalen

Vice President, Marketing: Jennifer Baker

Marketing Director: Wendy Mapstone

Senior Marketing Manager: Nancy Bradshaw

Marketing Coordinator: Piper Huntington

Production Director: Wendy Troeger

Production Manager: Andrew Crouth

Content Project Manager: Thomas Heffernan

Senior Art Director: Jack Pendleton

Media Editor: William Overocker

Cover Image Source: © www.Shutterstock.com

For product information and technology assistance, contact us at
Cengage Learning Customer & Sales Support, 1-800-354-9706
For permission to use material from this text or product,
submit all requests online at **www.cengage.com/permissions.**
Further permissions questions can be e-mailed to
permissionrequest@cengage.com

Library of Congress Control Number: 2012939649

ISBN-13: 978-1-4180-4092-5

ISBN-10: 1-4180-4092-4

Delmar
5 Maxwell Drive
Clifton Park, NY 12065-2919
USA

Cengage Learning is a leading provider of customized learning solutions with office locations around the globe, including Singapore, the United Kingdom, Australia, Mexico, Brazil, and Japan. Locate your local office at:
international.cengage.com/region

Cengage Learning products are represented in Canada by Nelson Education, Ltd.

To learn more about Delmar, visit **www.cengage.com/delmar**

Purchase any of our products at your local college store or at our preferred online store **www.cengagebrain.com**

Notice to the Reader

Publisher does not warrant or guarantee any of the products described herein or perform any independent analysis in connection with any of the product information contained herein. Publisher does not assume, and expressly disclaims, any obligation to obtain and include information other than that provided to it by the manufacturer. The reader is expressly warned to consider and adopt all safety precautions that might be indicated by the activities described herein and to avoid all potential hazards. By following the instructions contained herein, the reader willingly assumes all risks in connection with such instructions. The publisher makes no representations or warranties of any kind, including but not limited to, the warranties of fitness for particular purpose or merchantability, nor are any such representations implied with respect to the material set forth herein, and the publisher takes no responsibility with respect to such material. The publisher shall not be liable for any special, consequential, or exemplary damages resulting, in whole or part, from the readers' use of, or reliance upon, this material.

Printed in the United States of America
1 2 3 4 5 6 7 16 15 14 13 12

DEDICATION

So many people touch you as you go through life, both professionally and personally and each one, in their way, has had an impact

I would like to dedicate this text to those people-
- Who believed in me, even when I didn't believe in myself.
- who gave me opportunities I might not have had or envisioned

And to my family
- my daughters, their husbands, and of course the grandkids who provide me with endless joy and blessings
- To my husband, my rock, who has always supported me in my many endeavors with unconditional love.
- And to my mom, who has always believed in me, and who has been an inspiration.

You have all touched me and made a difference in my life.

With love to all,
Debby

TABLE OF CONTENTS

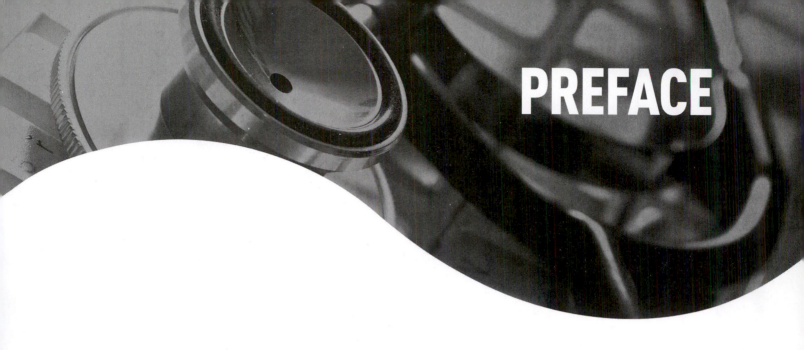

PREFACE

INTRODUCTION

You can be a manager!

To be a successful manager, you need to understand the fundamentals of the roles of the staff within the health care facility. *Introduction to Medical Practice Management* is written for those students enrolled in a management course who want to learn the aspects of management in a variety of health care facilities. The text uses a unique two-tiered approach in each unit to help students become a successful manager in any medical office setting. Learning is enhanced by activities directed toward the students' "practice," which they create through the "Think Like a Manager" feature found at the end of each unit. Units are organized into two chapters: The first chapter discusses the fundamentals of the topic, and the second chapter covers the manager's role in relation to each topic. Students will first learn the basics of medical practice management and the roles of each staff member within a health care facility and then they will learn about the skills and responsibilities of the manager in this setting.

PURPOSE OF THIS TEXT

I wrote this text because when teaching health care management courses, I came to realize that these students were from a variety of medical fields and settings and not every student had taken fundamental courses. Therefore, the essentials chapters can be used to teach basic information or review skills learned from previous training. By understanding the fundamentals, students will be better equipped to teach their staff, train new personnel, and monitor or audit procedures that occur in everyday practices.

As a manager, the student's responsibilities include creating new policies and procedures or updating existing ones to remain compliant. A policies and procedures manual is a guideline for all activities that happen within a health care facility. All policies and procedures need to be compliant with the appropriate regulatory agencies, such as the Office of Inspector General (OIG), the Centers for Medicare & Medicaid Services (CMS), and The Joint Commission, as well as many future laws and regulations. Therefore, in each unit students will learn to:

- Recognize applicable state, federal, and reimbursement laws.
- Create policies and procedures by following the partially completed templates in the chapters.

ORGANIZATION OF THIS TEXT

This book will walk students through the different aspects of running a health care facility. Each unit will include an introduction that defines important terminology, explains laws, and gives an overview of the unit content. The first chapter in each of the seven units will review the fundamentals of that department or area. The second chapter in a unit will provide the tools to manage that department or area.

Unit 1 covers medical personnel and their requirements for licensure and registration. Unit 2 discusses the responsibilities of the human resources department. The manager is responsible for the staff during employment; thus, the manager and human resources department work side by side to understand crucial activities that occur in placing personnel. In Unit 3, students will learn about the elements of the revenue cycle as well as how to perform audits as part of the role of a health care facility manager. Medical records are discussed in Unit 4, as they are vital to all health care settings. Students will learn about various policies and procedures for documenting, maintaining, and organizing medical records. Unit 5 explains audits and why they are necessary to avoid inaccuracies with coding and billing, including the linking of codes correctly. In Unit 6, students will learn about compliance with regulatory agencies. Identifying compliance and understanding the expectations are part of the daily routine for management. Finally, Unit 7 covers aspects of advertising and marketing, such as how to conduct a market analysis when determining advertising needs, managing choices on marketing techniques based on expenses, and managing advertising campaigns, designs, and costs.

In the appendices, students will find how-to documents and tools to help locate current rules and regulations so they will always be able to have the most current policies. Starting with Chapter 2, students will first create the dynamics of their practices as they complete the section "Think Like a Manager." In each of the management activities, they will be asked to perform management functions that pertain to each of the chapter topics. The student will create a cover for their practice by using the practice information provided and then add each of the activities to it. It creates a great visual tool when they are on an interview and seeking that management job!

Appendix A will guide students in creating their own practices, including the setting, specialty, number of physicians and other staff, and whether the practice is in the city or suburbs. The student is the manager of that facility.

Appendix B has templates to use for the activities in each chapter. These activities include the hiring process, conducting a background check, creating an employment advertisement, engaging in collection activities, and developing in-service or teaching activities.

Appendix C provides common medical abbreviations.

Appendix D has a table on specialties—physician and nonphysician.

Appendix E includes a list of useful medical websites.

FEATURES

Each chapter opens with a list of key terms and learning objectives. Numerous examples of letters, procedural policies, and medical forms are included throughout the book for hands-on learning. Critical thinking activities are provided at the end of each chapter in order to demonstrate how the material applies in an actual medical office setting. Review exercises challenge students to recall and employ the important concepts discussed in each chapter and improve their comprehension of the content. Students will learn to "Think Like a Manager" by creating their own practice. They will use templates from the back of the book to choose the dynamics for their practice, the personnel, and the setting. By completing tasks, such as writing policies and procedures, they will gain real-world practice in management and prepare for their future career.

ANCILLARIES

INSTRUCTOR'S MANUAL (ISBN: 978-1-4180-4093-2)

The instructor's manual includes answers to all the end-of-chapter review materials, including the review questions, critical thinking activities, and foundation exercises. Notes to the instructors give ideas on how to use the material to involve the student in assessment and learning.

ABOUT THE AUTHORS

Debby Montone is the dean emeritus of Eastwick College/HoHoKus schools. During her 27 years at the HoHoKus School of Business and Medical Science, she served as the director of continuing education, dean of medical sciences, and lead instructor and curriculum designer. She also spent more than 15 years as an office manager for a small physician's office. Debby is a current member of the American Health Information Management Association (AHIMA) and the American Nurses Association (ANA) and is the author of the Power Building Series of learning tools from Elsevier. Debby received her RN degree from the Hackensack Hospital School of Nursing and her BS degree in health care administration from St. Peter's College. She also has a graduate certificate in nursing and health care education and is a certified coding specialist (CCS-P) and an ICD-10 trainer through AHIMA.

Michelle Lenzi is owner and director of Lenzi Office Solutions, a medical coding school in Nashua, New Hampshire. She is a certified Professional Medical Coding Curriculum (PMCC) instructor for the American Academy of Professional Coders (AAPC), which allows her to teach students medical billing and coding while preparing them for the Certified Professional Coder (CPC) and Certified Professional Coder–Hospital (CPC-H) certification exams. Michelle is also an adjunct instructor for the medical assisting department at Hesser College and Kaplan University Online. She is the past president (2010) of the AAPC Derry chapter. Michelle has a bachelor's degree in business management from the University of Lowell and a master's degree in adult education from the University of Phoenix. She is also a certified professional coder (CPC) and a certified professional coder-hospital (CPC-H) through the AAPC.

ACKNOWLEDGMENTS

I want to thank Michelle Lenzi for her expertise and contributions to this project, and, of course, it would never have happened without the continued support of our product manager, Natalie Pashoukos.

REVIEWERS

Gerry A. Brasin, AS, CMA, (AAMA), CPC
Premier Education Group
Springfield, MA

Jennifer Claire, CMA, BA, MSHS
Kaplan University
Fort Lauderdale, FL

Anne M. Conway, CMA
National Career Education
Citrus Heights, CA

Susan Lewis, MBA, CMA
The University of Akron – Wayne College
Navarre, OH

Wilsetta McClain, NCICS, RMA, NR-CMA, NCPT, MBA, ABD
Baker College of Auburn Hills
Auburn Hills, MI

Michelle C. McCranie, CPhT
Ogeechee Technical College
Statesboro, GA

Lynn Meacham
Institute of Technology, Inc.
Modesto, CA

Alma D. Philpott, NRCMA
Kaplan Career Institute
Brooklyn, OH

Shelley C. Safian, MAOM/HSM, CCS-P, CPC-H
Herzing College
Winter Park, FL

Lori Warren Woodard, MA, RN, CPC, CPC-I, CCP, CLNC
Spencerian College
Louisville, KY

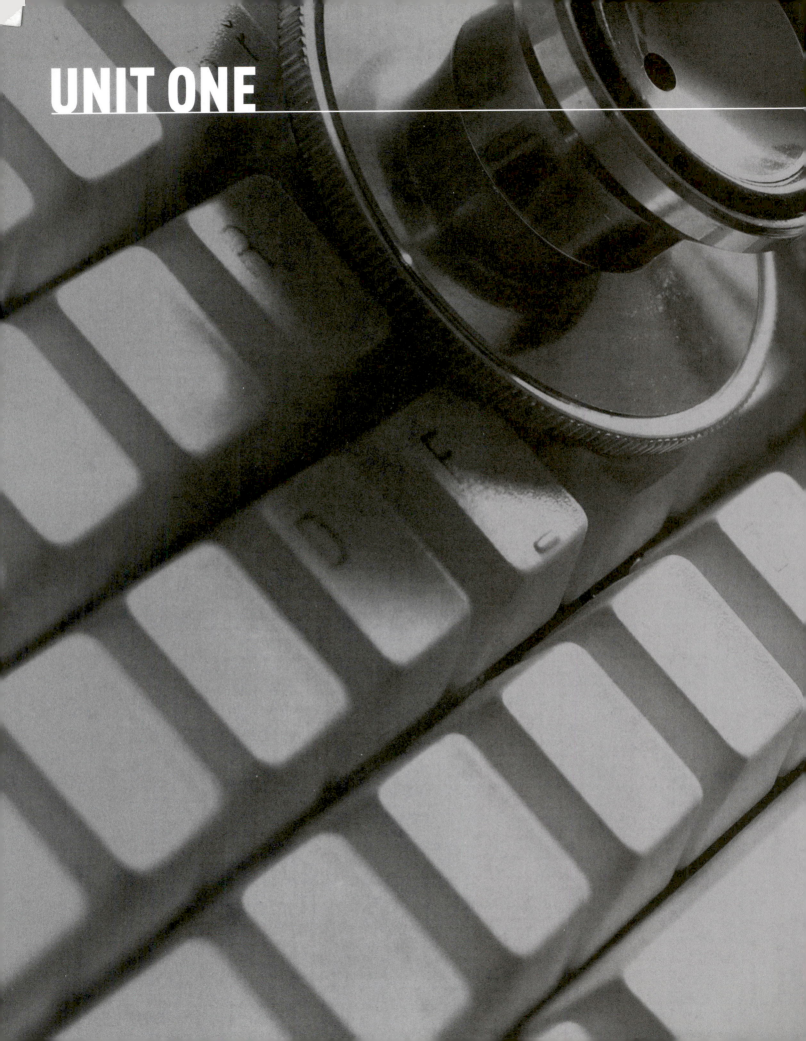

UNIT ONE

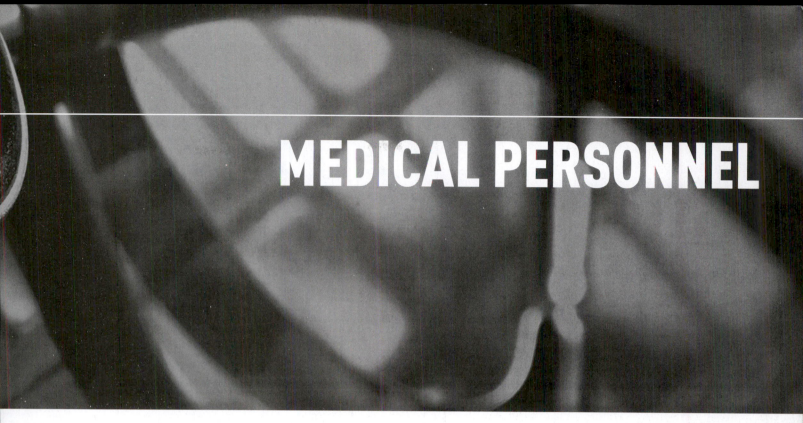

MEDICAL PERSONNEL

THERE ARE MANY health care settings and as many personnel that work within each setting. Discussed in this unit will be the different employees and their requirements for licensure and registration. Employment qualifications are important in the health care facility for clinical staff and administrative staff. Acknowledgment and compliance are the responsibility of the health care facility's manager.

CHAPTER 1 Fundamentals: Medical Personnel

CHAPTER 2 Managing: Medical Personnel

PROFESSIONALISM

- Display behaviors of a professional medical administrative specialist.
- Identify the diverse healthcare settings and the personnel that work within them
- Perform within limits under license and registration requirements.
- Demonstrate high standards of patient quality care.
- Create policies and procedures for the triage of phone calls and appointments
- Audit the everyday activities of a facility

CHAPTER 1

MEDICAL PERSONNEL

FUNDAMENTALS

Chapter 1 will discuss the fundamentals of the different personnel in a medical setting. Responsibilities of each type of personnel are reviewed.

OBJECTIVES

Upon completion of this chapter, the student will be able to:

- Look at different health care settings in which medical personnel may be employed.

- Review the categories of personnel within different specialties.

- Describe the varied responsibilities of each medical professional.

KEY TERMS

- Advanced beneficiary notice (ABN)
- Asthma
- Authorization
- Cardiologist
- Cardiology
- Chronic obstructive pulmonary disease (COPD)
- Dermatologist
- Dermatology
- Electronic health record (EHR)
- Explanation of benefits (EOB)
- Gastroenterologist
- Gastroenterology
- Gerontologist
- Gerontology
- Health Insurance Portability and Accountability Act (HIPAA)
- Health information technician (HIT)
- Notice of privacy
- Pediatrician
- Pediatrics
- Primary care physician (PCP)
- Pulmonologist
- Pulmonology
- Referral
- Registration
- Scope of practice
- Security
- Subscriber
- Specialist
- Specialty
- Surgeon
- Surgery
- Triage
- Urologist
- Urology

HEALTH CARE SETTINGS

Each health care facility has a distinct medical care it provides. Health care facilities have created a network to allow for different treatment and care to be performed at certain locations. Two primary distinctions are inpatient and outpatient facilities. Patients will have different diagnostic and treatment options available at each facility, and appropriate staffing is important at both facilities.

HOSPITALS

Many types of personnel and many specialties exist in hospitals. Hospitals also have specialty floors, such as cardiology, surgery, pediatric, cancer centers, and orthopedic floors. Licensed clinicians, technicians, and businesspeople perform functions vital to patient care and the operation of the hospital.

Clinicians include such licensed professionals as physicians, physician assistants, and nurses. Nurse practitioners, registered nurses (RNs), and licensed practical nurses (LPNs) are found in all areas of the hospital. Technicians are specialists with specializations that have additional education in their specific areas, and they are found in radiology and laboratories. Administrative personnel are found in outpatient departments, and business personnel work in billing and other administrative departments. Health information technicians (HITs) work in areas that use computers to process and store data.

OUTPATIENT SETTINGS AND PHYSICIAN OFFICES

Personnel can be employed in many different outpatient settings. Physician offices are the most prevalent type of outpatient setting, and they are specialty related and employ clinicians, technologists, and businesspeople familiar with that specialty. The type of specialty determines the type of personnel needed. For example, cardiology employs cardiovascular technicians, surgeons utilize surgical technicians, and orthopedics need x-ray personnel. Some personnel are employed in other types of outpatient settings, including freestanding radiology or laboratory facilities; physical therapy centers and clinics; and radiology treatment centers. One of the newest outpatient settings are clinics set up in stores that may be used for screening purposes, immunizations, or emergency care.

LONG-TERM CARE FACILITIES, ASSISTED LIVING, AND ADULT DAY CARE SETTINGS

In the long-term care, assisted living, and adult day care settings are clinicians, nurses, physical therapists, and medical administrative personnel. Physicians oversee the care of the patients. Nurses and LPNs carry out the care and treatments on the care plan. Certified nurse aides (CNAs) provide the daily care to patients, ensuring their safety and providing their daily living and nutritional needs. They also assist with restoration and mobility as well as admission and discharge when needed. Physical, occupational, recreational, and speech therapy are a part of most long-term care facilities. The medical administrative personnel role ranges from answering phone calls from family members to health care providers. The medical administrative personnel serve as a liaison between patient and family and often keep track of appointments and when the patient arrives and leaves a facility.

HOME SETTINGS

Many patients prefer to stay in their homes. Their care is prescribed by clinicians, assessed by nurses, and carried out by nurses, aides, home health aides, personal care assistants, and therapists.

The administrative medical person's part of home care would be done in the office of the home care agency. The responsibilities of frontline medical personnel in this setting include taking calls from families, calling home care personnel for assignments, contacting insurance carriers, and handling calls from physicians and therapists. This would be in addition to filing and maintaining medical records.

SPECIALTIES AND SPECIALISTS

Common specialties and specialists include:

- Cardiology and cardiologist
- Dermatology and dermatologist
- Family practice and family practitioner
- Gastroenterology and gastroenterologist
- Gerontology and gerontologist
- Gynecology and gynecologist and obstetrics and obstetrician
- Orthopedics and orthopedist
- Pediatrics and pediatrician
- Pulmonary and pulmonologist
- Surgery and surgeon
- Urology and urologist

Appendix D has a detailed look at the specialties, the body systems and their parts, common prefixes, and roots and suffixes to know. Common diseases, procedures, and treatments are also highlighted.

CARDIOLOGY AND CARDIOLOGIST

Cardiology is the study of the heart and its structures, and a **cardiologist** is someone who practices in the specialty of cardiology. This specialty would employ physicians who first specialized in internal medicine and then have had additional training in the field of cardiology. Nurses employed would have additional experience in cardiology treatments and procedures. Registered cardiovascular technicians would have specialty training in such procedures as echocardiograms and stress testing. General personnel, such as the medical administrative personnel, would need to understand the specific diseases, disorders, and emergencies for this specialty.

DERMATOLOGY AND DERMATOLOGIST

Dermatology is the study of the skin and its structures, and the **dermatologist** is someone who practices in the field of dermatology and has had specialized training in the diseases and disorders affecting the skin and its parts. A dermatologist may also have a subspecialty in the areas of derma pathology and pediatric dermatology. General personnel, such as the medical administrative personnel, would need to understand the specific diseases, disorders, and emergencies for this specialty, including infections, tumors, and other systemic diseases.

FAMILY PRACTICE

This specialty deals with the common disorders affecting all members of a family—from children through the elderly. This physician is often the **primary care physician (PCP)**. The physician has had additional training and experience in the care of many disorders. This physician can choose additional subspecialties, such as concentrating on adolescent medicine, sports medicine, or geriatric care. The staff in this practice also needs a broad range of experience in the many diseases affecting a family. General personnel, such as the medical administrative personnel, would need to understand the specific diseases, disorders, and emergencies for this specialty.

GASTROENTEROLOGY AND GASTROENTEROLOGIST

This specialty deals with the stomach, the small and large intestines, and mouth-to-anus disorders. As with the other specialties, the physician specialty is internal medicine and then will have additional training in this field, as will the nurses and other personnel. General personnel, such as the medical administrative, would need to understand the specific diseases, disorders, and emergencies for this specialty.

GERONTOLOGY AND GERONTOLOGIST

This specialty deals with the health of seniors and the normal and abnormal conditions people endure as they age. This specialist will have additional training in the normal and abnormal aging processes. Nurses as well as other personnel should also have knowledge of these aging processes.

GYNECOLOGY AND GYNECOLOGIST AND OBSTETRICS AND OBSTETRICIAN

These physicians have had additional training in the female reproductive system as well as pregnancy, labor, and delivery. They can also choose a subspecialty in gynecologic oncology as well as maternal and fetal disorders. General personnel, such as the medical administrative personnel, would need to understand the specific diseases, disorders, and emergencies for these specialties, such as dealing with pain and bleeding during pregnancy.

ORTHOPEDICS AND ORTHOPEDIST

Orthopedics is a specialty that treats diseases and disorders of the musculoskeletal system, including bones and muscles. The **orthopedist** is someone who has trained for this specialty. An orthopedist can also choose a subspecialty by concentrating on just one body part, such as the hand. One of the other personnel that would work in orthopedics would be an x-ray technician. General personnel, such as the administrative medical assistant or medical administrative personnel would need to understand the specific diseases, disorders, and emergencies for this specialty.

PEDIATRICS AND PEDIATRICIAN

Pediatrics is the study and practice of growth and disorders of children—usually from newborn to adolescents. A **pediatrician** is someone who has trained in this specialty. They must be aware of all types of medical and surgical conditions for children. The additional staff should also have experience with child disorders, normal immunizations, and childhood diseases. General personnel, such as the medical administrative personnel, would need to understand the specific diseases, disorders, and emergencies for all ages.

PULMONOLOGY AND PULMONOLOGIST

Pulmonology is the study of diseases and disorders of the lungs. The **pulmonologist** is someone who is a specialist in internal medicine and who has additional training in the lungs and its disorders. Respiratory therapists are personnel with training in the treatment of lung disorders. General personnel, such as the medical administrative personnel, would need to understand the specific diseases, disorders, and emergencies for this specialty, such as **asthma** and **chronic obstructive pulmonary disease (COPD)**.

SURGERY AND SURGEON

Surgery is a specialty that removes all or part of an organ. Many specialties exist within surgery. The **surgeon** is someone who has had additional training in operative procedures under sterile conditions. General personnel, such as the medical administrative personnel, would need to understand the specific diseases, disorders, and emergencies of patients needing surgery or after surgery. The staff in this specialty needs to understand the different types of anesthesia and the legal importance of consents.

UROLOGY AND UROLOGIST

Urology is the study of the urinary system and its parts, including the bladder and kidney. The **urologist** is someone who has had additional training in diseases and disorders of the urinary system. General personnel, such as the medical administrative personnel, would need to understand the specific diseases, disorders, and emergencies for this specialty, such as infections or kidney stones.

CATEGORIES OF PERSONNEL

Personnel can be thought of as:

- Licensed medical physicians and physician assistants
- Nursing personnel, including RN, LPN, and nurse practitioner
- Clinical personnel, including clinical medical assistants, laboratory personnel, x-ray technologists, cardiovascular technicians, and other specialty trained people
- Administrative personnel, including billers, coders, and medical administrative assistants or medical administrative personnel and data entry
- Health information technicians
- The medical manager

CLINICAL OR LICENSED PERSONNEL

Physicians and their staff undergo different training with respect to their duties in patient care—whether clinical or licensed. Requirements are specific to the type of license the staff members hold, authorizing them to perform their specific duties.

Physicians and Physician Assistants

Physicians and physician assistants are all licensed by a state and/or a board. The license must be maintained and renewed by achieving continuing education units per year. A code of conduct and code of ethics must be followed. These clinicians usually go into a specialty by accumulating additional training, education, and experience.

Nurse Practitioners, RNs, and LPNs

Nursing personnel are also licensed by a state and/or a board. They must also maintain their license by achieving continuing education units and following a code of conduct.

TECHNOLOGISTS

Technologists can receive their training at community colleges or vocational schools. Some personnel must also be licensed by a state or organization, such as x-ray technologists, cardiovascular technicians, or medical assistants, who can be certified by the American Association of Medical Assistants (AAMA) or registered by the American Medical Technologists (AMT).

ADMINISTRATIVE PERSONNEL

Administrative personnel usually go to vocational schools or community colleges for training and receive a diploma or certificate. Additional experience is acquired through internships and on-the-job training. They are responsible for a broad range of activities, such as receptionist, biller, coder, or data entry, and their training shows the diversity and broad range of responsibilities that are applied to all settings and specialties.

This role can be as diverse as it is critical. The responsibilities of this person are far greater than most realize. This person is the first person a patient has contact with, so it is critical that the medical administrative personnel always remain calm, professional, and reassuring, explaining as necessary the information requested. For example, the patient or family member can be anxious or even angry. If a patient or family member has a serious illness, money or insurance may be a concern. When the patient is asked for information about insurance, the patient may not understand why and how important it is.

HEALTH INFORMATION TECHNICIANS

Health information technician (HIT) is an emerging professional who is involved with data and electronic communication and is a link between documentation and coding. Qualifications include training at the technical or college level, and the knowledge can be as diverse as understanding computers, coding, and medical records.

MEDICAL MANAGER

This person should have management experience. This individual can be a nurse, a business-trained person, or someone with a management degree. The medical manager is a liaison, a coordinator, and a link between all personnel in all settings. This person must have knowledge about specialties and personnel as well as keep a health care setting functioning at its optimal level.

FUNDAMENTALS OF MEDICAL PERSONNEL ACTIVITIES

The employees in the medical field have many duties and must be trained in all areas of patient care. Staff members should work as a team and know what responsibilities they have during the patient encounter. Some of the general duties are outlined and explained in the following sections.

CHARACTERISTICS

The characteristics of any personnel, especially including the medical administrative personnel or medical administrative assistant, should include a positive attitude. A positive attitude is reflected in their verbal and nonverbal communications, particularly body language. Generating a warm and caring attitude makes the patient feel that he or she is not a patient number but is a person who deserves attention. Professionalism in actions and appearance are also important characteristics of the medical administrative personnel.

Characteristics of a medical administrative personnel or medical administrative assistant:

- Positive attitude
- Warm
- Caring
- Professional
- Knowledgeable
- Respectable

GREETING THE PATIENT

A person should be greeted with a title, such as Mr., Mrs., Dr., etc., unless the patient has instructed the staff differently:

"Good morning, Mr. Payne," not "Hi, Chet."

The medical personnel need to be aware of the cultural differences in health care and know the fundamentals of the cultures in your geographical area. Attitudes toward physical examinations, illness, treatments medications, and hospitalizations can vary greatly from culture to culture. Cultural diversity has become so important that government agencies, such as The Joint Commission and the American Nurses Association, and some states have created performance standards that include the importance of cultural diversity in the United States. In New Jersey, in 2005, the state legislature enacted a bill requiring New Jersey medical schools to include cultural competency training. We must also understand cultural diversity not only because of our patients but also because of our health care personnel.

Cultural diversity is recognized as important to the health care field by:

- The Joint Commission
- The American Nurses Association
- Individual states

TELEPHONE SCREENING OR TRIAGE

Telephone screening or **triage** is the ability to prioritize the urgency of phone calls and make appropriate decisions. This could be the responsibility of the medical administrative personnel or the medical administrative assistant or nurse. This person needs to be able to distinguish an emergency from a request for an appointment as well as determine that a billing question needs to be directed to other personnel in the health care facility. Phone calls that are an emergency would be patients who are having chest pains or difficulty breathing. Other urgent phone calls would be those from emergency rooms or from hospitals concerning the physician's patient. These phone calls need to be directed to the physician. Questions about a balance owed or whether insurance has paid can be directed to the billing department. Calls concerning renewals for medication, or results from lab

Emergency	Urgent	Billing	Appointments	Other
• Chest pain • Difficulty breathing • Asthma attack • Severe abdominal pain • Hospital emergency room	• Hospital calling on a patient • A Doctor calling about a patient	• Patients calling about insurance coverage • Insurance company	• Making appointments • Changing appointments • Canceling appointments	**Pharmacy** **Patients or family members** **Other health care personnel**
⇓	⇓	⇓	⇓	⇓
Direct to physician	Direct to physician	Direct to billing or account personnel	Receptionist can handle	Forward to nurses, or if not urgent leave for physician with chart attached

© Cengage Learning 2013

FIGURE 1-1 Screening or Triaging of Telephone Calls

TABLE 1-1: Calls that come in together

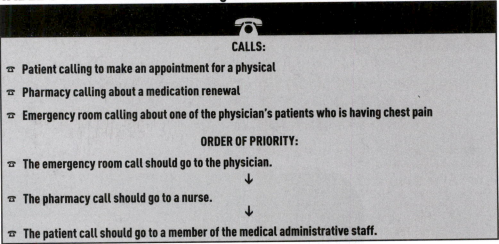

CALLS:

☎ **Patient calling to make an appointment for a physical**

☎ **Pharmacy calling about a medication renewal**

☎ **Emergency room calling about one of the physician's patients who is having chest pain**

ORDER OF PRIORITY:

☎ **The emergency room call should go to the physician.**
↓
☎ **The pharmacy call should go to a nurse.**
↓
☎ **The patient call should go to a member of the medical administrative staff.**

or x-ray tests should be directed to a nurse, physician, or other designated personnel. The medical administrative personnel then need to apply the appropriate action depending on the policies and procedures of the health care facility. When multiple calls come in at the same time, emergencies should be handled first and then urgent calls, appointments, billing, and other situations, respectively.

Figure 1-1 lists the situations that fall into emergency, urgent, billing, appointment, and other categories. See Table 1-1 an example of screening or triage calls.

APPOINTMENTS

Making, changing, and confirming appointments correctly, professionally, and according to the health care provider's **scope of practice** are essential tasks. Appointments are made either in a written appointment book or in a computer system (see Figures 1-2A and 1-2B). You should know who you are making appointments for and how many physicians, nurses, lab personnel, or x-ray personnel work on which days. Knowing what days each staff member is available as well as the types of procedures each staff person handles is necessary to ensure issues are handled by the proper person. This includes knowing the types of appointments as well as any preparations needed for them. Once you know this information, scheduling can be done. Several methods of scheduling exist. The type of practice, specialty, or setting is a factor in determining which method is best for the physician and staff. For example:

Enter physicians' names

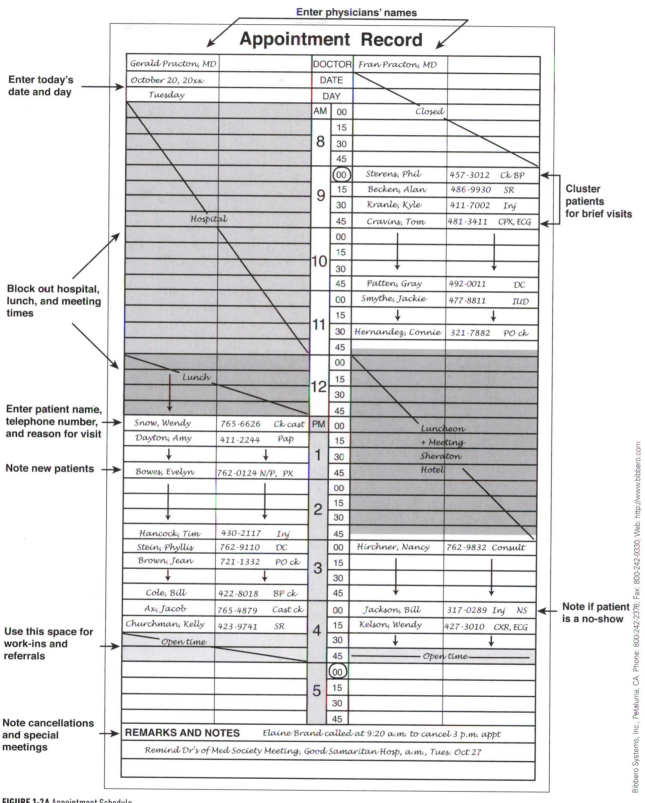

Appointment Record

| Gerald Practon, MD | | DOCTOR | Fran Practon, MD | |

Enter today's date and day → October 20, 20xx | DATE
Tuesday | DAY

		AM	00	Closed
			15
		8	30
			45
			00	Sterens, Phil	457-3012	Ck BP
		9	15	Becken, Alan	486-9930	SR
Hospital			30	Kranle, Kyle	411-7002	Inj
			45	Cravins, Tom	481-3411	CPX, ECG
			00
		10	15
			30
			45	Patten, Gray	492-0011	DC
			00	Smythe, Jackie	477-8811	IUD
		11	15
			30	Hernandez, Connie	321-7882	PO ck
			45
			00
Lunch		12	15	Luncheon
			30	+ Meeting
			45
Snow, Wendy	765-6626	Ck cast	PM	00
Dayton, Amy	411-2244	Pap		15	Sheraton
			1	30	Hotel
Bowes, Evelyn	762-0124	N/P, PX		45
				00
			2	15
				30
Hancock, Tim	430-2117	Inj		45
Stein, Phyllis	762-9110	DC		00	Hirchner, Nancy	762-9832	Consult
Brown, Jean	721-1332	PO ck	3	15
				30
Cole, Bill	422-8018	BP ck		45
Ax, Jacob	765-4879	Cast ck		00	Jackson, Bill	317-0289	Inj NS
Churchman, Kelly	423-9741	SR	4	15	Kelson, Wendy	427-3010	CXR, ECG
Open time				30
				45	Open time
				00
			5	15
				30
				45

REMARKS AND NOTES   Elaine Brand called at 9:20 a.m. to cancel 3 p.m. appt

Remind Dr's of Med Society Meeting, Good Samaritan Hosp, a.m., Tues. Oct 27

Annotations (left side):
- **Enter today's date and day**
- **Block out hospital, lunch, and meeting times**
- **Enter patient name, telephone number, and reason for visit**
- **Note new patients**
- **Use this space for work-ins and referrals**
- **Note cancellations and special meetings**

Annotations (right side):
- **Cluster patients for brief visits**
- **Note if patient is a no-show**

FIGURE 1-2A Appointment Schedule

Bibbero Systems, Inc., Petaluma, CA. Phone: 800-242-2376; Fax: 800-242-9330; Web: http://www.bibbero.com

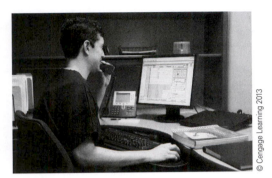

FIGURE 1-2B Medical Assistant Making an Appointment for a Patient using an Electronic Schedule

© Cengage Learning 2013

FIGURE 1-2C Electronic Appointment Schedule

© Cengage Learning 2013

Cluster: Scheduling groups of patients according to illness or procedures to be done. Pediatricians often use this method for well-baby visits and sick child visits. Other physicians may use this for such procedures as administering flu injections.

Open hours: No assigned times. When patients arrive, they sign in and are seen in the order in which they arrived. This type of appointment scheduling is seen in urgent centers, freestanding health centers, and in-store clinics.

Single booking: Similar to the traditional streaming approach and is used by the majority of physicians in which patients are assigned times in increments of 15 minutes. Longer visits are blocked off in additional 15-minute blocks.

Double booking: Assigns two people or more to one time, with the first one who arrives being seen first. This technique is good when the expected visit is to be quick or occasionally in the day to ensure no gaps in appointments.

Wave or modified wave: Best used for practices or settings in which other personnel, such as radiologists or nurses, can perform part of the exam or the diagnostic test.

Figure 1-2A shows how an appointment page should look after all the variables are in place. The variables in this schedule include hospital rounds, lunches, and meetings. They can also include vacations. In the first column, Gerald Practicum, MD has the morning blocked out because he is in the hospital. After his lunch, he begins to see patients. Some patients have 15-minute appointments; others have one-hour appointments. Figure 1-2B shows how this looks on the computer in the form of an electronic appointment schedule.

REGISTRATION

A patient **registration** is a form that has a number of parts that need to be completed the first time a patient goes to a health care facility (see Figure 1-3). Information from this registration is used for many different reasons. The patient's insurance information is used for billing an insurance carrier. The history is used as a foundation for the physician's assessment. These signatures are necessary to comply with confidentiality and the release of information.

Insurance cards copied ❑
Date: Feb 20, 20XX

**Patient Registration
Information**
Please PRINT AND complete ALL sections below!

Account # : _62153_
Insurance # : _572-XX-8966A_
Co-Payment: $ _____

Is your condition a result of a work injury? YES (NO)   An auto accident? YES (NO)   Date of injury: _____

PATIENT'S PERSONAL INFORMATION   Marital Status ❑ Single ☒ Married ❑ Divorced ❑ Widowed Sex: ❑ Male ❑ Female

Name: _Peterson_ (last name) _Mayze_ (first name) _F._ (initial)

Street address: _851 So. Adams_ (Apt # _12_) City: _Woodland Hills_ State: _XY_ Zip: _12345_

Home phone: (_555_) _289-4413_   Work phone: (___) _____ Social Security # _572_ - _XX_ - _8966_

Date of Birth: _Aug._/_07_/_1936_ (month/day/year) Driver's License: (State & Number) _XY VO45369X_

Employer / Name of School _Retired_   ❑ Full Time ❑ Part Time

Spouse's Name: _Peterson_ (last name) _Roy_ (first name) _T._ (initial) Spouse's Work phone: (___) _Retired_

How do you wish to be addressed? _____ Social Security # _572_ - _XX_ - _6022_

PATIENT'S / RESPONSIBLE PARTY INFORMATION

Responsible party: _Roy Peterson_   Date of Birth: _March 03, 1937_

Relationship to Patient: ❑ Self ☒ Spouse ❑ Other _____ Social Security # _572_ - _XX_ - _6022_

Responsible party's home phone: (_555_) _289-4413_   Work phone: (____) _____

Address: _851 So. Adams_ (Apt # _12_) City: _Woodland Hills_ State: _XY_ Zip: _12345_

Employer's name: _Retired Pasadena School District_ Phone number: (____) _____

Address: _44185 West Colorado Blvd._ City: _Woodland Hills_ State: _XY_ Zip: _12345_

Your occupation: _Retired Teacher_

Spouse's Employer's name: _____ Spouse's Work phone: (___) _____

Address: _____ City: _____ State: _____ Zip: _____

PATIENT'S INSURANCE INFORMATION   Please present insurance cards to receptionist.

PRIMARY insurance company's name: _Medicare_

Insurance address: _____ City: _____ State: _____ Zip: _____

Name of insured: _Mayze Peterson_ Date of Birth: _____ Relationship to insured: ❑ Self ❑ Spouse ❑ Other ❑ Child

Insurance ID number: _572-XX-8966A_   Group number: _____

SECONDARY insurance company's name: _Blue Cross_

Insurance address: _P.O. Box 1022_ City: _Woodland Hills_ State: _XY_ Zip: _12345_

Name of insured: _____ Date of Birth: _____ Relationship to insured: ❑ Self ❑ Spouse ❑ Other ❑ Child

Insurance ID number: _572-XX-8966_   Group number: _00276A_

Check if appropriate: ☒ Medigap policy ❑ Retiree coverage

PATIENT'S REFERRAL INFORMATION   (please circle one)

Referred by: _Glenda Marshall (Mrs. T.K.)_ If referred by a friend, may we thank her or him? (YES) NO

Name(s) of other physician(s) who care for you: _Gerald King, M.D._

EMERGENCY CONTACT

Name of person not living with you: _Kathryn Miller_ Relationship: _Cousin_

Address: _691 So. Brand_ City: _Woodland Hills_ State: _XY_ Zip: _12345_

Phone number (home): (_555_) _362-5711_ Phone number (work): (_____) _____

Assignment of Benefits • Financial Agreement

I hereby give lifetime authorization for payment of insurance benefits to be made directly to _Dr. G. Practon_ , and any assisting physicians, for services rendered. I understand that I am financially responsible for all charges whether or not they are covered by insurance. In the event of default, I agree to pay all costs of collection, and reasonable attorney's fees. I hereby authorize this healthcare provider to release all information necessary to secure the payment of benefits.

I further agree that a photocopy of this agreement shall be as valid as the original.

Date: _Feb 20, 20XX_   Your Signature: _Mayze Peterson_

Method of Payment: ❑ Cash ☒ Check ❑ Credit Card

FORM # 58-8423 • BIBBERO SYSTEMS, INC. • PETALUMA, CA. • TO ORDER CALL TOLL FREE : 800-BIBBERO (800-242-2376) • FAX (800) 242-9330   (REV. 7/94)

Bibbero Systems, Inc., Petaluma, CA. Phone: 800-242-2376; Fax: 800-242-9330; Web: http://www.bibbero.com

FIGURE 1-3 Registration Form

The parts of this form must include:

- Patient information
- Insurance information
- Health history
- Privacy information
- Signature, which give permission for treatment and billing

The patient needs 15 to 20 minutes to complete the patient registration form.

Patient information includes name, address, and employment information. Insurance information will include the name of the carrier, who the insured person is, and the ID number. Many registrations include a health history section, which is later reviewed with the patient by clinical staff. The registration form has become a crucial step in maintaining compliance with **Health Insurance Portability and Accountability Act (HIPAA)** regulations, as the patient indicates on the form how the health care facility can communicate with the patient. This includes who

---

Dear Patient:

Please answer the following questions so that we can communicate with you and still maintain your privacy rights.

You can call my home phone.

☐ Yes ☐ No Comments _____

You can leave a message on my answering machine.

☐ Yes ☐ No Comments _____

You can leave a message with a family member.

☐ Yes ☐ No Comments _____

You can call my work phone.

☐ Yes ☐ No Comments _____

You can call my cell phone.

☐ Yes ☐ No Comments _____

You can E-mail information to me.

☐ Yes ☐ No Comments _____

Your name _____

Signature _____

Date _____

Telephone number _____

Cell phone number _____

Work Number _____

E-mail address _____

FIGURE 1-4 Patient Preferences in Communication

	Overview:
	Insurance Portability
	Accountability
	Administration Simplification
Notice of Privacy	Privacy
	Security
For	Consent
	Authorization
	Right to have a copy
Multi Physician Practice	Right to request an amendment
	Electronic Data
	Business Associates
	Psychotherapy Notes
	The right to file a complaint
	Sanctions

© Cengage Learning 2013

FIGURE 1-5 Notice of Privacy

the facility can talk to and how much information can be left on answering machines or with family members (see Figure 1-4). Part of this process is also to provide the facility's **notice of privacy** to patients, which among many things notifies patients of their rights and informs them how their information is protected, who it is shared with, and how it is stored or destroyed (see Figure 1-5).

USING THE COMPUTER

As the push toward the **electronic health record (EHR)** becomes a reality, every health care setting will need to have a computer system that complies with new rules. The computer will be used for every aspect of running a facility—from registration to documentation to medications ordered.

The medical administrative personnel enter information into the computer, changing and updating information as necessary. This information can be on insurance, appointments, and payments. It will be important for the frontline medical administrative personnel to understand the new **security** regulations that are part of the HIPAA regulations and with what measures they need to comply.

The security regulations include:

- **Administrative safeguards:** The responsibilities of maintaining security at the workplace should be delegated to an individual who has received additional training on the many aspects of security and the relationship to privacy.

- **Technical safeguards:** A means to protect information should be in place. This includes access by individuals and authenticating that it is the correct person. It also includes maintaining a list of passwords. A password is assigned to each individual, and attached to the password is the employee's name, job description, and the type of information the employee is entitled to receive. The password also enables the identification of who accessed a medical record when a list is printed out.

- **Physical safeguards:** These include maintaining the work area around the computers so patient information remains confidential and is restricted to authorized users. Backing up information should be done on a regular basis based on the facility's policies and procedures. Information on the screen must be kept private. Some of the simplest things to do are to use privacy screens and to ensure everyone has his or her password rather than using a shared password.

GATHERING INSURANCE INFORMATION

An insurance card is asked for when a patient is seen in the office or another setting, such as the registration areas in hospitals, radiology centers, and laboratories. Copies are made of both the front and back of the card (see Figure 1-6). They should be compared to information given on the patient registration form. Insurance cards contain important information, such as:

- The patient's name
- The **subscriber**
- The name of the PCP
- The ID number for the insurance coverage
- Copay information for:
  - Office visits
  - Hospital visits
  - Emergency room services
  - Specialists
  - Preventative services
- What services might need preauthorization

By copying the front and back of the insurance card, personnel at the health care facility can confirm insurance coverage as well as the accuracy of information on the types of insurance a patient has, copayments, preauthorization requirements, and addresses and phone numbers to contact the carrier.

APPLYING CORRECT CODES AND SUBMITTING SERVICES TO INSURANCE COMPANIES

Clinicians and technicians who perform diagnostic tests and who document them in a patient's medical record as well as the coders who assign the correct codes work together so procedures and diagnoses are accurate and the codes reflect what has been documented. Once this step is done, a claim is generated and submitted to the insurance company.

IC Ideal Insurance Company	The following procedures need prior authorization:
	Surgery
	CAT scans
Subscriber: Jane Doe	Experimental procedures Telephone: 1 800 123-9876
ID no: 12345678 Group No: ABC	
Co pay: PCP $ 20	
ER $ 25	Send claims to: Ideal Insurance Co
Specialist $ 40	007 Main Street Chicago, Pa xxx09
Hospital $ 10	

© Cengage Learning 2013

FIGURE 1-6 Insurance Cards Front and Back

COLLECTION OF PAYMENTS

A payment is the monies that are collected by providers for services rendered. Practices and other health care facilities should keep a positive cash flow to pay for the expenses associated with the running of the practice or facility. Fees for services are usually predetermined through negotiated contracts or other formulas. Payments are received from a patient, from insurance carriers, and other third-party payers. These payments are credited to the patient's account—either manually in a patient ledger card (see Figures 1-7A and 1-7B), in a computerized system, or in a system that uses both methods. Payments can be for a previous service or in conjunction with a service performed. When payment is received, the medical administrative personnel record the date of payment, the amount of the payment, and the check number. The amount of the check is subtracted from the balance owed by the patient. Any balance remaining is inserted in the current balance column. If payment is in conjunction with the service just performed, then the amount of that service is recorded in the description column.

HANDLING REFERRALS

A **referral** is required by many insurance companies. It is a process of notifying the insurance company of planned procedures, services, and surgery as well as getting **authorization** for those services. This authorization or approval may have a referral number assigned to it. This number is affixed to the claim form sent to the insurance company for payment after the service or procedure. Although authorization may be given, it is not always a guarantee of payment, although the services are usually paid. If no authorization or referral occurs and it was required, the insurance carrier will not pay the claim. The new patient may present the medical administrative personnel with the referral information. This information needs to be given to the billing personnel. In another case, a patient may need a referral after being examined by the physicians of the facility. Obtaining the referral may be the responsibility of the medical administrative personnel or a referral specialist.

				Balance Forward
Date	Service	Charge	Payment	

Mary Jane Smith
123 Anystreet
My Town, USA

ID Number _____ Insurance _____

© Cengage Learning 2013

FIGURE 1-7A Blank Patient Ledger

Mary Jane Smith
123 Anystreet
My Town, USA

ID Number   SMJ1112223 _____   Insurance   Allcare _____

				Balance Forward
Date	Service	Charge	Payment	00.00
6/11/12	Office exam	$65.00	$15.00	$50.00

FIGURE 1-7B Completed Patient Ledger

© Cengage Learning 2013

TABLE 1-2: An appointment schedule

9:00	Chet Payne
9:15	consult
9:30	↓
9:45	↓
10:00	

The patient who makes an appointment for a referral needs to have the time blocked off in the appointment schedule, as shown in Table 1-2.

When a new patient comes to the office with a referral slip, the slip needs to be attached to the patient's medical record so the physician has that information. Previous diagnostic tests or a letter from the referring physician may accompany the patient or may have been sent previously. The billing department should also have the information from the referral slip (see Figure 1-8.)

The referral slip needs to be filed in the patient's medical record as well as reference the information in the physician's note.

In another situation, the patient may be told he or she needs a procedure or needs to see a specialist, which then requires giving the patient a referral slip or getting authorization from the patient's insurance company prior to the patient exam. The medical administrative personnel need to document the information in the patient medical record that will include the specialist or exam, the diagnosis, and the authorization number.

Consultation Referral Form

Date of Referral:	Payer Information:

Patient Information:

Name:

Name (Last, First, MI)

Address:

Date of Birth (MM/DD/YYYY)   Phone:
(   )

Member #:   Phone Number: (   )

Site #:   Facsimile / Data #:   (   )

Primary or Requesting Provider:

Name: (Last, First, MI)   Specialty:

Institution / Group Name: Provider ID #:   1   Provider ID #:   2 (If Required)

Address: (Street #, City, State, Zip)

Phone Number: (   )   Facsimile / Data Number: (   )

Consultant / Facility / Provider:

Name: (Last, First, MI)   Specialty:

Institution / Group Name: Provider ID #:   1   Provider ID #:   2 (if Required)

Address: (Street #, City, State, Zip)

Phone Number: (   )   Facsimile / Data Number: (   )

Referral Information:

Reason for Referral:

Brief History, Diagnosis and Test Results: _____

_____

Services Desired: Provide Care as indicated:	Place of Service:
☐ Initial Consultation Only	☐ Office
☐ Diagnostic Test: (specify) _____	☐ Outpatient Medical/Surgical Center*
☐ Consultation with Specific Procedures: (specify) _____	☐ Radiology ☐ Laboratory
_____	☐ Inpatient Hospital*
☐ Specific Treatment: _____	☐ Extended Care Facility*
☐ Global OB Care & Delivery	☐ Other: (explain)
☐ Other: (explain) _____	*(Specific Facility Must be Named)
Number of visits: (If blank, 1 visit is assumed) Authorization #: (If Required)	Referral is Valid Until: (Date) (See Carrier Instructions)
Signature: (Individual Completing This Form)	Authorizing Signature (If Required)

Referral certification is not a guarantee of payment. Payment of benefits is subject to a member's eligibility on the date that the service is rendered and to any other contractual provisions of the plan.

White: Payer • Yellow: Primary or Requesting Provider • Pink: Consultant / Facility / Provider • Goldenrod: Patient

See Carrier/ Plan Manual For Specific Instructions.

© Cengage Learning 2013

FIGURE 1-8 Medical Record for Referral on Chet Payne

Patient referred to Dr. Carl Dio because of a recent episode of chest pain. The patient's insurance called, and the authorization number for the consultation is #123098.

COMMUNICATIONS AND OPENING AND SORTING MAIL

Depending on the health care setting, communications can be in the form of regular mail or electronic mail delivered to a health care facility. Mail can be sorted according to personnel, department, or task (see Table 1-3). Medical administrative personnel need to understand

TABLE 1-3: Sorting mail

PERSONNEL				
Physicians	Nurses or Clinical Staff	Billing Personnel	Ancillary Staff: Compliance Officers	Office Manager
Professional journals	Meeting notices Journals	Insurance payments from insurance companies	Legal notices Journals	Credentialing forms Requests for disability on staff
X-ray reports on patients		Insurance payments from patients	New regulations	Payroll benefits
Lab reports on patients		Check payments from patients		Bank statements
Meeting notices		Explanation of benefits (EOB) from insurance companies		Bills on office supplies

the importance of each type of mail that is delivered. Lab reports on patients must be opened and attached to a patient's file that day. These reports are what a physician needs to determine a patient's diagnosis, course of treatment, and prognosis. Recognizing mail that includes payments from patients or insurance carriers must be sent to the billing department for the financial stability of a health care facility.

Electronic mail is becoming a large part of the communication system in this twenty-first century. A clear understanding of how this message is to be reviewed and forwarded to the proper personnel of the facility is required. The electronic mail can take several forms. E-mail is the most common, with communication from one person, organization, or company to another.

Electronic Mail

- Patient to physician
- Physician to patient
- Hospital to physician
- Medical organization to physician
- Insurance company to billing department

ADVANCED BENEFICIARY NOTICE

The frontline medical administrative personnel needs to recognize situations that require an **advanced beneficiary notice of noncoverage (ABN)** to be signed by the patient. An ABN is needed for Medicare patients and provides a written notice when a service may not be covered or when it is believed to not be covered (see Figure 1-9). This notice allows the patient to decide whether he or she still wants the service. On its Medicare Learning Network, Medicare publishes

A. Notifier:

B. Patient Name: **C. Identification Number:**

Advance Beneficiary Notice of Noncoverage (ABN)

NOTE: If Medicare doesn't pay for **D.** _____ below, you may have to pay.
Medicare does not pay for everything, even some care that you or your health care provider have good reason to think you need. We expect Medicare may not pay for the **D.** _____ below.

D.	E. Reason Medicare May Not Pay:	F. Estimated Cost

WHAT YOU NEED TO DO NOW:
- Read this notice, so you can make an informed decision about your care.
- Ask us any questions that you may have after you finish reading.
- Choose an option below about whether to receive the **D.** _____ listed above.
   Note: If you choose Option 1 or 2, we may help you to use any other insurance that you might have, but Medicare cannot require us to do this.

G. OPTIONS: Check only one box. We cannot choose a box for you.

☐ **OPTION 1.** I want the **D.** _____ listed above. You may ask to be paid now, but I also want Medicare billed for an official decision on payment, which is sent to me on a Medicare Summary Notice (MSN). I understand that if Medicare doesn't pay, I am responsible for payment, but **I can appeal to Medicare** by following the directions on the MSN. If Medicare does pay, you will refund any payments I made to you, less co-pays or deductibles.

☐ **OPTION 2.** I want the **D.** _____ listed above, but do not bill Medicare. You may ask to be paid now as I am responsible for payment. **I cannot appeal if Medicare is not billed**.

☐ **OPTION 3.** I don't want the **D.** _____ listed above. I understand with this choice I am **not** responsible for payment, and **I cannot appeal to see if Medicare would pay.**

H. Additional Information:

This notice gives our opinion, not an official Medicare decision. If you have other questions on this notice or Medicare billing, call **1-800-MEDICARE**(1-800-633-4227/**TTY:**1-877-486-2048).
Signing below means that you have received and understand this notice. You also receive a copy.

I. Signature:	J. Date:

According to the Paperwork Reduction Act of 1995, no persons are required to respond to a collection of information unless it displays a valid OMB control number. The valid OMB control number for this information collection is 0938-0566. The time required to complete this information collection is estimated to average 7 minutes per response, including the time to review instructions, search existing data resources, gather the data needed, and complete and review the information collection. If you have comments concerning the accuracy of the time estimate or suggestions for improving this form, please write to: CMS, 7500 Security Boulevard, Attn: PRA Reports Clearance Officer, Baltimore, Maryland 21244-1850.

Form CMS-R-131 (03/11)   Form Approved OMB No. 0938-0566

FIGURE 1-9 Advanced Beneficiary Notice of Noncoverage (ABN)

a decision tree to help office and/or lab personnel when an ABN is needed. Examples of when an ABN form is needed are listed in a notice of exclusions from Medicare.

Some of exclusions listed in 2011 include:

- Personal comfort items
- Hearing aids
- Orthopedic shoes
- Health care received outside the United States
- Services paid by a governmental entity that is not Medicare
- Dental care
- Routine foot care

- Services by immediate relatives
- Services as described as uncovered by **national coverage determination (NCD)**

FILING SYSTEMS

The frontline medical administrative personnel needs to recognize the different types of filing systems used when information is stored in the paper form in order to correctly retrieve a file, such as in the case of handing a file to the physician for an incoming phone call or to file a report in a patient's chart. A number of different filing systems exist, including alphabetical systems, numerical systems, color-coded systems, and bar-coded systems. In some cases, a combination of systems is used.

Alphabetical systems are the most common, especially in smaller outpatient settings. In this system, a combination of letters from the last and first names of a patient are used. Color is also commonly used, with letters having different colors. This makes it very easy to find a misfiled chart. For example, if the letter B is red and the letter D is yellow, spotting a file with a yellow letter D and the last name of Davis will be easy to see in the files with last names starting with B in the color red. Numerical systems are often used in conjunction with computer systems. This system is used in health care facilities with a large volume of patients, such as in hospitals. As it usually used in conjunction with computer systems a cross-reference with a patients name should be used to find the bar code number. Bar-coded filing systems assign a unique bar code to a patient. This bar code is inputted into the computer and applied to all reports and pages within the patient's file, as shown in Figure 1-10. Labels can be printed out to apply to a laboratory or x-ray requisition, which helps to identify the patient. Filing systems by subject are used for filing **explanation of benefits (EOB)**, bills to be paid, medical information, or third-party payer guidelines.

MAINTAINING THE RECEPTION AREA

The reception area must be clean and safe from hazards at all times. Current reading material is always appreciated by patients and accompanying family or friends.

Maintaining patient privacy can be done by limiting the sign-in sheet to patient name, time, and physician to be seen. Not using the phone to call patients, physicians, and other health care facilities in an open area where patients can hear diagnoses and test results is also recommended. A glass window that can be opened or closed as necessary would ensure some privacy. Having the checkout and check-in areas in different locations is also helpful. Keeping charts and open computer screens away from other patients and family members maintains the confidentiality of information.

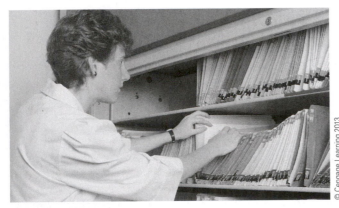

FIGURE 1-10 A Bar Coded Patient File

FIGURE 1-10 B

Sign in please:

SIGN-IN SHEET

Name	Time	Physician
Chet Payne	8:30	Dr. Carl Dio

OPENING AND CLOSING A FACILITY EACH DAY

As with every medical facility, certain requirements need to be fulfilled every day. Upon arrival and at the end of the day, personnel need to follow a checklist of items as patients are seen. Be sure each job is completed accurately and completely in a timely manner.

OPENING A FACILITY EACH DAY

Beginning each day, the role of the frontline medical administrative personnel includes:

- Checking messages:
  - From patients who need an appointment
  - From patients cancelling appointments
  - From physicians or specialists
  - From patients or insurers concerning bills or payments
- Checking the printed schedule for changes and adjusting files pulled
- Opening and sorting any mail

CLOSING A FACILITY EACH DAY

At the end of each day, medical administrative personnel should fulfill various requirements, including:

- Straightening the reception room as needed
- Printing schedules for the next day and pulling corresponding medical records
- Reviewing important messages with the manager

SUMMARY

- Health care settings include hospitals, physician offices, outpatient settings, long-term care settings, and patients' homes.
- Many specialties and specialists exist in the field of medicine.
- Categories of medical personnel include clinicians, technicians, and clinical and administrative personnel that work within different health care settings.
- You should know the qualifications for each type of person that works in a health care setting.

- The responsibilities of health care personnel are as diverse as the settings in which they can work.

- Activities for personnel are many and cross over categories of personnel.

- Processing and prioritizing telephone calls are essential duties.

- Making appointments involves knowing what personnel appointments are made for as well as how much time the different types of appointments need.

- The registration process involves completing paperwork and determining insurance coverage.

- Understanding regulations, such as HIPAA, is an integral part of all medical administrative personnel.

- The medical administrative personnel need to process some payments, such as copayments. Collecting the correct amount and crediting the patient's ledger require training and accuracy.

REVIEW EXERCISES

TRUE OR FALSE

1. _____ A medical administrative personnel can be found working in hospitals and outpatient setting.

2. _____ The frontline receptionist should be aware of cultural differences.

3. _____ Telephone screening is important to eliminate personal calls for employees.

4. _____ Patient payments get sorted to the physician.

5. _____ An urgent phone call would be from the emergency room.

6. _____ Dental care, hearing aids, and personal comfort items may need an ABN signed for a Medicare patient.

7. _____ You should check messages before the start of each day.

8. _____ The registration process includes verifying insurance.

9. _____ To make appoinments, the medical administrative personnel need to know who is working.

10. _____ Daily schedules are printed out each morning.

MATCHING

A   ABN

B   EOB

C   Subscriber

D   Triage

E   Scope of practice

F   Specialist

G   Patient registration form

H   Referral

I   PCP

J   Alphabetical system

1. _____ A combination of letters from patient names used for filing.

2. _____ A method of prioritizing the importance of phone calls.

3. _____ A physician who has additional education in a specific area.

4. _____ An explanation of benefits from an insurance company.

5. _____ The process of notifying an insurance company of a planned procedure and getting authorization or preapproval.

6. _____ A form for Medicare patients to complete for a service that is believed to not be covered by Medicare.

7. _____ The person who has the insurance.

8. _____ Completed by the patient at the first visit.

9. _____ Defines the role of health care personnel.

10. _____ The patient's physician who directs other care.

FOUNDATIONS EXERCISES

Write what diseases or disorders you might consult the following specialists about. Hint: Look in Appendix D if you are not sure.

Cardiologist _____

Dermatologist _____

Family practitioner _____

Gastroenterologist _____

Gerontologist _____

Gynecologist _____

Obstetrician _____

Orthopedist _____

Pediatrician _____

Circle the correct answer for each statement.

1. The patient has a skin rash; he would see a dermatology/dermatologist.

2. The patient needs to have her appendix removed; she would see a pathologist/surgeon.

3. The patient had a heart attack; he needs to go to a gerontologist/surgeon.

4. The patient has a stomach ulcer; the physician he is seeing is a gastroenterologist/gerontologist.

5. The patient has a broken bone; he needs to see a obstetrician/orthopedist.

CRITICAL THINKING ACTIVITIES

ACTIVITY 1

Sort the following pieces of mail to the correct person or department.

Medical society journal _____

Lab report _____

Payment from a patient _____

Bill from a medical supply company on supplies purchased _____

Insurance EOB _____

Request for additional information from an insurance carrier _____

ACTIVITY 2

Complete a patient ledger.

Mary John, a patient in the practice, is responsible for her own bill. She pays $50 for her exam on October 16, 2011. The total visit's fee is $150. The exam was $50, the EKG was $50, the blood tests were $25, the urinalysis was $10, and the flu shot was $15. Credit her account by using this ledger format:

DATE	SERVICES	TOTAL FEE	PAYMENT	BALANCE

ACTIVITY 3

A Medicare patient calls to make an appointment for what you know is cosmetic care. You also believe that Medicare will not cover this service. Discuss what you would tell the patient regarding an ABN.

CRITICAL THINKING QUESTIONS

1. Debate the pros and cons of working in different health care settings.

2. Discuss the role of working on the pediatric floor of a hospital or at a pediatrician's office.

3. Explore what role an HIT should have in a hospital setting and in an office setting.

WEB ACTIVITIES

1. Go to Medicare's Learning Network website at https://www.cms.gov/MLNGenInfo. Research ABNs and then list the current services not covered by Medicare that require the completion of an ABN.

2. Visit the Occupational Outlook Handbook website at http://www.bls.gov/oco. Research the different categories of jobs in health care.

CHAPTER 2

MEDICAL PERSONNEL

MANAGING

Chapter 2 will discuss the managing of a health care facility. Now that you have reviewed the fundamentals of medical personnel, you can develop the skills to effectively manage personnel in a medical facility.

OBJECTIVES

Upon completion of this chapter, the student will be able to:

- Develop an understanding of how to effectively manage health care personnel.
- Create policies and procedures that outline responsibilities for each category of personnel.
- Develop job descriptions for different personnel.

KEY TERMS

- Advanced beneficiary notice (ABN)
- American Association of Medical Assistants (AAMA)
- American Association Professional Coders (AAPC)
- American Health Information Management Association (AHIMA)
- American Medical Technologists (AMT)
- Audit
- Emergency Medical Treatment and Labor Act (EMTALA)
- Medicare is a secondary policy (MSP)
- National Center for Competency Testing (NCCT)
- Privacy
- Receptionists

DEFINING ROLES

In order to effectively manage medical personnel, a medical manager first needs to understand the diverse responsibilities of each position. Chapter 1 briefly reviewed these responsibilities. The manager of a health care facility will have many responsibilities. One of these roles is to understand the whole, meaning the role and responsibilities of each personnel and the importance of different specialties and specialists. One important role is to create, implement, revise, and teach personnel about facility policies and procedures.

Let us take a closer look at what each of these roles needs and how you, the manager, can ensure that your personnel are performing these roles correctly and efficiently for the health care facility. First, you need to know what the educational requirements are for each category, what the scope of practice is, and what their responsibilities are. Then, formal job descriptions can be developed. A template for creating job descriptions is found in Appendix B. These job descriptions can also serve as the basis for the annual evaluation of employees. Information to help define these roles can be obtained from the Department of Labor's Occupational Outlook Handbook as well as individual boards in each state, such as the board of nursing.

CLINICIANS OR LICENSED PERSONNEL

Licensed personnel, such as physicians, physician assistants, and nurse practitioners, have extensive education that included clinical rotations. Those who become specialists or specialized have had additional clinical experience in that specialty. Physicians, physician assistants, and nurse practitioners may see a patient, determine a diagnosis, and prescribe treatments. For this process to take place, all personnel within the health care setting work together—clinical people who perform diagnostic tests and administrative personnel who schedule appointments, determine insurance, record information in the computer/medical record, and bill the patient. A medical manager must ensure that these clinicians have the documentation and requirements to practice. Periodic review of their roles and responsibilities should take place.

CLINICAL PERSONNEL

Such clinical personnel as lab technicians and x-ray and ultrasound technicians have graduated from approved programs at colleges, universities, and other schools. They have such credentials as Registered Vascular Technologist (RVT), Registered Cardiovascular Technologist (RCVT), and Radiation Therapy (RT), and they have documentation of their licensure. The tests they perform are important for clinicians to diagnose an illness and successfully treat that patient.

ADMINISTRATIVE PERSONNEL

Such administrative personnel as medical administrative assistant, medical biller, and receptionist have usually had training at a community college or vocational school. They are responsible for a broad range of functions that are important for any setting. They make appointments, check patients in and out, gather information, maintain medical records and are responsible for gathering payments. They can have credentials for clinical certification from the **American Association of Medical Assistants (AAMA)**, the **American Medical Technologists (AMT)**, or the **National Center for Competency Testing (NCCT)** as well as the certification for the medical coding and billing from the **American Association Professional Coders (AAPC)** or the **American Health Information Management Association (AHIMA)**. The medical manager needs to know the needs of the health care facility to know which of these personnel will meet them.

LOCATION OF THE FRONTLINE RECEPTIONIST

The location of the frontline **receptionist** is extremely important because he or she is the first contact with the patient upon arrival. To ensure that the medical facility is conducive to patient treatment, the frontline receptionist must be located in an easily accessible area that is also private and confidential.

HOSPITALS

In a hospital setting, the medical administrative personnel could be located in:

- A central area, such as outpatient or inpatient registration
- A part of one department or service, such as radiology, laboratory, or cardiology
- Administrative offices, such as in patient billing or financial services

The medical manager is responsible for training and managing these personnel and ensuring they know the responsibilities for the setting.

LONG-TERM CARE, ASSISTED LIVING, AND OTHER ADULT HEALTH CARE SETTINGS

The frontline medical administrative personnel are usually responsible for greeting visitors and answering phone calls from family, physicians, and other health care personnel. These medical administrative personnel could be located in:

- The reception area
- The administration area
- Part of a manager's office

PHYSICIAN OFFICES AND OTHER OUTPATIENT SETTINGS

The frontline medical administrative personnel will be the one greeting patients and their families, answering the phones, making appointments, and even accepting payments. (see figure 2-1) The mail and other deliveries are delivered to the front desk.

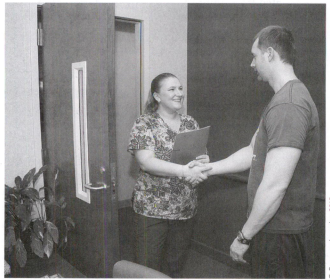

© Cengage Learning 2013

FIGURE 2-1 Medical Administrative Personnel Talking with a Patient

TELEPHONE SCREENING AND TRAINING

To effectively handle all types of telephone calls, a manager needs to review with the medical administrative personnel the types of personnel working in the health care facility.

An office setting could include:

- Physician(s) and physician assistants
- RNs, LPNs, and nurse practitioners
- X-ray technicians and technologists
- Ultrasound technicians
- Laboratory personnel
- Medical assistants
- Billing personnel
- Insurance specialist
- Referral specialist

Additional personnel within specialties could include:

- Respiratory therapists in the pulmonary practice
- Physical therapists in hospitals, freestanding centers, and rehabilitative centers
- Speech therapists in hospitals, speech centers, and rehabilitative centers
- Recreational therapists in assisted living and long-term care centers
- Surgical technicians in hospitals or outpatient surgical suites
- Diabetic counselors
- Nutritionists
- Cardiovascular technicians in hospitals or cardiology practices

TELEPHONE TRAINING

The manager should outline the role of each personnel, the types of phone calls that should be routed to each, and the time constraints or the designated times they can receive or handle calls.

Some examples could include:

- A medical administrative personnel in the outpatient department may set appointments for personal in that department.
- A medical administrative personnel in a long-term care nursing home can route phone calls to the nurses' station, the social worker, the occupational therapist, or other personnel.
- A medical administrative personnel in a physician's office can route phone calls to the billing department or nurse.

No matter who the call is for, proper telephone etiquette is important.

Some general guidelines to teach personnel about answering the phone include:

- Answer the phone promptly and by the third ring.
- Identify yourself and the facility or department you are in.
- If you are currently on another call, ask that caller if it is okay to put him or her on hold.
- Answer the phone professionally and with a "smile" in your voice.
- If the call must then be transferred to another department or individual, also tell the caller what you are doing.

- Get complete information on the caller, including name, the name of the patient if different, the telephone number where the individual can be reached, and a brief description of the nature of the call.
- Conclude the call professionally and pleasantly.

CALLS FOR THE PHYSICIAN

A physician could receive telephone calls from other physicians, from hospitals, from nursing homes, and from health care professionals involved in the care of the physician's patients. The manager needs to review with the medical administrative personnel the level of importance and priority for these types of telephone calls. In addition, if phone calls cannot be immediately forwarded to the physician, this needs to be established. An example of this is when the physician is performing a diagnostic exam, a procedure, or is engaged in an important family conference.

CALLS FOR THE NURSE

If nurses are part of the health care facility that the medical administrative personnel triages call, the responsibilities and roles of the nurses need to be outlined. Some nurses handle medication renewals. Other nurses provide patient education or act as a liaison between patient and physician. Others assist the physician with procedures. As with the physician, medical administrative personnel need to be aware of when the nurses are available to receive telephone calls and when calls need to be held.

CALLS FOR BILLING DEPARTMENT STAFF

The personnel in this department can include coding personnel, billing personnel, and account personnel. The organization of this area can be by function or account. Telephone calls can be forwarded to a specific individual, who then refers it to the appropriate person or to the account manager. The types of phone calls that would be forwarded to this department include calls from insurance carriers regarding additional information needed. Patients will call regarding balance due, overdue payments, inquiries about insurance payments, or the need to update information about their insurance coverage. The medical manager should understand the workings of this department and teach the medical administrative personnel the policies to be followed.

CALLS FOR OTHER PERSONNEL

Other personnel in the health care facility will need to be determined and the importance of receiving phone calls discussed. Examples of different personnel within a health care facility and the types of phone calls include:

- Radiology personnel—either technician or physician—may receive calls from other physicians about the results of x-rays.
- Laboratory personnel may receive phone calls from other physicians or from other floors of a hospital.
- Therapists may receive phone calls regarding a new patient who needs therapy, such as physical therapy, speech therapy, or occupational therapy, or a patient currently undergoing treatment.
- Dieticians may receive phone calls from new patients needing guidance or from established patients following a diet plan.

TYPES OF PHONE CALLS AND PRIORITIZING

The manager should teach the medical administrative personnel the levels of importance when receiving phone calls (see Figure 2-2). Table 2-1 can be used as a guide when teaching personnel how to answer phone calls in their department.

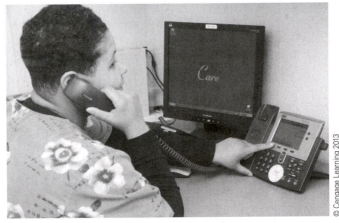

© Cengage Learning 2013

FIGURE 2-2 Learning to Prioritize Phone Calls

TABLE 2-1: Prioritizing phone calls in your department

Personnel	Phone Calls Received	Order of Importance	When Not to Disturb
Physician	Other physicians Hospital departments Long-term care facilities Pharmacies Patients and patient families Physician family	Hospital about a patient Physicians concerning new or established patients Emergencies Long-term care facilities for one of the physician's patients Pharmacy Other	During some diagnostic exams Invasive procedures, such as office surgery Family conference
Nurse	Medication renewals Patient education Some emergencies Patient updates on illnesses	Emergency screening New illness Update current illness Medication Patient education	Assisting with procedures On another call Providing patient education to patient or family
Billing department, including billers, coders, insurance specialists, and referral coordinator	Insurance companies Patients Other health care facilities	In Order Received Patient with outstanding balance Insurance company regarding denied claim	When dealing with another patient Sometimes if posting payments or finding a posting error.

What an Emergency Is in Specialties:

Cardiologist	heart attack, severe chest pain
Dermatologist	severe infection, severe outbreak of hives
Family Practice	high fever in an adult

(Continues)

Gastroenterologist	vomiting blood
Pediatrician	vomiting uncontrollably
Pulmonologist	difficulty breathing
Surgeon	severe bleeding after surgery
Urologist	difficulty and bleeding with urination

Table 2-2 demonstrates how to answer phone calls for personnel in other settings.

APPOINTMENTS

After the medical administrative personnel has an understanding of how many personnel they are making appointments for, what the time frame is per day for appointments, and the types and length of appointments are, the manager must then assure that the system is functioning smoothly. Table 2-3 shows what personnel should get what type of phone call.

TABLE 2-2: Prioritizing phone calls in other settings

Personnel	Phone Calls Received	Order of Importance	When Not to Disturb
Radiologists	From physicians From staff within hospital departments	Physicians Other departments	When taking x-rays or on call with physicians
Laboratory	From physicians From staff within hospital departments	Physicians Other departments	When on the phone or speaking with physicians
Dietician/nutritionist	From physicians From staff within hospital departments Patients or caregiver	Long term care facilities about current patient Patients with diabetes or other diseases having a health emergency	When on the phone or speaking with family or caregivers
Respiratory therapist	From physicians From staff within hospital departments	Physicians hospitals	When performing procedures When on calls
Social services or discharge planner	From physicians From staff within hospital departments Patient or caregiver	Inpatient at a hospital Family member	When on phone with family, patient, caregivers, or physicians

TABLE 2-3: Setting appointments for health care personnel

Personnel Title	Types of Appointments
Physician	Patient appointments
	Emergencies
	Drug representatives
Nurse	Routine blood pressure checkups
	Flu shots
	Other designated functions based on degrees and scope of practice
Radiologist	X-rays
Ultrasound technicians	Ultrasound exams
	Certification and scope of practice
	Determine what type of appointments/exams
Laboratory	Blood, urine, and culture tests
	Venipuncture
Therapists	Evaluations and treatment
Managers	Family conferences
	Insurance referrals
	Interviews

Policies and procedures must be created so making appointments is consistent. These policies and procedures include:

- Emergencies
- Routine appointments
- Illness
- Handling no-shows

The manager should ensure the efficiency of the system by periodically reviewing or auditing the system. This can be done by:

1. Review one day's appointment schedule.
2. Note start and end times of the day.
3. Survey patients for satisfaction.
4. Determine if a pattern exists when appointments take longer than scheduled, to determine if a problem has occurred in information gathering, scheduling, time allotment, etc.

Figure 2-3 shows an auditing form to check the efficiency of setting appointments.

A review of the audit form shows how a schedule can get backed up by not allotting enough time for exams. A review of the triage or screening process with the medical administrative personnel would be the recommended action.

Appointment schedule of people, times and reason:

9:00	Amy Apple	15 minutes for cold
9:15	Betty Bananan	15 minutes for blood pressure check
9:30	Carlie Cerlz	15 minutes for possible joint pain
9:45	Debby Dancer	15 minutes for possible sprain ankle
10:00	Ellie Eastman	15 minutes for dizziness
10:15	Frank Fella	30 minutes for brief physical
10: 10:30	George Ginger	30 minutes -bleeding

Audit Form

Patient name	Actual Time	Actual Time	In line with time assigned		reason
	in	out	Yes	No	
A	9:00	9:15	✓		
B	9:15	9:30	✓		
C	9:30	9:45	✓		
D	9:45	10:30		✓	More extensive exam needed to determine a fracture
E	10:30	11:15		✓	Blood test had to be performed. Delay in time also due to longer than scheduled appointment before this one
G	11:15	12:00		✓	Delay in start because of previous appointments. More extensive exam needed.

FIGURE 2-3 Auditing an Appointment Schedule

NO-SHOWS

With the frontline medical administrative personnel, the manager needs to follow-up with patients who do not show for appointments. The reason for the appointment needs to be reviewed, and if the patient's illness requires a follow-up, the medical administrative personnel needs to first attempt to call the patient to set up a new appointment. If the patient cannot be reached by phone, then he or she needs to be notified in writing. This must be documented in the patient's chart. You should know, for the different specialties, what has a greater urgency when a patient does not show. For example:

- In cardiology, the patient who has just had a heart attack and does not show is critical to follow up with.

- In dermatology, the patient with skin cancer is equally important.

- The patient scheduled for surgery who does not show for a preoperative exam could mean the surgery would have to be cancelled. The manager must train and monitor the staff who handles calls and appointments to understand this importance.

DOCUMENTATION FOR PATIENTS AND APPOINTMENTS

The manager needs to teach the medical administrative personnel the importance of documentation as it pertains to appointments and telephone calls. Document calls from patients who cancel appointments, who do not show for appointments, or who may repeatedly change an appointment.

This will show that the facility has been diligent in monitoring a patient, especially if the patient develops a new or more severe illness. As with no-shows, you need to know the importance of documentation for conditions within specialties.

DOCUMENTATION FOR EMERGENCIES

When a patient, family member, or caregiver calls a health care facility indicating an imminent emergency, the screener or triage person must ask appropriate questions, document responses, and ask the manger or physician for advice. Each specialty has different situations that constitute emergencies, as indicated earlier.

Documentation might look like this:

Mmddyyyy   **Time: 9 AM**   **Patient: Nicole Smith**

Mary Smith called and stated that her daughter is in severe pain, is having difficulty urinating, and doesn't want to move. Mother instructed to bring child in immediately.

Signed: Nurse S. Raschet

Mmddyyyy   **Time: 11 AM**   **Patient: Nicole Smith**

Mother has not come with daughter. Tried to call mother. No one answers phone.

Signed: Nurse S. Raschet

Mmddyyyy   **Time: 2 PM**   **Patient: Nicole Smith**

Mother called. Took daughter to urgent center. Has kidney stone.

Signed: Nurse S. Raschet

DOCUMENTATION FOR ROUTINE APPOINTMENTS

Documentation for routine appointments should include:

- Date
- Follow-up appointment to be given
- Instructions during the period of time, such as diet and medication
- Instructions for the next visit, such as fasting for a blood test

Documentation would look like this:

> Mmddyyyy   Patient to follow up in one month. Take new medication and follow diet provided. At that time, check cholesterol and blood sugar. Patient needs to come fasting.
>
> Signed: Dr. Smith

DOCUMENTATION FOR PATIENTS WHO CALL WITH A NEW ILLNESS

Documentation for a new illness should include:

- Date called
- Information provided on this new illness
- Instructions given, such as making an appointment

Documentation would look like this:

> Mmddyyyy   Patient called with complaints of cough and a fever of 101.8 F. Patient instructed to come to the office at 4 PM.
>
> Signed: Nurse S. Raschet

DOCUMENTATION FOR PATIENTS WHO DO NOT SHOW FOR AN APPOINTMENT

Documentation for patients who do not show for an appointment and who did not call to reschedule should include:

- Date of missed appointment
- Date called
- Reason to make a new appointment

Documentation would look like this:

> Mmddyyyy   This is Nurse S. Raschet from your physician's office. You missed your appointment today following your heart attack, and we must follow up with your new medications. Please call this office so you can reschedule your appointment for this week.
>
> Signed: Nurse S. Raschet

Note: A HIPAA privacy law protects the inappropriate release of a patients' personal health information and to keep the release to the minimum necessary for a person in healthcare to do their specific job.

REGISTRATION

The manager must review with the medical administrative personnel the purpose of the patient registration process. You should gather correct demographics for each patient, including address and telephone numbers. Insurance information is also gathered in this process. This information should also be updated on a regular basis. Part of the registration process is gathering information about the patient's illnesses—past and present. The medical administrative personnel must ensure that this information is completed by the patient before the patient is seen by the physician. The frontline medical administrative personnel need to recognize situations that may not be covered by the patient's insurance. In the case of a Medicare patient, an **advanced beneficiary notice (ABN)** is a document required by Medicare to inform the patient when it is believed a service will not be covered. It must be filled out and signed by the patient. The following scenario demonstrates when to have a patient complete an ABN.

(Refer back to Figure 1-9.)

A Medicare patient wants a cosmetic procedure done. You know this is an uncovered procedure, but the patient still wants it anyway. You need to provide an ABN to the patient to sign after you put it in the information.

USING THE COMPUTER

Many computer programs are used in the health care industry. Most programs provide the health care facility with the function to enter patient information, enter appointments, and make notations on a financial ledger. Programs usually provide a database of codes used for completing claim information and submitting insurance claims. Many also provide other functions, such as letters and accounts aging. Since the implementation of the HIPAA regulations in 2003 (see Table 2-4), there must be restrictions on access to each function of the computer. Personnel are assigned passwords, which helps to control the access of information. As medical administrative personnel are usually positioned where patients and family members wait for their appointment, the computer screen should be positioned so information entered cannot be seen by other people. The manager is responsible for having personnel select a password. When the password is selected, the manager must also instruct the employee about why we have a password, which is to limit access of information to those authorized to see it. Different categories of personnel have different types of information they need, such as billers needing insurance information about diagnoses and procedures, while the medical assistant may only need access to progress notes. The importance of not sharing

TABLE 2-4: Summary of HIPAA regulations

Component	Brief Description
Privacy and Security	Applies to covered entities, such as providers and health plan clearinghouses that transmit health information in an electronic form.
	Facilities need a designated privacy and/or security officer.
	Use and disclosure of information in either the paper or electronic form
Transaction standards and code sets	Code sets
	Standardizing for diagnoses, procedures, and drug codes

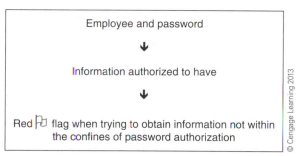

FIGURE 2-4   Shows the Flow of Information

it with anyone else and the implications when sharing it improperly must be stressed. Sharing it improperly might result in access of information you should not have. The manager must also explain that a password might be changed anywhere from 14 days to 30 days as required by the facility. Figure 2-4 shows the flow of information.

GATHERING INSURANCE INFORMATION

In this function, the manager needs to instruct the medical administrative personnel how to gather insurance information. Asking for the insurance card is of paramount importance and the first step in identifying the patient's insurance carrier. Not every health care facility or physician participates with every insurance company. The patient needs to be informed if the physician is not a participating provider. Some insurance providers, such as Medicare, do not cover all procedures. An ABN is required by Medicare when it is known that a procedure will not be covered. The patient may choose not to have that procedure or must sign an ABN if he or she wants it done. However, the manager needs to be aware that routine signing of this document can be viewed as a violation of the law and may result in an audit of the facility's practices.

Asking the patient if he or she has another secondary policy is also important. Never assume the patient will tell you without prompting. Illness and age may cloud their memory. Some patients may have coverage with two insurers, making one primary and one secondary. With Medicare patients, you just determine if the patient has a primary insurer as well as a secondary insurer. With Medicare patients, you must also determine if **Medicare is a secondary policy (MSP)** (see Figure 2-5).

Developing policies and procedures for use of an ABN and identifying patients for whom Medicare is the secondary insurance will ensure consistent policies as well as compliance with the law.

1. Is the illness or injury due to a work related accident or illness covered under a workers' compensation plan?

2. Was the illness or injury due to an auto accident or injury?

3. Is the patient employed and covered by the Employers Group Health Plan?

4. Is the patient's spouse employed which covers the patient under the groups' health plan?

If the answer to any of these questions is yes, that indicates that another insurance is primary and Medicare is secondary. A yes also means additional information is needed on the insurance carrier including the name of the policy, the ID number and insured's name.

FIGURE 2-5 MSP Questionnaire

COLLECTION OF PAYMENTS

The manager must review with the medical administrative personnel policies and procedures for collecting payments. One policy should be on the collection of copayments. A patient may have a copayment that facilities collect either prior to the visit or after. The patient's insurance card will list the type of facility and the amount of copay on it. For example, the card may say an emergency department visit has a copay of $25; an inpatient stay has a copay of $100; a visit to the PCP has a copay of $20; and a visit to a specialist has a copay of $50. This underscores the importance of checking insurance cards for new patients and at least once a year for established patients. Many practices routinely ask to see the patient's insurance card each visit.

Other monies received may be from the patient who is paying on balances due or payments a patient receives from insurance and is brought to the facility. Policies must be in place for these situations, which the manager can review with the medical administrative personnel or as employees take on additional roles.

REFERRALS

Those medical administrative personnel working in an emergency department as well as those managing personnel in the emergency department must understand the requirements of the **Emergency Medical Treatment and Labor Act (EMTALA)**. EMTALA is a federal law that was passed in 1986 and is also known as the Patient Anti-Dumping Statute. The law was enacted by Congress to prevent emergency rooms or departments who participate in Medicare from turning away poor or uninsured patients or from transferring patients before they have been evaluated for emergency conditions and stabilized. (Refer to Figure 2-6 for a brief summary of EMTALA components.)

AUDITS

In order to ensure that the facility is operating within the law and not engaging in fraudulent activities, the manager of the health care facility must learn how to **audit** the facility's everyday practices.

Review denials from insurance companies for services not covered by Medicare. If these denials are from services not covered and an ABN was not signed, then the manager knows as a result of this audit that the staff needs education on recognizing services needing a signed ABN and how to complete one.

Review the process of registration. For new patients, review the chart for completion of the registration form. In the audit, the manager should review:

- The completeness of the registration form
- A copy of the insurance card
- The attestation that the patient received the notice of privacy
- Whether a health history was completed

Brief summary of the responsibilities of Hospitals which treat Medicare patients and which have an Emergency Room Department.

The Hospital must provide to a patient who presents to a dedicated emergency room or has presented on hospital property or is in an ambulance owned or operated by the hospital:

1. An appropriate medical screening examination to determine if a medical emergency exists
2. The examination must be conducted by a qualified individual as determined by rules and regulations
3. If an emergency exists, stabilizing treatment must be provided before the patient is transferred
4. An emergency medical condition is one which:
   a. Places the health of an individual, or unborn child in serious jeopardy
   b. serious impairment to bodily functions
   c. serious dysfunction of a body organ or part
   d. inadequate time to effect a safe transfer
   e. the transfer will pose a serious threat to life.

FIGURE 2-6 Brief Summary of EMTALA Components

SUMMARY

- The manager must know the diverse roles and responsibilities of the different personnel within his or her medical setting in order to define their roles.

- The manager must define each role and responsibility according to each person's education, credentials, and scope of practice.

- The manager needs to train all medical personnel to effectively triage phone calls to the proper personnel in the health care facility.

- The manager must also train other personnel how to make appointments, review patient registration forms, use the computer, gather insurance, and collect payments.

- Administrative personnel working in a hospital setting need to recognize the components of the EMTALA and situations that apply.

- The manager needs to have policies and procedures in place to ensure that all personnel in those roles are consistent and correct as they perform their job.

- Personnel need to recognize emergency situations within specialties.

REVIEW EXERCISES

TRUE OR FALSE

1. _____ Proper telephone etiquette includes identifying yourself and the office when you answer.

2. _____ All phone calls asking for the physician should be put through.

3. _____ The medical administrative personnel must know how many personnel they are making appointments for.

4. _____ When a patient does not show for an appointment, cross out the date in his or her medical record.

5. _____ Documentation is not necessary for routine appointments.

6. _____ Documentation for patients who call with a new illness includes date, information on the illness, and any instructions.

7. _____ A job description is important for all employees.

8. _____ Always pick up the phone by the third ring.

9. _____ If another call comes in while you are talking to a patient, immediately put the first caller on hold to answer the second call.

10. _____ The manager will tell all employees what the office password is for the computer.

MATCHING

A   Audit

B   Privacy

C   ABN

D   MSP

E   Password

F   No-Show

G   Transactions/ Code Sets

H   Telephone Etiquette

I   Registration

J   EMTALA

1. _____ A process for gathering information on a patient and his or her insurance.

2. _____ Antidumping statute; a federal law passed in 1986.

3. _____ Patients who do not call when they are not going to keep an appointment.

4. _____ Requires a covered entity to have a privacy officer.

5. _____ Required by Medicare for noncovered services or procedures.

6. _____ When Medicare is the secondary insurer.

7. _____ Answering the phone in a professional manner.

8. _____ Checks the efficiency of procedures in place, such as appointment scheduling.

9. _____ Components of HIPAA.

10. _____ Limits access of information to those who are authorized.

CRITICAL THINKING ACTIVITIES

ACTIVITY 1

Physicians are not able to take every telephone call that comes into the office. A protocol is needed as to what a physician should take and what other staff, including nurses and office managers, should take. Mark the following with the appropriate letter to represent the following:

P – Physician   C – Clinical   M – Manager

1. _____ Prescription refill request.

2. _____ Angry patient upset about bill.

3. _____ Hospital lab with normal results.

4. _____ Potential employee for interview.

5. _____ Patient with an appointment.

6. _____ Pharmacist with concern about prescription.

7. _____ Nurse from another office about clinical results.

8. _____ Newspaper about an advertisement that was submitted.

9. _____ Hospital radiology with stat results.

10. _____ Complaint about a bill and does not want billing.

ACTIVITY 2

Certain steps are taken when a patient calls with a question for the physician or provider. Label the steps with 1 through 10, with 1 being the first step and 10 being the last step.

_____ Take a detailed message, including time, date, and what they need.

_____ Contact patient with provider response.

_____ Let patient know when someone will call back.

_____ Pull file and put with message.

_____ Follow provider directions for patient request.

_____ File chart—electronic or paper.

_____ Answer telephone within three rings.

_____ Document complete message in patient file, including date and signature.

_____ Ask patient what he or she needs.

_____ Speak with provider about the message.

ACTIVITY 3

Documentation is essential to the health care facility, including appointment information. List five types of documentation that pertains to appointments and are required to be documented in the patient's records.

1. _____

2. _____

3. _____

4. _____

5. _____

CRITICAL THINKING QUESTIONS

1. As the manager, what would you do if your administrative personnel were not following up on missed or no-show appointments?

2. Discuss what action you would take if your clinicians were not accurately documenting.

3. Debate the pros and cons of cross-training administrative and clinical personnel in the outpatient setting.

WEB ACTIVITY

1. Further research a hospital's responsibility for treating emergencies and advisory bulletins on the antidumping law statutes (EMTALA) on the Office of Inspector General's website: www.oig. hhs.gov/fraud. Link to compliance guidance and alerts and bulletins on antidumping. Report on specific examples of abuse of this statute.

THINK LIKE A MANAGER

CREATE YOUR PRACTICE

It is now time to create your own practice, for which you will complete activities throughout each of the management chapters. Refer to Appendix A. You will first create the dynamics for your practice, the personnel you have, and the setting you choose. In each of the "Think Like a Manager" sections, you will have an activity in which you will complete a task that goes with the topics of the chapter, such as job descriptions or writing policies and procedures. These activities will provide real-world practice in managing and prepare you for your future career. In Appendix D, you will have a guide for different specialties, their body systems, diseases, diagnoses, illnesses, tests, and procedures found within that specialty.

Using the templates found in Appendix B and the information presented in this unit, complete the following interactive exercises:

1. Write a policy and procedure for the use of advanced beneficiary notices.

2. Write a policy and procedure for when to use an MSP questionnaire.

3. Write a policy and procedure for triaging or screening phone calls.

4. Write a policy and procedure for collecting copayments.

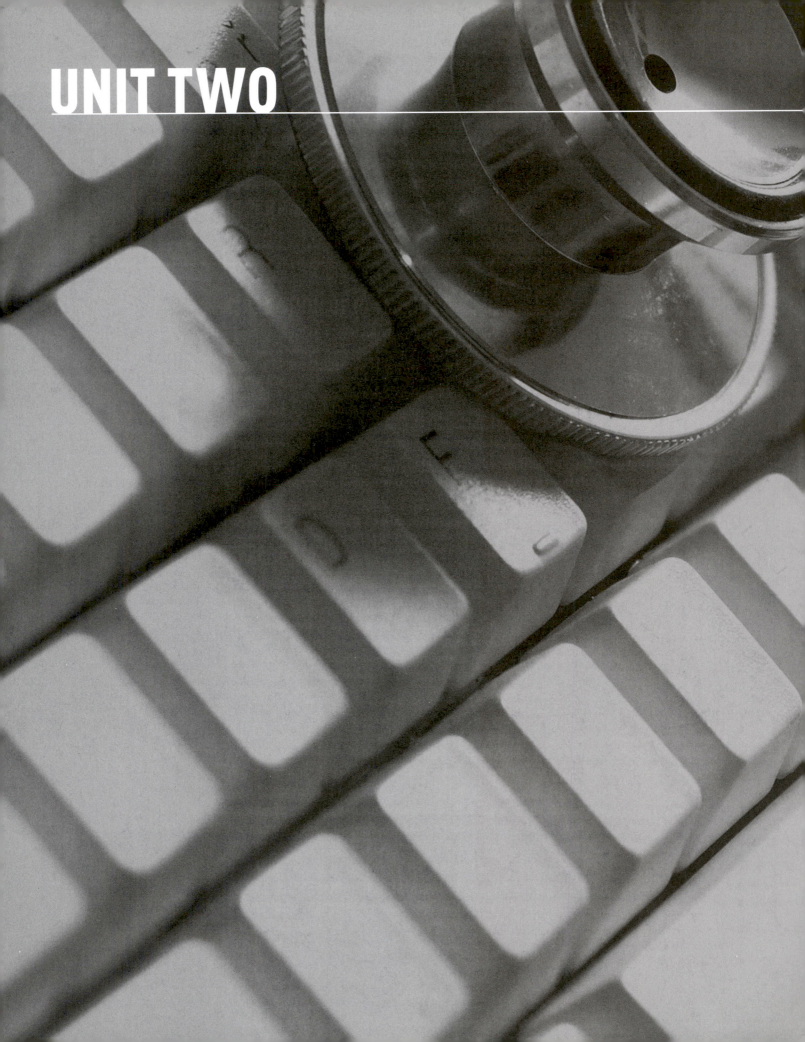

UNIT TWO

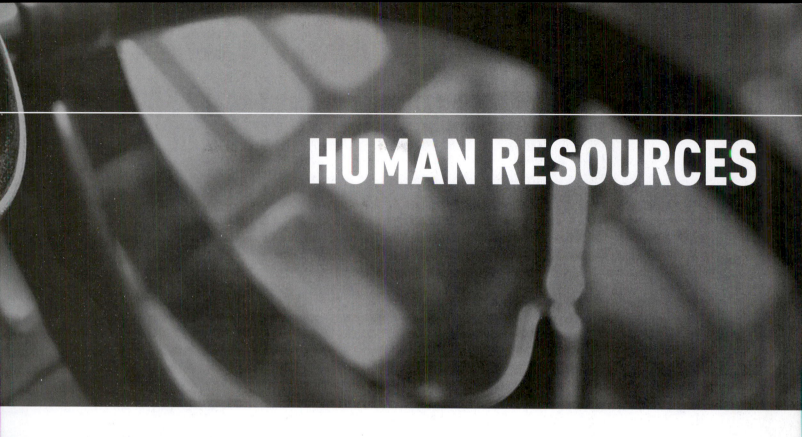

HUMAN RESOURCES

HUMAN RESOURCES IS the department responsible for hiring new medical personnel, interviewing and screening potential employees, arranging follow-up interviews with appropriate departments, administering background checks, managing benefits, and educating new hires about the rules and regulations of the health care facility. These functions may be the responsibility of one generalist or, in larger facilities, is divided into recruitment, benefits, and training. The manager and human resources department must work side by side to understand the fundamental activities that occur in placing personnel because the manager will be responsible for the staff during employment.

CHAPTER 3 Fundamentals: Human Resources

CHAPTER 4 Managing: Human Resources

HUMAN RESOURCES

- Manage/supervise medical office employees.
- Manage the parts of the hiring process
- Conduct performance reviews and administer disciplinary action.
- Maintain the office's policy manual.
- Manage the compliance procedure manual.
- Manage employee scheduling.
- Manage employee recruiting in compliance with state and federal laws.
- Train new employees and conduct orientation procedures
- Manage employee benefits.

CHAPTER 3

HUMAN RESOURCES

FUNDAMENTALS

Chapter 3 will discuss the fundamentals of the human resources department from the applicant's perspective by reviewing the parts of the résumé, the contents of a portfolio, how to compose a cover letter, the interview process, and sending a thank-you letter after the interview. Evaluating educational requirements and licensing will also be reviewed.

OBJECTIVES

Upon completion of this chapter, the student will be able to:

- Identify all steps in the employment process.
- Review the format of a résumé.
- Create a cover letter.
- Identify methods of applying for a job.
- Know how to complete an application for employment.
- Evaluate an advertisement and determine if he or she meets the qualifications for the position.
- Know the importance of sending a thank-you letter.

KEY TERMS

- Application for employment
- Cover letter
- Credentials
- The Joint Commission
- Licensure
- Mission statement
- Objective
- Portfolio
- Résumé
- Thank-you letter

THE EMPLOYMENT PROCESS

Before one can manage or work with the human resources department, one must be familiar with a résumé and cover letter, including format and content. When creating an appropriate résumé and cover letter, you must understand what these entail. Online websites and local agencies, such as a career center or an unemployment agency, can assist you in writing résumés. The entire process of employment from an employee's perspective includes creating a résumé, deciding if you have the qualifications for the job description as described in the classified ad, see Figure 3-1, responding to a job opening, and then preparing for an interview. You may have to submit an application for employment in addition to submitting a résumé and cover letter. Once you are chosen for an interview, you will set up a time to meet, obtain appropriate attire, bring a copy of your résumé and portfolio, arrive early for your interview, and write a follow-up thank-you note. Let us take a closer look at these areas.

THE RÉSUMÉ

A **résumé** is a summary of important information about a person (see Figure 3-2). It is an important tool when seeking an interview for employment. When someone submits a résumé, he or she is presenting a story about him or herself, and the potential employer should be impressed immediately. The résumé should be well written and easy to read and must include education, past employment, and licensure. Avoid errors when completing a résumé, as this is a representation of you and the hiring manager will be looking for perfection. In order to include all the appropriate information, the format of a résumé should include a heading, objective, education, skills, work experience, and other activities.

Once you know a job's requirements, you can change your résumé to fit what the employer is searching for. As you find available jobs, the résumé objective can change. One way to prepare for these changes is to maintain several types of résumés that coincide with the job for which you are applying. For example, a medical secretary position and medical billing position require different qualities. If you hold an interest in both positions, you can apply to both but change the résumé to reflect the job for which you are submitting the résumé. In addition to changing the objective, you can also change key qualifications, and highlight **credentials** or past experience. When the hiring manager reviews the résumé, you want the related qualifications to be apparent in the first few seconds he or she reviews your résumé so yours stands out among the other résumés.

HEADING

A heading should include the applicant's name, address, telephone numbers, and e-mail address. Make sure your résumé has all current information. The résumé should be reviewed yearly and updated as often as necessary. The applicant should ensure that any answering machine and/or voice mail greetings are professional and that e-mail addresses are also professional, as e-mail might be the first contact a potential employer has with an applicant. You should also include any credentials you use with your name. The first impression should be positive.

OBJECTIVE

Some formats include an **objective** or goal. This should be appropriate for the job for which the applicant is applying. Read the job description to use words that coincide with the expectations. When applying for the position of a medical office manager, the objective should incorporate why the applicant would be a good candidate. Examples of good and bad objectives are:

- **Good Objective:** Apply my education of health care management and office manager experience in a physician's office that encourages personal and professional growth.
- **Bad Objective:** I have no formal management education, but I am willing to learn.

Medical
BILLER/CODER
For MSO in Woodland Hills.
Exp required. Detail oriented,
computer skills. *ICD-9, CPT*
knowledge. Fax resumé to
555-878-1913.

ADMIN MEDICAL ASSISTANT
FT for busy OB-GYN group. Pleasant,
friendly team player with patient
skills in modern office– needs
bright, motivated person to perform
varied clerical duties. Competitive
salary, bonuses, benefits. Fax
confidential resumé to 555-430-6789.

MEDICAL
Fast-paced Woodland Hills med
facility has F/T evening/wknd shift
and day shifts available. Exp req'd.
Possible weekend and evening hrs.
Fax resumé 555-552-7030.

DATA ENTRY F/T busy ins agency.
Computers, Microsoft. M-F 9–5 pm.
555-457-5092.

**MEDICAL FRONT &
BACK OFFICE
P/T TO F/T**
Good computer and
people skills, insurance
billing experience.
555-486-8710

**MEDICAL ASST/MEDICAL
BILLER/CODER**
Exp'd only. F/T, poss PT/job share
Woodland Hills FP/OB practice.
Fax resumé to 555-527-0783.

MEDICAL ADM ASSISTANT
USA's premier provider of
electrotherapy products
has an opportunity for an
experienced medical administrative assistant. We need
someone to support the
Woodland Hills area. The job
includes performing home-
based administrative functions
and traveling to physicians'
offices. The ideal candidate
will be detail oriented,
energetic, possess great
communication skills and be
bilingual (Spanish). One day
a week will be spent working
in a suburb. Competitive salary,
full company benefits and all
travel expenses offered.
Expected start date is May 6,
20XX. If interested, please
fax your resumé to 555-575-9429.

MEDICAL
NOW HIRING
Busy FP/IM med facility in
Woodland Hills has the following
FT positions avail for exp., energetic
candidates with positive attitudes.
Fax resumé: 555-370-3776.
• **Medical Receptionist**
• **Medical Records Clerk**

Medical Assistant
Cardiology Associates Medical
Group in Woodland hills seeks
an energetic front office medical
asst. to perform administrative
duties. Exp and/or MA training req'd.
If you have a team player attitude
and care about patients, fax resumé
to Sara at 555-641-0434.

FIGURE 3-1 Examples of Classified Advertisements

Deanna Crumm
123 Clay Street
Mitown, NJ 00000
123-222-1234
dk@emailaddress.com

Objective   Desire an entry level position in a medical office as a medical Assistant

Education   **2006 Diploma in Medical Assisting, Mitown vocational school**

EKG certified
CPR and First Aid certified
National Phlebotomy certification
RMA-registered medical Assistant
2005 HS Diploma in Mitown H S, NJ 00000

Skills   **Administrative skills**

Schedule appointments
Maintain medical records
Open and sort mail
Complete insurance claim forms
CPT and ICD coding

Clinical Skills
Perform vital signs: BP Pulse, Respirations and Temperature
EKG
Venipuncture

Computer
Word
Powerpoint
Excel
Medical software

Work Experience   **2006– externship, Mitown Medical Physicians Practice**
2004–5 Hospital volunteer, Mitown Medical Center

References available upon request

FIGURE 3-2 Résumé

EDUCATION

Schooling and education should be listed next, starting with the most recent. This section must include at minimum a high school diploma or GED. When presenting education, the applicant should include the year he or she received his or her education. All degrees, certifications, and registries should be presented in this section. If appropriate, include vocational school certificates. When acknowledging your education, include the program of study for each one. Identify the type of acknowledgment you received, such as certification, licensure, or degree. Licenses, registries, and certificates that are not part of an educational program should also be listed and should be current. You must maintain membership and requirements that coincide with the license, registration, and/or certification. The applicant can list identification numbers on the résumé that pertain to his or her credentials, especially if they are required for the job description. For example, a physician would include his or her medical license dates with the medical license identification number so potential employers can confirm the information. The following are categories of personnel and their educational requirements as well as settings of employment:

LICENSED CLINICIANS

Physician

Educational Requirements	Complete four years of undergraduate school. Complete four years of medical school. Complete three to eight years of residency depending on the specialty.
Licensing Requirements	Pass an MD or DO license exam. Complete one to seven years of medical school.
Settings of Employment	Physicians are involved in all health care settings with patient care.

Physician Assistant

Educational Requirements	Complete two years of college in a health care field. Complete a physician assistant program—usually two years.
Licensing Requirements	Pass a PA licensing exam.
Settings of Employment	Physician assistants are involved in a health care setting under the direction of a physician.

Nurse Practitioner

Educational Requirements	Complete a five-year master's degree program with a supervised clinical experience in a specialty.
Licensing Requirements	Pass a registered nurse license exam with additional certification in an advanced nursing specialty.
Settings of Employment	Nurse practitioners are involved in most health care settings.

Registered Nurse

Educational Requirements	Three degree paths exist for becoming a registered nurse. Each leads to an entry-level position as an RN. Complete an associate's degree in nursing. Complete a bachelor's of science degree in nursing. Complete a diploma program—usually at a hospital.

Licensing Requirements	Pass a registered nurse license exam in each state you practice.
	All states require graduation from an accredited school or college and the passing of a licensing examination to work as a registered nurse.
Settings of Employment	Registered nurses are involved in hospitals, offices, long-term care, and home care settings.

Licensed Practical Nurse

Educational Requirements	Completion of an approved LPN program—usually offered at a vocational school, community college, or hospital.
Licensing Requirements	Pass a licensed practical nurse exam after graduation from an approved program.
Settings of Employment	Licensed practical nurses are involved in hospitals, offices, long-term care, and home care settings.

CLINICAL

Laboratory Technicians

Educational Requirements	Complete a two-year associate degree from a community college.
	Complete a certificate program from a vocational school.
	Complete a four-year bachelor's degree with a major in medical technology.
Licensing Requirements	Pass a medical technologist exam.
	Certifications can be through the American Medical Technologists (AMT) or the Board of Registry of the American Society of Clinical Pathology or the National Credentialing Agency for Laboratory Personnel. Exams vary from state to state.
Settings of Employment	Laboratory technicians are involved primarily in hospitals, outpatient labs and large physician practices.

X-Ray Technicians

Educational Requirements	Complete a two-year associate's degree.
	Complete a four-year bachelor's degree.
Licensing Requirements	Pass an x-ray technician license exam. Different states have different licensing requirements. The American Registry of Radiologic Technologist (ARRT) offers voluntary certification for radiologic technologists.
Settings of Employment	X-ray technicians are involved primarily in hospitals and outpatient radiology settings as well as physician practices, such as an orthopedist.

Ultrasound Technicians

Educational Requirements	Complete training in a hospital, college, or technical school.
Licensing Requirements	No state licensing regulations exist, but ultrasound technicians can get credentialed.
	The American Registry for Diagnostic Medical Sonography (ARDMS) and the Registered Diagnostic

Medical Sonographers as well as the Cardiovascular Credentialing International (CCI) provide registries for cardiac and vascular sonography. Diagnostic medical sonographers can specialize in obstetrics and gynecology sonography; abdominal sonography, where one inspects the organs located within the abdominal cavity, such as the liver and the gallbladder; or neurosonography, which visualizes the nervous system.

Settings of Employment	Ultrasound technicians are involved in hospitals, radiology centers, and physician practices, such as an echocardiologist working in a cardiologist office.

Medical Assistant

Educational Requirements	Complete medical assistant training at a vocational school or community college. The training includes administrative and clinical functions that are performed in physician offices and other settings.
Licensing Requirements	No licensing requirements exist; however, medical assistants can become registered by the American Medical Assistants as an RMA or certified through the American Association Medical Assistants as a CMA.
Settings of Employment	Medical assistants are involved primarily in medical offices, although they can work in other settings.

Certified Nurse Aide

Educational Requirements	Complete a certified nurse's aide course, which varies by state.
Licensing Requirements	Pass a certified nurse's aide license exam in each state you practice. Varies by state; usually, an application is made to that state with a background check.
Settings of Employment	Certified nurse aides are primarily involved in long-term care settings, assisted living, and similar settings.

Home Health Aide

Educational Requirements	Complete a home health aide class. Varies by state. Requirements usually fall under the state's board of nursing.
Licensing Requirements	Pass a home health aide license exam. Varies by state; usually, after the training is completed, an application is made to the board, along with a background check.
Settings of Employment	Home health aides are primarily involved in a patient's home or in assisted living facilities.

ADMINISTRATIVE

Receptionist

Educational Requirements	They learn via on-the-job training. Complete education in office skills, communication, and computers.
Licensing Requirements	No licensing requirements exist.
Settings of Employment	Receptionists are involved in the physician office, hospital department, radiology and laboratories, and long-term care.

Data Entry

Educational Requirements	Complete education or gain on-the-job experience with computers, including such software programs as Excel and Access.
Licensing Requirements	No licensing requirements exist. Microsoft certification would be an asset but is not required.
Setting of Employment	Data entry employees are involved with computers and the access of data.

Health Information Technology

Educational Requirements	Complete a two-year degree in an accredited school in health information technology. Complete a four-year degree in an accredited school in health information technology.
Licensing Requirements	No licensing requirements exist; however, certification is available as a registered health information technologist (RHIT) through the American Health Information Management Association (AHIMA) or as a registered health information administrator (RHIA).
Settings of Employment	A health information technologist is involved in any health care facility in which health information is gathered, stored, released, and used for patient care.

Medical Manager

Educational Requirements	Complete a degree in health services, health care management, or an equivalent. Undergo on-the-job training to gain strong knowledge about all aspects of the medical community.
Licensing Requirements	No licensing requirements exist; however, certification can be obtained as a certified medical manager (CMM), which is recommended but not required by smaller practices, and is available from the Professional Association of Medical Office Managers or as a certified medical administrative specialist (CMAS) through the American Medical Technologists (AMT).
Setting for Employment	Medical managers are involved in any health care facility.

Do my educational and licensing requirements meet the job for which I am applying?

- Title of job
- Education requirements
- Licensing or certification requirements
- Applicable previous experience to the current potential job

SKILLS

When applying for a skill-oriented profession, skills should appear next on the résumé. Information regarding occupations, areas of expertise, or accomplishments could appear in this place. List skills that will complement the job you are applying for because previous experience demonstrates a strong knowledge and expertise. A combination of skills and accomplishments is also appropriate. Skills can be listed by category, such as:

- Clinicians
- Clinical
- Administrative
- Information technology
- Managerial

Skills can also be listed under each previous employment position.

An example of listing skills under a previous employment could be:

Medical Assistant	Answered phones, entered data into the computer system, created letters, and prepared patients for exams.
Medical Manager	Responsible for overseeing daily operations, including managing accounts receivable, instructing staff, orienting new employees, and evaluating staff annually. Retention of staff was nearly 100%.

The skills should be kept short and not put into paragraph format. You may also want to combine skills if they are similar in description to allow for different skills to be listed. You want the hiring manager to notice your skills immediately, and having to read a paragraph can take too long to recognize information. When providing skills, keep in mind that the hiring manager will identify the skills he or she is searching for and will decide to read further if they are present. Thus, providing appropriate skills can capture the attention of the reader, creating an interest in you as a potential candidate.

WORK EXPERIENCE

In the work experience section, you must portray your life experience and relate it to the job description at hand. The primary goal is to create an image of a knowledgeable and experienced applicant for the hiring manager as he or she reviews your past experience. When the hiring manager reads the résumé, your résumé should grab his or her attention in the first minute if you want him or her to call you for an interview. Otherwise, he or she will go to another applicant's résumé instead. Every potential employer is interested in your work experience because life experience demonstrates good qualities and it is easier to train someone who has experience. The applicant should use this section to highlight the qualities the hiring manager is searching for. However, if your past experience does not relate to the current position, it is still appropriate to outline what you have done because this will portray life experience and employers will still view work experience as it pertains to longevity, organization, leadership skills, and maturity. It is here that you would list the name of previous employers, their locations, dates of employment, titles, and duties or responsibilities. List the most current work experience first, and include starting and ending dates for each.

For example:

2010–present   General Hospital, your town, state   Ultrasound Technician

Duties include: Preparing the patient, recording the patient history, performing examinations, performing measurements, and working as a member of a health care team.

Or

2001–present   Dr. LaBeste,   Utopia, ST   Office Manager

Duties include: Managing a staff of 12, including credentialing physicians, scheduling staff, evaluating accounts payable and receivables, and preparing and updating policies and procedures.

Instituted orientation for new employees and monthly in-service presentations.

Reason for leaving: physician retired

Or

5/09 to 2/11   Orthopedic Center, Utopia, ST

Office Manager: AP/AR, HR, payroll, benefits, 401K.

Billing, financial reports, fee schedules, end of month close.

Worked closely with practice manager.

Administrative Assistant: Staffing, billing, assisting office manager.

Medical Records: Transcription and record storage.

***Billing:* Coding (ICD-diagnostic coding and CPT), AR, aged balances, patient statements, collections**.

Claims: Third party, Medicare, Medicaid, HMOs, private, workers' compensation and auto, etc.

Reception/Secretary: Registering patients, referrals, scheduled surgery, tests, etc.

OTHER ACTIVITIES

When reviewing a résumé, the employer will view all areas to determine the integrity of the potential employee. If you have activities that are not listed in the main categories, be sure to include a category for other activities. In this section, you should include volunteer service, military service, and other activities that represent you as an organized and professional individual. In addition, it is customary to list professional affiliations and continuing education activities, if appropriate. When you are credentialed or licensed, this area allows you to include memberships, licensure, publications, awards, recognitions, and accomplishments. The applicant's qualifications are represented, and this section can assist in the decision for a hiring manager to call you for an interview.

REFERENCES

A list of people who can serve as references should be available, including their name, address, telephone number, and their relationship to you. References should include personal and work related. With references, you can include them on your résumé, attach a separate sheet with references, or provide references upon request. The job you are pursuing usually dictates how you provide references. Professional positions will usually require references, and they can be included with your submission. When applying for entry-level positions, references will usually be requested if the employer is interested in hiring the employee.

In preparing your reference list for employment, be sure to contact your listed references and request permission to use them as a reference. Ask if they are willing and able to provide a potential employer with information regarding you. If they agree to be part of your reference list, obtain accurate information from them to be placed on your reference list and be sure to thank them for allowing you to use them. If you have not contacted your references recently, you may want to check with them again as a courtesy to your reference. When a potential employer has indicated he or she is going to contact references, you may decide to alert your references of the potential for the phone call so they can prepare accordingly. With all interviews, you should always expect to provide references and have references contacted in an effort to impress the potential employer.

COVER LETTER

Every résumé should be sent with a dated **cover letter** (see Figure 3-3). The cover letter should reference the source of the job posting and include a brief description of your qualifications, including how you would fit with the position available. In addition, you should include some of the key words found in the job posting to demonstrate your understanding of the expectations. A job description will include the title of the position, posting date, job duties and special requirements, experience required, and credentials required. Locating these key requirements and including them in your cover letter will let the hiring manager know you are serious about the position.

When writing a cover letter, you are reflecting on your qualities and you should not submit a cover letter with errors. As the hiring manager reads your cover letter, he or she is creating an image of you through your writing and you must ensure your information relates to the position and that you are accurate. Be cautious of what you write, and do not present yourself as someone different.

LOOKING FOR THE JOB

Many ways exist to look for employment opportunities. The classified sections in the newspaper organize jobs by profession, such as medical, receptionist, and manager, and they are denoted as being part-time or full-time positions. The newspaper will list jobs in the counties the paper serves. It will be important to read the classified advertisement carefully and write the objective on the résumé as well as create the cover letter in response to what the advertisement is asking for (see Table 3-1).

EMPLOYMENT AGENCIES

Another avenue for seeking employment is through employment agencies. The employment agency is responsible for identifying potential employees who might match with employers. Using an employment agency is voluntary, and they will charge a fee to the employer for using this

Deanna Crumm
123 Clay St
Mitown, NJ 00000

June 25, 200x

Multi-Physician Practice
123 Main St
Your Town, NJ 00003
Att: Ms. Monty

Dear Ms, Monty,

I am responding to the Ad in the Mitown Chronicle on June 24, 200x for a Medical
Assistant.

I have graduated from the Mitown Vocational School in June 200x with a diploma in Medical Assisting.
I have both administrative and clinical skills that you are looking for, as stated in the Ad. I have had practical
experience in an externship that was part of my training and before that was a volunteer at Mitown Medical
Center.

I would like the opportunity to meet with you and discuss the position available.

Thank you,

Deanna Crumm

FIGURE 3-3 Cover Letter

TABLE 3-1: Creating a cover letter for a classified advertisement

What the Classified Advertisement States	What the Cover Letter States
Job title or job number or code (such as: Medical biller, code no. 1234	I am applying for the job of medical biller, code no: 1234, as listed in . . .
Job requirements require a detailed individual and a problem solver who has worked with CPT, ICD- diagnostic codes, and HCPCS codes in a medical facility.	I am a detailed individual who has been able to solve problems as they pertain to the use of CPT, ICD-diagnostic codes and HCPCS code in a medical facility.
Experience required: Two years Credentials required: CCS and CPC	I have three years in the field of medical billing. My credentials related to the field include.
Respond to Ms. Done, office manager	Dear Ms. Done: . . .

service. To use an employment agency, look in your local county in the phone book or online for medical staffing agencies. Some staffing agencies are general, while others specialize in particular settings, such as health care. Although employment agencies will cost the employer, the network opportunities and pre-employment interviewing will help the employer with potential candidates. The need for an employment agency depends on the job that needs to be filled. Whenever an employer uses an employment agency, he or she must select the one that fits the company's goals. The hiring employer should investigate the employment agency and also get references on them.

ONLINE SITES AND TRADE ORGANIZATIONS

A number of online sites allow employers to list job openings and employees to post résumés. Because job boards are usually free to access, an abundance of information is provided. Employers have begun listing their jobs in several places, especially where advertising job openings is free. One method of finding openings is going directly to employers' websites, such as hospitals. Another location for free advertising is professional agency websites, which employees are affiliated with because of their credentials. Trade magazines also list job opportunities in various fields, sorted by county or state. Knowing where to locate job openings is sometimes difficult and can take up a lot of time. When you begin your research, be sure to bookmark websites that offer job listings. Some of these websites have filters, allowing you to sort by preference, such as full time or part time, which makes it easier to find only the job openings that are appropriate for you. However, filters can also be limiting if you are open to different opportunities. Some employers with online job postings require online applications also to be filed. Review Table 3-2 for a listing of trade magazines, journals, and websites that may aid in a job search.

TABLE 3-2: List of organizations and trade magazines

Organization or Trade Magazine	Contact Information
Advance magazine. Editions for: ☎ Health information professionals ☎ RNs, LPNs, nurse practitioners, and physician assistants ☎ Imaging and radiation therapy ☎ Laboratory medicine ☎ Respiratory care professionals ☎ Other health care professionals	Published by Merion Publications 2900 Horizon Drive King of Prussia, PA 19406 800-355-6504 Job hotline: 800-355-5627 Website: http://www.advanceweb.com
American Academy of Professional Coders	2480 S. 3850 W., Suite B Salt Lake City, UT 84120 800-626-CODE Website: http://www.aapc.com
American Association of Medical Assistants	233 N. Michigan Ave., 21st Floor Chicago, IL 60601-5809 Website: http://www.aama-ntl.org
American Health Information Management Association	P.O. Box 97349 Chicago, IL 60690-7349 800-335-5535 Website: http://www.ahima.org
American Medical Technologists	10700 West Higgins, Suite 150 Rosemont, IL 60018 847-823-5169 Website: http://www.americanmedtech.org/default.aspx

(continued)

TABLE 3-2: continued

Organization or Trade Magazine	Contact Information
Association for Healthcare Documentation Integrity	4230 Kiernan Ave., Suite 130 Modesto, CA 95356 800-982-2182 Website: http://www.ahdionline.org
Nurse.com: Offers links to various nursing magazines as well as job listings	Published by Gannett Healthcare Group 1721 Moon Lake Blvd., Suite 540 Hoffman Estates, IL 60169 Website: www.nursingspectrum.com
Professional Association of Health Care Office Management	1576 Bella Cruz Drive, Suite 360 Lady Lake, FL 32159 800-451-9311 Website: http://www.pahcom.com
Monster.com	Website: www.monster.com
Careerbuilder.com	Website: www.careerbuilder.com

SENDING THE RÉSUMÉ

Once an applicant has found a job that matches his or her interests, educational background, and certifications, then he or she should send a cover letter and résumé. Some employment advertisements specify that the résumé and cover letter should be sent through the mail. Others request the résumé to be faxed or sent via e-mail. If the job opening was found on the employer's website, the employer may request that you file an application and résumé via the website and not through another form of submission. This is usually a safe and secure method of submission and will require you to set up a username and password. Some websites will show you the status of your application at any time. Whichever method you use to send your résumé, be sure to follow up with a phone call to the human resources department to ensure someone received your résumé. Some employers wait until many applicants have sent résumés before deciding who to interview. Some employers will send a postcard or an e-mail to acknowledge the receipt of a résumé. If you do not hear from a prospective employer, you can call after a week to see if someone received your résumé and you can also try to set up an interview.

THE INTERVIEW PROCESS

When an employer decides to interview an applicant, a time and date are set that are mutually agreeable to the applicant and employer. The applicant should always arrive before the scheduled time and allow extra time for traffic delays. In the initial interview, you should present yourself as a professional by dressing appropriately. Your goal is to present yourself as an individual who is organized, professional, detail oriented, and eager for the position. Your first impression is a lasting one, and you want the hiring manager to remember you. Knowing the employer you are interviewing with is important during the interview process. If you research information about the company, you will know what to expect during the interview and be better prepared. For example, knowing that the company has eight providers in the facility will increase your knowledge of how busy the practice is and what your expectations may include. With the availability of the Internet, you can do this via a web search in some cases. It is also advisable to do a search on the Internet for directions if the area is unfamiliar. If you have time, taking a trial run is also a good idea. In the interview, you will meet with one or more representatives in the health care facility. In this interview, your credentials will be reviewed, previous positions discussed, and questions asked that determine how you react to different situations.

Interview Checklist Information

- ☐ Date
- ☐ Time
- ☐ Address
- ☐ Telephone number
- ☐ Position
- ☐ Person to ask for on arrival

PORTFOLIO

The applicant should bring a **portfolio** to the interview. A portfolio is a visual picture of all education, credentials, accomplishments, awards, and skills possessed by the applicant. The portfolio should include additional copies of the résumé that may be distributed if you are asked to interview with additional people, managers, or departments. The portfolio should also include a list of references, letters from references, copies of diplomas or certificates, and other pertinent items for the field.

Order of Portfolio:

- Résumé
- List of references
- Letters of reference
- Copies of diplomas
- Copies of certificates, licenses, and registries
- Awards
- Other items representative of the position you are applying for

RESEARCH THE FACILITY

Knowing about your potential employer is pertinent to the interview. Prior to the interview process, spend some time locating information about the health care facility to be sure this is somewhere you are comfortable working. If the health care facility has a website, review the information on that website. This will help you during the interview to ask pertinent questions as well as answer questions appropriately. When viewing the website of the health care facility, the **mission statement** on the website will indicate the philosophy of the facility. The names of the president, vice president, physicians, and other officers of the health care facility may also be listed. Health care facilities might also post results of the last accreditation, such as hospitals or long-term care facilities accredited by **The Joint Commission** accrediting agency. In essence, be familiar with where you are interviewing and then prepare appropriately for the interview.

APPLICATION FOR EMPLOYMENT

You may be given an **application for employment** to fill out before the interview (see Figure 3-4). An application for employment asks for the same information that is on your résumé. Employers use applications as a formality and will request one be filled out to go in your employee file. If you are uncomfortable filling something out, ask the hiring manager how important that information is for the application during the interview process or leave the area blank and then explain your reason for not answering, such as salary information.

Read the application thoroughly before filling it out. This will avoid errors when completing the form and will eliminate the appearance of being sloppy or disorganized. Use your résumé so the information on the résumé is the same on the application.

Name_____

Address_____

Home phone: _____   Work phone: _____   Cell phone:_____

Position you are applying for_____

Current work history starting with the most recent

Start date	End date	Position	Company name

FIGURE 3-4 Application for Employment

Education

Start date	End date	Degree or certification or courses taken	Name of institution

References

Name	Relationship	Telephone number	Year(s) known

I attest that this information is correct   initial _____

I authorize this facility to verify the above
information   initial _____

Date _____ Signed _____

To be completed by interviewer:

Interviewed by: _____

Comments:

FIGURE 3-4 continued

Deanna Crumm
123 Clay Street
Mitown, NJ 00000

July 1, 200x

Ms. Monty
Manager
Multi Physician Practice
Your town, NJ 00003

Dear Ms. Monty,

I want to thank you for the opportunity to meet with you today and discuss the opening in your multi-physicians practice. After meeting with you, I feel I would very much like the opportunity to work in your office. I would welcome the opportunity to utilize the skills I have learned in my training and to continue to grow in your practice.

Yours truly,

Deanna Crumm

FIGURE 3-5 Thank-You Letter

AFTER THE INTERVIEW

After the interview is over, acknowledge the hiring manager's time spent with you and let him or her know you appreciate his or her consideration of your desire for employment with this company. When exiting, you can inquire about the hiring process and ask when a final decision will be made. In addition, you can also ask that someone contact you either way to let you know what decision was made. If the information about the final decision is unclear, then after some time has passed, you can call and check with the hiring manager for an update. During this time, a **thank-you letter** should be sent to the person(s) who conducted the interview (see Figure 3-5). In this letter, you should thank the interviewers for their time and you should reiterate why you are the best candidate for the job. In some cases, the thank-you letter can be the determining factor for hiring the candidate.

SUMMARY

- A résumé is a tool that summarizes all education, skills, and work experiences into a one- or two-page document.

- A portfolio is a visual picture of what you state in your résumé. It will include such items as certificates, diplomas, and letters of recommendation.

- A cover letter introduces you to a prospective employer and states what in your background would be important to this position. The job description posted should be included in the cover letter.

- An application for employment is a handwritten form given to a prospective employee before an interview begins.

- A mission statement describes the philosophy of the facility.

- A thank-you letter is sent after the interview to reinforce your qualifications for the position and how you see yourself as an asset in this position.

REVIEW EXERCISES

TRUE OR FALSE

1. _____ A summary of important information about a person is called a résumé.

2. _____ A good objective on a résumé asks a prospective employer for a chance at a job.

3. _____ A résumé includes educational background.

4. _____ It is not necessary to send a cover letter unless it is requested.

5. _____ If applying to an advertisement, the job description should be referred to.

6. _____ An employment agency matches employees to employers.

7. _____ Jobs can only be posted online.

8. _____ You should show up on time for an interview.

9. _____ A portfolio is for pictures.

10. _____ It is appropriate to write "See résumé" when you fill out an application for employment.

MATCHING

A   Heading

B   Résumé

C   Portfolio

D   Mission
    Statement

E   Cover Letter

F   Thank-You
    Letter

G   *Advance*

H   Spectrum

I   Objective

J   Application for
    Employment

1. _____ A visual picture of a candidate's accomplishments and skills.

2. _____ A statement of the philosophy of the health care facility.

3. _____ Sent with a résumé when applying for a job.

4. _____ Sent after an interview for a job.

5. _____ A magazine for people in the nursing profession.

6. _____ A magazine for people in the health care profession.

7. _____ A stated goal at the top of a résumé.

8. _____ Where the name, address, and telephone numbers go on a résumé.

9. _____ Includes a heading, objective, educational background, and work experience.

10. _____ To be completed at the time of the interview.

CRITICAL THINKING ACTIVITIES

ACTIVITY 1

Create a résumé.

A. Use the following guide to list your education and experiences:

Objective _____

_____

Education

Licenses and/or Certifications _____

_____

Skills _____

_____

Work Experience _____

_____

Other Activities _____

_____

_____

References _____

_____

B. Using the previous guide, create a résumé with a heading, an objective, education, skills, work experiences, and other activities.

C. Create a separate reference list with personal and work-related people.

ACTIVITY 2

Look in your local newspaper in the classified section to find a job you are interested in. Paste the advertisement in this box.

Potential Job

ACTIVITY 3

Create a cover letter to accompany your résumé, addressed by using the information in the advertisement. Be sure to include information directly related to the job description in the advertisement as your basis for being qualified.

ACTIVITY 4

Write a sample thank-you letter to be sent after your interview. Be sure your dates for the letters are consistent with the advertisement and the time frame.

CRITICAL THINKING QUESTIONS

1. You have finished your 18 months of schooling in echocardiography. You had extensive hands-on practice in your school, and you completed an 800-hour externship. You find an advertisement that asks for two years of experience in the field. Describe how would you word your cover letter to demonstrate the extent of your experience?

2. Explain how trade organizations can play a role in promoting a job search. Describe a trade organization in the area that you may be familiar with or research one you can network with.

3. Discuss the role of the portfolio during the interview process. Identify what you would include in your portfolio and when you would present it as a tool for interviewing.

WEB ACTIVITY

1. Research an employment advertisement through one of the online job site(s). Refer to Figure 3-2 as a guide.

    *   What is different about the search, the advertisement, and the submission of your résumé?

    *   What is the same about the search, the advertisement, and the submission of your résumé?

    *   Write a cover letter specifically for an advertisement found on the online site.

2. Research templates for résumés online. Choose two different ones that may be something you are interested in. Save them for future use in your job search as a manager. Consider two options that pertain to different positions you may apply for, such as a hospital or a physician's office.

CHAPTER 4

HUMAN RESOURCES

MANAGING

Chapter 4 will discuss a manager's responsibilities as they relate to the functions of the human resources department. Policies and procedures form the basis of the hiring, orientation, and termination processes. A set policy ensures standardizing the process for all employees. In the area of human resources, creating, revising, and/or deleting policies and procedures is an ongoing process. Policies and procedures are needed for:

- The hiring process
- Background checks
- Credentialing physicians
- The content of orientation
- Termination procedures

OBJECTIVES

Upon completion of this chapter, the student will be able to:

- Create an employment advertisement.
- Review résumés from applicants.
- Conduct interviews of prospective employees.
- Begin an employee manual.
- Outline an orientation presentation for your practice.
- State termination procedures.
- Create policies and procedures.

KEY TERMS

- Americans With Disabilities Act (ADA)
- Continuing education units (CEU)
- Credentialing
- Curriculum vitae (CV)
- Electronic data interchange (EDI)
- HIPAA
- I-9
- Job description
- Mission statement
- Orientation
- OSHA
- W-4

INTRODUCTION TO THE HIRING PROCESS

The responsibility for recruitment falls to the person or persons in the department of human resources. The size of the health care facility will dictate whether the responsibilities fall to one person (called a generalist) or whether the responsibilities are divided among several people with roles in employee relations, recruitment, benefits, and training. In a small practice, all the responsibility will fall to the office manager. The hiring process is the same regardless of who does the hiring.

CATEGORIES OF EMPLOYEES

For outpatient settings as well as hospital or long-term care settings, the first step in recruitment is to know the category of employee needed. With several tasks in the medical facility requiring fulfillment, employees are needed for clinical and administrative duties. All positions must have appropriate personnel who meet the requirements for the duties at hand. For each employee, the hiring manager must consider educational requirements as well as licenses or certifications. Administrative positions have fewer requirements than clinical positions because working with patients requires appropriate training and standards as required by law in some states. For the hiring manager, having knowledge of all potential categories for which he or she will be recruiting is pertinent.

JOB DESCRIPTIONS FOR ADVERTISEMENT

For each of these categories, human resources staff needs to know the qualifications for each position. A **job description** is a written explanation of an employee's responsibilities. It is directly related to the expectations of the employer. Achieving expectations and performing the job well are often the basis of the employee's yearly evaluations. The job description's format includes the job title, the department in which the job falls, and all duties under that job title. Table 4-1 shows different job titles that would need a job description. The direct line manager would be a part of this description as well as detailing the responsibilities and expectations.

Reviewing a job description for a position will be necessary, so the wording of advertisements for the job represents the position you want to hire for. Job descriptions and qualifications can

TABLE 4-1: Job titles

Certified Nurse Aide (CNA)
Home Health Aide
Laboratory Technician
Licensed Practical Nurse (LPN)
Licensed Vocational Nurse (LVN)
Medical Assistants (MA)
Medical Record Technicians
Nurse Practitioner (NP)
Pharmacists
Physician Assistants (PA)
Physicians (all specialties)
Radiology Technologists
Registered Nurse (RN)
Respiratory Therapists
Speech Therapists

be found through professional associations and publications. The Bureau of Labor Statistics also includes information about occupations in their Occupational Outlook Handbook, which describes the nature of the work, training and qualifications, and average salary requirements. Information can be found by going to the bureau's website at http://www.bls.gov.

When creating policies and procedures for hiring personnel, you will need to define what type of position you want to hire for. Is the employee part of the medical staff, clinical staff, or ancillary personnel? Define the tasks of this position. Some state laws define the scope of practice, such as in nursing or for medical assisting, and the tasks need to fall within that scope of practice. What educational requirements or work experience does the position require? Is the position a part-time or full-time position? Define the hours of work that is expected. If the position requires a certification or registration in your state, a policy needs to define this. Attach the specific job description to this policy as well as your state's scope of practice. A good reference is the Department of Labor, the Bureau of Labor Statistics' website (http://www.bls.gov), or the Occupational Outlook Handbook (http://www.bls.gov/oco).

PLACING AN EMPLOYMENT ADVERTISEMENT

To place an advertisement, you must include:

- The name of the position
- Educational requirements
- Credentialing requirements
- Job responsibilities
- Whether the position is part time or full time
- Benefits
- How to submit an application: fax, e-mail, or postal mail
- Who the hiring contact is

Information to know when placing a job advertisement includes:

- Job title
- Department and company
- Education
- Licenses or registries required
- Full time or part time
- Hours
- Qualifications
- Benefits
- Who to send a résumé to
- Fax number
- Telephone number
- E-mail address

> Medical Assistant
>
> Administrative and Clinical skills. RMA or CMA preferred.
>
> Full-time Mon–Fri One Saturday per month
>
> Benefits after 3 months available
>
> Please mail resume to Ms.Monty, Multi physician practice, Yourtown, NJ 00003

© Cengage Learning 2013

FIGURE 4-1 Sample Advertisement Ad for Employment

Figure 4-1 shows a sample advertisement for employment.

Once the advertisement has been created, you must decide the method of placing the advertisement. An advertisement can be placed in the classified sections of the area's newspapers, employment agencies, trade journals and magazines, or Internet websites. Some popular Internet websites are Monster.com (www.monster.com) and CareerBuilder (www.careerbuilder.com).

An example of a trade journal is *Advance* magazine. This magazine has different editions for different professions, such as RNs, LPNs, and radiology technicians. When placing the advertisement, keep in mind the cost involved and how many candidates will have access to the advertisement. More viewers are on larger forums, so the chance of getting a qualified candidate improves. Beginning the advertising process on a free forum is sometimes feasible if you have time and the position does not need to be filled immediately. Otherwise, paid advertising is a better method when you need a larger network.

REVIEWING RÉSUMÉS

In Chapter 3, the parts of a résumé were reviewed. The human resources staff and the manager are responsible for reviewing résumés and choosing candidates for the position. When reviewing résumés, consider the following:

- **Overall Impression:** Is the format of the résumé professional? Are the font, margins, and paragraphs consistent? Are there obvious spelling mistakes? This simple review can differentiate candidates who review their work and demonstrate proficient computer skills.
- **Objective:** If the résumé or **curriculum vitae (CV)**, which is a more comprehensive résumé, includes an objective statement, is the objective consistent with the job that the applicant is applying for?
- **Education:** Is the applicant's education consistent with the requirements of the job or profession?
- **Certification:** Does the candidate hold appropriate and current licenses or certifications? Has he or she kept up his or her **continuing education units (CEU)** (credits toward certification)?
- **Employment History:** Is the applicant a new graduate or does he or she have prior work experience? Is the work experience in line with the needs of the open position? Has the applicant stayed at a job for two or more years or changed jobs every year or so?

It will be important to discuss these topics with the applicant. If the applicant has changed jobs frequently, you may need to weigh the time it takes to train or orient a new hire to your facility.

Checklist for reviewing résumés

- ☐ Overall impression
- ☐ Objective in line with the job the candidate is applying for
- ☐ Education appropriate for the job
- ☐ Appropriate licenses or certifications
- ☐ Employment history
- ☐ Other observations

THE HIRING PROCESS

Once the résumés have been reviewed and applicants are chosen to be interviewed, contact potential applicants to set up interviews. Interviews may have to be set up either before work hours or after work hours for the interviewee who is still working at another job. When contacting the interviewee, leave a detailed message so the applicant can make appropriate arrangements prior to returning your call (Figure 4-2).

When the applicant comes in for the interview, you may have him or her complete an application for employment. The completion of this form demonstrates accuracy and neatness, and the information should be compared to the résumé. Applications can also allow you to view reasons for leaving companies, reasons for gaps in employment, and salary requirements, if listed. (Refer back to Figure 3-3.)

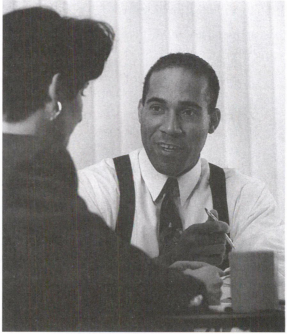

© Cengage Learning 2013

FIGURE 4-2 The Interview

TABLE 4-2: Questions not to ask in an interview

Questions Not to Ask During an Interview

1. Are you married?
2. Do you have children?
3. What kind of day care arrangements do you have for your children?
4. Have you been in the hospital? Why?
5. Do you have any illnesses? What are they?
6. What is your political party?
7. Do you have any debt?
8. Are you taking any prescribed medications? What are they?
9. Do you anticipate having to take time off under the Family Medical and Leave Act?

INTERVIEW QUESTIONS

The manager and human resources staff should be aware of the many laws and regulations that impact this department. Federal and state laws and the **American With Disabilities Act** (ADA) strictly prohibit discrimination in hiring based on disabilities, marital status, children, sexual preference, gender, age, and race. Questions should be prepared in advance to ensure you avoid questions that hint at those topics (see Table 4-2).

Questions should be directed to the candidate's qualifications, skills, education, and experience. Interviewers can ask situational questions concerning the job category for which they are hiring. Questions such as the following can be asked:

- What qualifications do you have for this job?
- What skills or experience can you offer to our health care facility?
- How would you handle such-and-such job-related situation?
- What questions do you have?
- Can we call your references?

An example of a situational question would be: "A fellow employee gets you aside and complains about a third employee. She further states she feels that the employee is not doing her share of the work. How would you handle that?"

THE OFFER

When the interview process has concluded and an applicant has been chosen, you should send an acceptance letter (see Figure 4-3). If salary was not discussed, you should direct the applicant to contact you to further discuss this information. This letter should state:

- The position being offered
- The department
- The management
- The starting date
- Orientation date
- Salary
- Agreed benefits and hours
- Contingency clause, pending results of a background check, credentialing, etc.

Multi-Physician Practice

123 Main At

Yourtown, NJ 0000x

Ms. D. Crumm

38 Clay Street

Mitown, NJ 00000

July 10, 200x

Dear Ms. Crumm,

We would like to offer you the position of Medical Assistant in our multi-physician practice at $15 per hour. Your starting date would be July 30, 000x. After the three month probationary period you can receive medical and dental benefits.

Please reply within one week of receipt of this letter.

We look forward to having you join our team.

Sincerely,

T. J Monty

Manager

Multi-Physician Practice

FIGURE 4-3 Offer Letter

BACKGROUND CHECKS

The request for a background check is now a part of many professions, such as banking, education, and health care. You must be aware of your state's laws as well as applicable federal laws with respect to background checks. The results of a background check may be a contingency requirement for some positions, and you should state that in an offer letter. If a background check is necessary, the applicant must be aware that he or she needs to sign for approval of a background check prior to being hired.

The "Request for Criminal History Background check" is a form that is part of a **States Bureau of Identification** (SBI) (see Figure 4-4). The position the applicant is hired for determines the extent of this background check. Senior-level management persons, such as a chief executive officer (CEO) or chief financial officer (CFO) requires a more extensive background check.

NEW JERSEY STATE POLICE, STATE BUREAU OF IDENTIFICATION (SBI)

REQUEST FOR CRIMINAL HISTORY RECORD INFORMATION
FOR A NONCRIMINAL JUSTICE PURPOSE
(TYPE OR PRINT ALL INFORMATION)

A. COMPLETE NAME AND ADDRESS OF REQUESTER

This will be used as a mailing label - Type/Print legibly

ADDITIONAL DATA (Optional)

B. SUBJECT OF THE REQUEST

NAME (Including Maiden Name)

SBI NUMBER (If Known)

(Last Name)	(Maiden Name)	(First Name)	(Middle)

ADDRESS

FBI NUMBER (If Known)

(Number)	(Street)	(City)	(State)

DOB	SEX	RACE	SOCIAL SECURITY NUMBER (If furnished)

(Month)	(Day)	(Year)

C. AUTHORITY AND PURPOSE OF THE REQUEST

(Check appropriate box to indicate the type of request and supply all other required information.)

☐ Noncriminal justice purpose by a governmental entity of this State, the federal government, or any other state for any official governmental purpose, including but not limited to employment, licensing, and the procurement of services pursuant to <u>N.J.A.C.</u> 13:59-1.2(a)(1).
(Authorization By Subject of Request And Privacy Act Notification; Certification of Requester <u>are required.</u>)

☐ Noncriminal justice purpose by a person or non-governmental entity of this State for purposes of determining a person's qualifications for employment, volunteer work, or other performance of services pursuant to <u>N.J.A.C.</u> 13:59-1.2(a)(2).
(Authorization By Subject of Request And Privacy Act Notification; Certification of Requester <u>are required.</u>)

☐ Noncriminal justice purpose by a private detective licensed by the Division of State Police pursuant to <u>N.J.A.C.</u> 13:59-1.2(a)(4) and <u>N.J.S.A.</u> 45:19-8 <u>et.seq.</u>, for purposes of obtaining information in furtherance of the performance of their statutorily authorized functions, as specifically enumerated by <u>N.J.S.A.</u> 45:19-9(A) 1 to 9.
(Certification of Requester <u>is required.</u> However, section D (3) and (4) <u>DO NOT</u> apply.)

(OVER)

FIGURE 4-4 Background Check Form

D. CERTIFICATION OF REQUESTER

I hereby **certify** that:

(1) I am authorized to receive and use New Jersey Criminal History Record Information pursuant to N.J.A.C. 13:59-2(a) (1), (2), or (4) as indicated under section "C" of this request.

(2) A. Any record(s) received shall be used solely for the authorized purpose for which it was obtained.

   B. Any record(s) received shall not be disseminated to persons not authorized to receive the record(s).

   C. The record(s) will be destroyed immediately after it has served its authorized purpose(s).

   D. In the case of a request not accompanied by fingerprints, I am aware that the SBIS cannot guarantee that the record(s) provided relates to the subject of the request.

   E. I am aware that the SBI will rely upon the accuracy and truthfulness of the information provided in this request.

(3) The subject of this record request will be provided with adequate notice to complete or challenge the accuracy of any record(s) provided by the SBI and, if requested by the subject of this record request, will be provided with a reasonable period of time to correct or complete any information provided by the SBI. (Does not apply to private detective requests.)

(4) The subject of this record request will not be presumed guilty of any pending arrest(s) or charge(s) indicated on any record(s) received from the SBI. (Does not apply to private detective requests.)

_____   _____
Type or print name of authorized person making **certification**   Signature of authorized person making **certification**

E. AUTHORIZATION BY SUBJECT OF REQUEST AND PRIVACY ACT NOTIFICATION

Supervisor, State Bureau of Identification:

I hereby authorize the release of any Criminal History Record Information maintained by your agency, meeting dissemination criteria, for the above indicated purpose to _____ .

(Insert name of agency you authorize to receive this information)

Pursuant to the Privacy Act of 1974 (P.L. 93-579), I realize the disclosure of my social security number is **voluntary.** I also realize my social security number will be used for the purpose of facilitating the security check authorized by the above referenced authority. Any information released as a result of this authorization, including the furnishing of my social security number, shall be used only for the express purpose of processing the above indicated application.

_____   _____
Signature of Applicant   Date

NOTE: The SBI **will not** process photocopies of this form. The current processing fee for this document is $18.00 pursuant to N.J.S.A. 53:1-20.6A and N.J.A.C. 13:59-1.3. A cashier's check, certified check, or money order payable to the Division of State Police - SBIS must be stapled to each SBI 212B Form.

If a fingerprint search is required, submit a completed state applicant fingerprint card and SBI 212B Form with a check for $30.00. Staple the check to the lower left corner of the applicant fingerprint card and then staple the applicant fingerprint card to the SBI 212B Form.

FIGURE 4-4 continued

© Cengage Learning 2013

This form will include:

- The name and address of the requestor
- The subject of the request
- The type of request, such as a noncriminal justice purpose by either a governmental entity, by a person, by a nongovernmental entity, or by a licensed private detective
- Certification by requestor attesting to his or her authority to receive and use the criminal history
- Authorization by the subject of the background check and privacy act notification through his or her signature
- Request for fingerprinting if indicated; each state and/or county has its own fingerprint forms.

In addition to this criminal history background, new employees with licenses, certificates, and/or registries need to be confirmed. For nurses, the state board of nurses would be contacted. For physicians, it would be the state medical board. The licenses and certifications can be checked for status as well as any complaints against the provider. All licensed and certified professionals should go through this process.

When creating the policies and procedures for background checks, you should define the employees who are required by facility rules or security levels to have this check. The purpose of such a policy can be defined as a standard requirement for a particular state. If the offer of employment is contingent on the outcome of the background check, then this statement needs to be included in the policy statement. The procedure needs to be defined according to state requirements as well as job requirements. This includes naming the type of documentation form your state requires, such as the "Request for Criminal History Background check." Some job titles or facilities also require fingerprinting. Included in this step is verifying licenses or certifications, such as for radiology technicians, RNs, or ultrasound technicians. Not only make a copy of these licenses but verify them with the appropriate board prior to an employee's start date.

CREDENTIALING PHYSICIANS

Credentialing physicians may be a function of a manager, the human resources department, or a separate credentialing department depending on the type and size of the health care facility. Credentialing is a process that confirms that a physician is indeed who he or she says he or she is. The credentialing process cannot officially begin until after a recommendation to hire is made. The process of credentialing has many parts.

In general, the process includes:

1. A report from a variety of databases that will include the applicant's full name, date of birth, gender, current location if he or she has been practicing, education, and any record of actions taken against the physician.
2. Any sanctions taken by a government agency. That agency can be The Joint Commission, the Food and Drug Administration, the Office of Inspector General (OIG), or a third-party carrier, such as Medicare.

After the initial credentialing, the physician may choose to participate with various insurance carriers. Additional forms and applications are then required.

If the physician chooses to participate with insurance carriers who pay the physician directly, forms for authorization for electronic funds transfer and an **electronic data interchange** (EDI) agreement are completed. By credentialing with insurance companies, the physician is allowed to submit claims and receive payments via paper or electronic transfer. Credentialing with insurance companies is important for physicians who will bill directly to the insurance and not get paid a salary. The credentialing process is a long one, and physicians and providers must be prepared to

TABLE 4-3: Checklist of errors to avoid in the process of credentialing

Checklist
☐ Has the applicant signed all forms as indicated?
☐ Does the name match the official documents?
☐ Has each form been dated?
☐ Are all attachments in order?
☐ Are all questions answered?
☐ Are dates of employment correct?
☐ Are dates of schooling correct?
☐ Is there any missing or vague information?

submit all necessary paperwork for a smooth application process. With the credentialing process, one must submit copies of CVs, diplomas, licenses, registrations, and credentials. Hospitals and larger facilities usually have a credentialing department that can help; if not, contact the insurance companies you wish to credential with, and they will guide you through the process.

You should be aware of a number of common errors that you need to avoid. Table 4-3 offers a checklist to help you avoid these mistakes.

Although the credentialing process is a lengthy one, it is necessary so physicians can treat patients and submit claims for payment. Different forms also exist for different third-party carriers. You should attach a copy of all forms to the policy and procedure manual, which will define the step-by-step process.

THE CONTENT OF ORIENTATION

Once an employee is hired, the **orientation** is the vehicle via which rules and regulations are given to the new employee (see Figure 4-5). These rules and regulations set the stage for employer regulations for internal issues, such as dress codes, hours of operation, vacations, and personal time. If

Note:

I would like a picture of an office manager conducting an orientation with several people in the audience. She (the office manager) will be pointing to a screen or blackboard which has the following listed on it:

Welcome to this healthcare facility

Employee manual

Policies and procedures

Forms

© Cengage Learning 2013

FIGURE 4-5 Orientation

TABLE 4-4: State and federal laws in the human resources area concerning hiring practices

Laws and Regulations	Description
American With Disabilities Act of 1990 (ADA)	This act prohibits discrimination in hiring qualified people because of disabilities.
Family and Medical Leave Act (FMLA)	This law provides up to 12 weeks of unpaid leave per year, without an employee losing his or her job or group benefits. Pregnancy and caring for a terminal relative are examples of applying this act.
Civil Rights Act (1964, 1991) (CRA)	This act prohibits the discrimination of hiring in the areas of employment and compensation because of race, religion, color, or gender.
Fair Credit Reporting Act (FCRA)	This act defines the tools that can be used to do background checks. This act also defines the disclosures and consents that are needed to conduct a legal background check.
The Fair Labor Standards Act (FLSA)	This act requires employers to pay a minimum federal wage and to also pay overtime at one-and-a-half times that regular wage.
The Employee Retirement Income Security Act (ERISA)	This act regulates a variety of benefit plans.

the health care facility is large, then the organizational framework, mission, goals, and outcomes from applicable accreditation review will also be examined.

The orientation may also include training that complies with state, federal, and occupational laws. Different categories of employees may need different orientations based on these laws. For example, such medical personnel as nurses, physicians, and laboratory and medical assistants will need training in **Occupational Safety and Health Administration (OSHA)** regulations as well as HIPAA privacy and security laws. As a manager, you might have to maintain paperwork and logos to comply with OSHA in case of hazardous materials or exposure to materials. Medical billers and coders will need orientation and training with regard to HIPAA, fraud and abuse, and insurance regulations.

The manager also needs to know state and federal laws concerning hiring practices. In order to meet all the necessary requirements of hiring, view Table 4-4, which lists state and federal laws in the human resources area concerning hiring practices. Keep note of the information and have it available at all times. Also, be sure to update the rules and regulations as they change.

COMPLETE PAPERWORK

Paperwork will need to be completed, such as a **W-4 form** (see Figure 4-6). A W-4 form is needed for the employer so the correct federal income tax can be withheld from your pay. In addition, an **I-9 form** is completed to document your identity and citizenship (see Figure 4-7). For all employees, regardless of position, they need to complete these two forms.

The orientation can be of a general format or specific to a department or job title. When creating the policy and procedure, indicate whether it is a general orientation under the human

Form W-4 (2005)

Purpose. Complete Form W-4 so that your employer can withhold the correct federal income tax from your pay. Because your tax situation may change, you may want to refigure your withholding each year.

Exemption from withholding. If you are exempt, complete only lines 1, 2, 3, 4, and 7 and sign the form to validate it. Your exemption for 2005 expires February 16, 2006. See Pub. 505, Tax Withholding and Estimated Tax.

Note. You cannot claim exemption from withholding if (a) your income exceeds $800 and includes more than $250 of unearned income (for example, interest and dividends) and (b) another person can claim you as a dependent on their tax return.

Basic instructions. If you are not exempt, complete the **Personal Allowances Worksheet** below. The worksheets on page 2 adjust your withholding allowances based on itemized deductions, certain credits, adjustments to income, or two-earner/two-job situations. Complete all worksheets that apply. However, you may claim fewer (or zero) allowances.

Head of household. Generally, you may claim head of household filing status on your tax return only if you are unmarried and pay more than 50% of the costs of keeping up a home for yourself and your dependent(s) or other qualifying individuals. See line **E** below.

Tax credits. You can take projected tax credits into account in figuring your allowable number of withholding allowances. Credits for child or dependent care expenses and the child tax credit may be claimed using the **Personal Allowances Worksheet** below. See Pub. 919, How Do I Adjust My Tax Withholding? for information on converting your other credits into withholding allowances.

Nonwage income. If you have a large amount of nonwage income, such as interest or dividends, consider making estimated tax payments using Form 1040-ES, Estimated Tax for Individuals. Otherwise, you may owe additional tax.

Two earners/two jobs. If you have a working spouse or more than one job, figure the total number of allowances you are entitled to claim on all jobs using worksheets from only one Form W-4. Your withholding usually will be most accurate when all allowances are claimed on the Form W-4 for the highest paying job and zero allowances are claimed on the others.

Nonresident alien. If you are a nonresident alien, see the Instructions for Form 8233 before completing this Form W-4.

Check your withholding. After your Form W-4 takes effect, use Pub. 919 to see how the dollar amount you are having withheld compares to your projected total tax for 2005. See Pub. 919, especially if your earnings exceed $125,000 (Single) or $175,000 (Married).

Recent name change? If your name on line 1 differs from that shown on your social security card, call 1-800-772-1213 to initiate a name change and obtain a social security card showing your correct name.

Personal Allowances Worksheet (Keep for your records.)

A Enter "1" for **yourself** if no one else can claim you as a dependent . . . . **A** _____

B Enter "1" if:
- You are single and have only one job; or
- You are married, have only one job, and your spouse does not work; or
- Your wages from a second job or your spouse's wages (or the total of both) are $1,000 or less.

. . . . **B** _____

C Enter "1" for your **spouse**. But, you may choose to enter "-0-" if you are married and have either a working spouse or more than one job. (Entering "-0-" may help you avoid having too little tax withheld.) . . . . **C** _____

D Enter number of **dependents** (other than your spouse or yourself) you will claim on your tax return . . . . **D** _____

E Enter "1" if you will file as **head of household** on your tax return (see conditions under **Head of household** above) . . . . **E** _____

F Enter "1" if you have at least $1,500 of **child or dependent care expenses** for which you plan to claim a credit . . . . **F** _____
(**Note.** Do not include child support payments. See **Pub. 503**, Child and Dependent Care Expenses, for details.)

G **Child Tax Credit** (including additional child tax credit):
- If your total income will be less than $54,000 ($79,000 if married), enter "2" for each eligible child.
- If your total income will be between $54,000 and $84,000 ($79,000 and $119,000 if married), enter "1" for each eligible child plus "1" **additional** if you have four or more eligible children. . . . . **G** _____

H Add lines A through G and enter total here. (**Note.** This may be different from the number of exemptions you claim on your tax return.) ▶ **H** _____

For accuracy, complete all worksheets that apply.
- If you plan to **itemize or claim adjustments to income** and want to reduce your withholding, see the **Deductions and Adjustments Worksheet** on Page 2.
- If you have **more than one job** or are **married and you and your spouse both work** and the combined earnings from all jobs exceed $35,000 ($25,000 if married) see the **Two-Earner/Two-Job Worksheet** on page 2 to avoid having too little tax withheld.
- If **neither** of the above situations applies, **stop here** and enter number from line H on line 5 of Form W-4 below.

- - - - - - - - - - Cut here and give Form W-4 to your employer. Keep the top part for your records. - - - - - - - - - -

Form **W-4**	**Employee's Withholding Allowance Certificate**	OMB No. 1545-0010
Department of the Treasury Internal Revenue Service	▶ **Whether you are entitled to claim a certain number of allowances or exemption from withholding is subject to review by the IRS. Your employer may be required to send a copy of this form to the IRS.**	**2005**

1 Type or print your first name and middle initial	Last name	2 Your social security number
Home address (number and street or rural route)	3 ☐ Single ☐ Married ☐ Married, but withhold at higher Single rate. Note. If married, but legally separated, or spouse is nonresident alien, check the "Single" box.	
City or town, state, and ZIP code	4 If your last name differs from that shown on your social security card, check here. You must call 1-800-772-1213 for a new card. ▶ ☐	

5 Total number of allowances you are claiming (from line **H** above or from the applicable worksheet on page 2) . . . . . **5** _____

6 Additional amount, If any, you want withheld from each paycheck . . . . **6** $ _____

7 I claim exemption from withholding for 2005, and I certify that I meet **both** of the following conditions for exemption.
- Last year I had a right to a refund of all federal income tax withheld because I had no tax liability and
- This year I expect a refund of all federal income tax withheld because I expect to have no tax liability.

If you meet both conditions, write "Exempt" here . . . . ▶ **7** _____

Under penalties of perjury, I declare that I have examined this certificate and to the best of my knowledge and belief, it is true, correct, and complete.

Employee's signature (Form is not valid unless you sign it.) ▶ _____ **Date** ▶ _____

8 Employer's name and address (Employer. Complete lines 8 and 10 only if sending to the IRS.)	9 Office code (optional)	10 Employer identification number (EIN)

For Privacy Act and Paperwork Reduction Act Notice, see page 2. | Cat. No. 102200 | Form **W-4** (2005)

FIGURE 4-6 W-4 Form

Form W-4 (2005)   Page **2**

Deductions and Adjustments Worksheet

Note. Use this worksheet *only* if you plan to itemize deductions, claim certain credits, or claim adjustments to income on your 2005 tax return.

1 Enter an estimate of your 2005 itemized deductions. These include qualifying home mortgage interest, charitable contributions, state and local taxes, medical expenses in excess of 7.5% of your income, and miscellaneous deductions. (For 2005, you may have to reduce your itemized deductions if your income is over $145,950 ($72,975 if married filing separately). See *Worksheet 3* in Pub. 919 for details.) . . . .   **1** $ _____

2 Enter: { $10,000 if married filing jointly or qualifying widow(er)
            $ 7,300 if head of household   } . . . .   **2** $ _____
            $ 5,000 if single or married filing separately

3 **Subtract** line 2 from line 1. If line 2 is greater than line 1, enter "-0-" . . . .   **3** $ _____

4 Enter an estimate of your 2005 adjustments to income, including alimony, deductible IRA contributions, and student loan interest   **4** $ _____

5 **Add** lines 3 and 4 and enter the total. (Include any amount for credits from *Worksheet 7* in Pub. 919) . . . .   **5** $ _____

6 Enter an estimate of your 2005 nonwage income (such as dividends or interest) . . . .   **6** $ _____

7 **Subtract** line 6 from line 5. Enter the result, but not less than "-0-" . . . .   **7** $ _____

8 **Divide** the amount on line 7 by $3,200 and enter the result here. Drop any fraction . . . .   **8** _____

9 Enter the number from the **Personal Allowances Worksheet,** line H, page 1 . . . .   **9** _____

10 **Add** lines 8 and 9 and enter the total here. If you plan to use the **Two-Earner/Two-Job Worksheet,** also enter this total on line 1 below. Otherwise, **stop here** and enter this total on Form W-4, line 5, page 1 . . . .   **10** _____

Two-Earner/Two-Job Worksheet (See *Two earners/two jobs* on page 1.)

Note. Use this worksheet *only* if the instructions under line H on page 1 direct you here.

1 Enter the number from line H, page 1 (or from line 10 above if you used the **Deductions and Adjustments Worksheet**)   1 _____

2 Find the number in **Table 1** below that applies to the **LOWEST** paying job and enter it here . . . .   2 _____

3 If line 1 is **more than or equal to** line 2, subtract line 2 from line 1. Enter the result here (if zero, enter "-0-") and on Form W-4, line 5, page 1, **Do not** use the rest of this worksheet . . . .   3 _____

Note. If line 1 is *less than* line 2, enter "-0-" on Form W-4, line 5, page 1. Complete lines 4–9 below to calculate the additional withholding amount necessary to avoid a year-end tax bill.

4 Enter the number from line 2 of this worksheet . . . .   4 . . . . . . _____

5 Enter the number from line 1 of this worksheet . . . .   5 . . . . . . _____

6 Subtract line 5 from line 4 . . . .   6 _____

7 Find the amount in **Table 2** below that applies to the **HIGHEST** paying job and enter it here . . . .   7 $ _____

8 **Multiply** line 7 by line 6 and enter the result here. This is the additional annual withholding needed . . . .   8 $ _____

9 Divide line 8 by the number of pay periods remaining in 2005. For example, divide by 26 if you are paid every two weeks and you complete this form in December 2004. Enter the result here and on Form W-4, line 6, page 1. This is the additional amount to be withheld from each paycheck . . . .   9 $ _____

Table 1: Two-Earner/Two-Job Worksheet

Married Filing Jointly						All Others	
If wages from **HIGHEST** paying job are —	AND, wages from **LOWEST** paying job are —	Enter on line 2 above	If wages from **HIGHEST** paying job are —	AND, wages from **LOWEST** paying job are —	Enter on line 2 above	If wages from **LOWEST** paying job are —	Enter on line 2 above
$0–$40,000	$0 – $4,000	0	$40,001 and over	30,001 – 36,000	6	$0 – $6,000	0
	4,001 – 8,000	1		36,001 – 45,000	7	6,001 – 12,000	1
	8,001 – 18,000	2		45,001 – 50,000	8	12,001 – 18,000	2
	18,001 and over	3		50,001 – 60,000	9	18,001 – 24,000	3
				60,001 – 65,000	10	24,001 – 31,000	4
$40,001 and over	$0 – $4,000	0		65,001 – 75,000	11	31,001 – 45,000	5
	4,001 – 8,000	1		75,001 – 90,000	12	45,001 – 60,000	6
	8,001 – 18,000	2		90,001 – 100,000	13	60,001 – 75,000	7
	18,001 – 22,000	3		100,001 – 115,000	14	75,001 – 80,000	8
	22,001 – 25,000	4		115,001 and over	15	80,001 – 100,000	9
	25,001 – 30,000	5				100,001 and over	10

Table 2: Two-Earner/Two-Job Worksheet

Married Filing Jointly		All Others	
If wages from **HIGHEST** paying job are —	Enter on line 7 above	If wages from **HIGHEST** paying job are —	Enter on line 7 above
$0 – $60,000	$480	$0 – $30,000	$480
60,001 – 110,000	800	30,001 – 70,000	800
110,001 – 160,000	900	70,001 – 140,000	900
160,001 – 280,000	1,060	140,001 – 320,000	1,060
280,001 and over	1,120	320,001 and over	1,120

© Cengage Learning 2013

FIGURE 4-6 continued

U.S. Department of Justice
Immigration and Naturalization Service

OMB No. 1115-0136
Employment Eligibility Verification

Please read instructions carefully before completing this form. The instructions must be available during completion of this form. **ANTI-DISCRIMINATION NOTICE.** It is illegal to discriminate against work eligible individuals. Employers CANNOT specify which document(s) they will accept from an employee. The refusal to hire an individual because of a future expiration date may also constitute illegal discrimination.

Section 1. Employee Information and Verification. To be completed and signed by employee at the time employment begins

Print Name: Last	First	Middle Initial	Maiden Name
Address *(Street Name and Number)*		Apt. #	Date of Birth *(month/day/year)*
City	State	Zip Code	Social Security #

I am aware that federal law provides for imprisonment and/or fines for false statements or use of false documents in connection with the completion of this form.	I attest, under penalty of perjury, that I am (check one of the following): ☐ A citizen or national of the United States ☐ A Lawful Permanent Resident (Alien # A _____) ☐ An alien authorized to work until ___/___/___ (Alien # or Admission # _____)

Employee's Signature	Date *(month/day/year)*

Preparer and/or Translator Certification. *(To be completed and signed if Section 1 is prepared by a person other than the employee.)* *I attest, under penalty of perjury, that I have assisted in the completion of this form and that to the best of my knowledge the information is true and correct.*

Preparer's/Translator's Signature	Print Name
Address *(Street Name and Number, City, State, Zip Code)*	Date *(month/day/year)*

Section 2. Employer Review and Verification. To be completed and signed by employer. Examine one document from List A OR examine one document from List B **and** one from List C as listed on the reverse of this form and record the title, number and expiration date, if any, of the document(s)

List A	OR	List B	AND	List C
Document title: _____		_____		_____
Issuing authority: _____		_____		_____
Document #: _____		_____		_____
Expiration Date *(if any)*: ___/___/___		___/___/___		___/___/___
Document #: _____				
Expiration Date *(if any)*: ___/___/___				

CERTIFICATION - I attest, under penalty of perjury, that I have examined the document(s) presented by the above-named employee, that the above-listed document(s) appear to be genuine and to relate to the employee named, that the employee began employment on *(month/day/year)* ___/___/___ and that to the best of my knowledge the employee is eligible to work in the United States. (State employment agencies may omit the date the employee began employment).

Signature of Employer or Authorized Representative	Print Name	Title
Business or Organization Name	Address *(Street Name and Number, City, State, Zip Code)*	Date *(month/day/year)*

Section 3. Updating and Reverification. To be completed and signed by employer

A. New Name *(if applicable)*	B. Date of rehire *(month/day/year)* *(if applicable)*

C. If employee's previous grant of work authorization has expired, provide the information below for the document that establishes current employment eligibility.

Document Title: _____   Document #: _____   Expiration Date *(if any)*: ___/___/___

I attest, under penalty of perjury, that to the best of my knowledge, this employee is eligible to work in the United States, and if the employee presented document(s), the document(s) I have examined appear to be genuine and to relate to the individual.

Signature of Employer or Authorized Representative	Date *(month/day/year)*

Form I-9 (Rev. 11-21-91) N

© Cengage Learning 2013

FIGURE 4-7 I-9 Form

resources department or specific to a department, such as medical billing or nursing. In the policy, include not just the general content but the job-specific inclusions, such as OSHA training for clinical and medical staff. In the procedure section, include each part of the orientation, what forms are needed, and what regulations the orientation is complying with and then attach a copy of each.

A sample agenda for orientation could look something like this:

> Welcome
>
> Mission Statement: What this organization is about
>
> Organizational Framework
>
> Polices and Procedures
>
> Review of Employee Manual

Additional parts of the orientation would depend on the category of personnel. If clinicians are in orientation, then a review of OSHA procedures will be conducted. If the employee is involved in billing and coding, then applicable rules and laws for billing and collection will be covered. Some of the orientation is similar for everyone, such as computer training, access codes for computers, parking permits, and security clearance for the building. The hiring manager or human resources department must plan strategically to orient new employees in a group when it is required. Orientation and training do take time, so organizing the process will save time.

EMPLOYEE MANUAL

An employee manual is one vehicle that can be used in new employee orientations.

This manual should be clear, concise, and pertinent. Relevant state, federal, and occupational laws should be a part of this manual and the policies and procedures within it. Parts of an employee manual may include:

- General information about the facility
- Employment at the facility
- Organizational framework of the health care facility
- Mission statement
- Job descriptions
- Benefits
- Employer expectations
- Pertinent policies and procedures
- Dress code
- Policies and procedures directly related to the jobs

ORGANIZATION OF A HEALTH CARE FACILITY

The organization of a health care facility depends on the type and size of that facility.

A physician's office can be organized as simply as:

- Physician
- Office Manager
  - Other personnel, such as receptionist, medical assistants, or billers

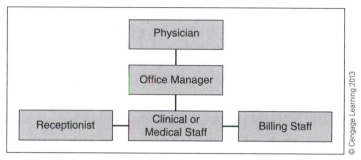

FIGURE 4-8 Organization of a Small Physician's Office

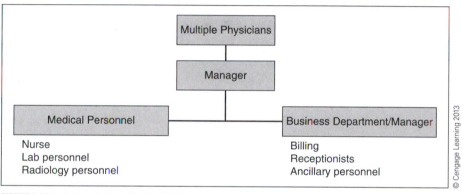

FIGURE 4-9 Organization of a Large Physician's Office

Figure 4-8 shows the organization of a small physician's office.

Or a larger facility:

- Physician(s)
- Medical personnel, such as physician assistants, nurses, and lab or radiology personnel
- Clinical manager and/or business manager
  - Clinical staff
  - Billing department personnel
  - Receptionists
  - Ancillary personnel

Figure 4-9 shows the organization of a larger physician's office.

Or a freestanding facility:

- Physician
- Office manager
  - Laboratory or radiology technicians
  - Billing personnel
  - Receptionists

Figure 4-10 shows the organization of a freestanding laboratory or radiology facility.

The organizational framework for a hospital would be much more complicated because it has a president/CEO, a board of directors and trustees, a medical department chairman, a nursing department director, and various department heads that oversee appropriate staff. When the facility has large departments that need to be managed, upper management is needed to operate appropriately and meet requirements for patient care.

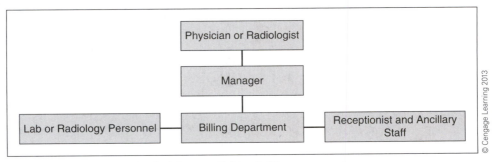

FIGURE 4-10 Organization of a Free-Standing Laboratory or Radiology Facility

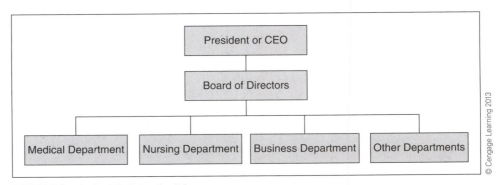

FIGURE 4-11 Organizational Charts for a Hospital

Figure 4-11 shows organizational charts for a hospital.

MISSION STATEMENT

A **mission statement** is one that clearly defines the purpose for the existence of the organization, what it intends to do, and who it serves. A mission statement plays an important role in large organizations as the company grows and they are unable to demonstrate their purposes through personal contact. Understanding the intent of the organization can guide employees through their employment as they attempt to fulfill the mission statement. Each facility determines its own need for a mission statement, and most mission statements can be viewed on each facility's website. Mission statements are not a requirement; however, they portray a positive image that employees can follow.

JOB DESCRIPTION

Job descriptions are an important detail of the hiring process. New employees want to know what they are expected to do when they begin. In addition, this is an ongoing process for them through their employment. Some facilities have job descriptions written out and presented to employees, and others present job descriptions verbally with the expectation that the employee will fulfill all requirements. Whether written or verbal, job descriptions play a role for employees, and their expectations must be clear and coincide with their experience or credentials. If a job requires an employee to have certain credentials, the facility must follow those guidelines in hiring the employee.

When jobs are posted for applicants, the job description is included and should represent the job description as presented at the facility. It is appropriate for job descriptions to be written; however, they must be followed regardless. When a new employee is hired, job descriptions are reviewed and that person's relationship to job performance evaluation and raises are discussed. Should the employee not follow his or her job description, raises can be held and the employee could potentially be released for noncompliance.

BENEFITS

Benefits offered often depend on the size of the health care facility. When employers offer benefits, employees are required to complete additional paperwork to apply for the benefits. Benefits are reviewed in the hiring process as well as in orientation. Employers will include appropriate forms on the first day of employment and submit appropriate applications in a timely manner on behalf of the employee.

Benefits can include:

- Medical plans
- Dental coverage
- Other insurance, such as life insurance, long-term care insurance, or disability insurance
- Personal time off (PTO) accruement of hours and holiday pay
- Vacations
- Personal days
- 401(k) plans

Employer Expectations

Employer expectations are important for the employee to know. Often times these expectations are the bases for performance evaluations leading to a raise of salary. Not following these expectations can also be the grounds for termination. These employer expectations include:

- Workplace rules and regulations
- Performance expectations, development, and evaluation
- Termination

POLICIES AND PROCEDURES

Policies and procedures can be general in nature related to the health care facility. They can also be related to a job description. Depending on the job and the category, the policies could be more extensive. All policies need to be outlined for employees by management and presented upon hiring or orientation.

Examples of policies and procedures that are general to all employees are:

- Vacations
- Pay raises
- Evaluations
- Dress code
- Personal days
- Holidays
- Sick days
- Bereavement
- Medical leave
- Schedules

Examples of policies and procedures that are job related for medical personnel (such as nurses or medical assistants) are:

- OSHA and the importance of safety in the workplace:
  - Blood-borne pathogens
  - Use of personal protective equipment
  - Preventing needle sticks

- Confidentiality
- HIPAA and the importance of maintaining confidentiality

Examples of policies and procedures that are job related to billing and coding personnel are:

- Collecting a copayment, which should include in this policy when to tell the patient the copayment must be paid
- Defining charity care, which should include in this policy who determines if the patient qualifies and what your states guidelines are
- Following up on denied claims, which should include in this policy whose responsibility it is and what the steps are for different reasons of denial. This topic will be covered more extensively in the next unit.
- Fraud and abuse related to billing and coding

After employees complete the policies and procedures review, the hiring or orientation process should include a final step to obtain a signature that verifies that the employees understand how important these policies and procedures are for the facility. When this signature is on file, the new employee has agreed that he or she has been notified of all policies and procedures, that he or she understands the policies and procedures, and that he or she will ask management about any information that he or she does not understand. When employees provide a signature, the employer must maintain the signature for the duration of employment.

PROBATION PERIOD

You should tell new employees about a probation period. A probation period is a designated time period, usually 3–6 months, in which the new employee becomes oriented to his or her new place of employment and exhibits competency in the area for which he or she was hired. It is a reasonable amount of time for a new employee to adjust to the health care facility and perform the job responsibilities he or she was hired to do.

The employee handbook should outline the steps that will be taken if the new hire does not achieve a level of competency upon completion of the probation period. The handbook should discuss whether the period will be extended or if the employee will be terminated. During the probation period, employees can be restricted from benefits until the probation period is over. This is a policy that needs to be clearly defined in the employee manual and during the orientation and/or hiring process.

REVIEWS AND RAISES

The frequency of reviews and raises needs to be stated in the employee handbook and reviewed during orientation. Are reviews annual? Are they automatic or based on performance? Reviews and raises are important parts of the application process because employees are motivated by raises. When reviews are done on a regular basis, employees appreciate this because it gives them the opportunity to make changes if they are doing something wrong, allowing them to improve and maintain a high level of performance. In return, they become eligible for a raise. When an employer has a specific protocol for review and raises, employees should be made aware so they are knowledgeable about the process and are able to prepare accordingly. Awareness of reviews and raises can increase morale and create a positive working environment.

HEALTH INSURANCE PORTABILITY AND ACCOUNTABILITY ACT (HIPAA)

HIPAA has components on privacy, security, electronic health care transactions, code sets, and the simplification of identifiers for providers and health plans. HIPAA discusses privacy and confidentiality as it relates to all areas of patient care. The medical record and billing are all covered under HIPAA, and the guidelines need to be followed by all employees.

Depending on the job category, an orientation to the standards and compliance with these standards will be important. For example, employees who use a computer to perform their jobs, complete claim forms, and input patient information need to understand security regulations as well as privacy rules. Most employees will need to understand the privacy rules as part of their orientation. For any employee accessing patient data—whether clinical or administrative—they will need to keep patient data confidential and not allow other employees to use their access codes. HIPAA plays a large role in the medical field in clinical and administrative areas, and all employees should have some training in HIPAA requirements.

TERMINATION PROCEDURES

Termination procedures are as important as orientation. Whether the employee leaves to relocate, takes another job, or is terminated, the employee must know the standard procedures involved in the termination process. Termination procedures may include retrieving keys and access cards, changing passwords, or deleting e-mail addresses. The employee needs to be reminded of legal, ethical, and confidentiality issues. Documentation of termination must be maintained in the employee file.

Policies and procedures for termination of employment are necessary. They can be general policies or, in larger facilities, designed by department or job description. In these policies, set out steps and a timetable to retrieve keys and access devices, to turn off e-mail addresses, and to change passwords. If you require a document that the terminated employee signs regarding laws and confidentiality, be sure to also attach that to the policy manual for employees to have during orientation.

Checklist for the hiring process

- ☐ Place employment advertisement.
- ☐ Review résumés.
- ☐ Set up interviews.
- ☐ Interview candidates.
- ☐ Make an offer.
- ☐ Check background.
- ☐ Check credentials.
- ☐ Offer orientation.
- ☐ Discuss employee manual.
- ☐ Review policies and procedures.

MANAGEMENT FUNCTIONS

Requirements for management are detailed and must be followed. The importance of following protocol in a medical facility is just as important for managers as it is for clinical personnel because they are responsible for all administrative and clinical employees. Human resources and office managers oversee every employee, and they must be trained in orientation procedures, including federal and state rules and regulations, such as HIPAA, coding compliance, and OSHA. Additional training for management would be in employment law, which requires knowledge of the hiring requirements, staffing needs, licensure and certification, and personnel laws at the state and federal levels.

Functions of the Manager

- Perform orientation and hiring requirements.
- Maintain updated employee manual.
- Maintain updated policies and procedures manual.
- Train regularly on all state and federal law requirements.
- Understand all personnel laws and regulations.
- Perform accounting duties regularly.
- Process payroll in a timely manner.
- Perform employee evaluations annually.
- Follow termination procedures.

ADD TO THE POLICIES AND PROCEDURES MANUAL

Understanding all state and federal regulations is important for human resources and management. All policies must be maintained and kept accessible to employees. In the medical facilities, the policies and procedures manual will include policies that pertain to job functions. These policies and procedures needed to be updated immediately when changes occur. The policies and procedures related to the medical field include OSHA, HIPAA, compliance in all departments, and any other pertinent policies or procedures that pertain to patient treatment. Human resources and management are required to maintain and identify a location to allow all employees to view all policies and procedures at all times. Following policies and procedures as they relate to laws and regulations is a requirement for all employees, and noncompliance should result in reprimand.

In order to stay current with changes, human resources and management may have to participate in workshops or obtain membership to groups that follow compliance in the medical field. Keeping up with the current changes is pertinent and a difficult process, and by creating a network for themselves, they can easily obtain information needed to stay current for their employees. Maintaining their policies and procedures has become easier with the Internet; however, a lot of work is still involved in finding the changes. Some ways to ensure you are current is to join compliance groups, set up e-mail alerts, create a network with neighboring managers, and attend workshops. Whatever method you chose to obtain information, be sure the source is credible and trustworthy.

CREATE AN EMPLOYMENT ADVERTISEMENT

Knowing the qualifications and type of employee you are searching for is the most important information when creating an employment advertisement. The advertisement must target the employee and give specifics about the requirements as well as preferences. The category of employee you are hiring is important to what you will create in order to be certain the appropriate candidates apply.

Specific employment advertisements can create less work for human resources or management. If you are detailed about your expectations, the résumés you receive will be more appropriate. Licensure or certification requirements should always be included if they are a requirement for the position. Past experience is another factor that plays a role in hiring and can be included in the employment advertisement to avoid résumés from candidates without life experience. In addition, education requirements will also be listed as they pertain to the position requirements. All these requirements can be listed as necessities or preferences depending on the nature of the position and the facility's expectations.

Other details to include in the employment advertisement would be hours, salary range, whether the job is part time or full time, and benefits. If these are listed, potential candidates can make a better decision as to whether they should submit an application based on their own requirements in an employer.

All employment advertisements should be customized based on the information for the position. When submitting a general advertisement, nonqualified candidates will apply, creating a submission of more résumés and more work for management or human resource. Creating a template for the basic information is appropriate, to be sure all the appropriate information is included. Be sure to check your employment advertisement after it is posted, and if possible, ask someone else to read the advertisement to be sure it is appropriate for the facility's employment needs.

START AN EMPLOYEE MANUAL

In addition to the policies and procedures manual, you are required to maintain an employee manual. Unlike the policies and procedures manual, which is usually updated when state and federal laws change, the employee manual is based on the facility's requirements, and updating the manual is a preference but can also be done annually. The employee manual is usually customized to the employer's needs and includes general and specific expectations of the facility and each new administrative and clinical employee.

An employee manual will outline all the expectations and requirements for each employee and department. However, if an employee manual has already been created, reviewing the manual and updating all pertinent information should be performed immediately. Included in the employee manual should be the mission statement, employer expectations, job descriptions and qualifications for administrative and clinical personnel, hours denoted for part-time and full-time employees, probation period explanations, termination procedures, discussions about reviews and raises, and explanations of benefits, including vacation, sick time, insurance, 401(k), and more. Human resources and management should create and maintain an employee manual that identifies all employees' expectations as they pertain to each position. If the employee manual is completed properly, employees will have fewer questions for human resources and management as they read their manuals during the hiring process or orientation.

SUMMARY

- The hiring process begins with understanding the roles of each of the personnel within the health care facility. The educational requirements, certifications, and/or registries required and the scope of practice are essential.

- Placing an advertisement for hiring personnel requires knowing what the position is, the hours and days for the position, whether the job is part time or full time, and what qualifications are sought.

- Résumés are the first step in the hiring process. The overall impression, including the format and appearance, should reflect professionalism. The requirements in the advertisement should be reflected in the applicant's résumé.

- The interview process is the next step. The potential employee is interviewed by the manager and/or by personnel in human resources.

- An offer is sent in an acceptance letter outlining the position being offered, the rate of pay, the starting date, benefits, and any contingency clauses, such as the results of a background check.

- The new employee goes through an orientation process. This orientation process will include the organizational framework and mission statement. A job description as well as policies, procedures, and benefits should also be discussed.

- An employee manual is given to each new applicant, and applicable areas are reviewed and explained, with questions being answered by the people conducting the orientation.

- Part of the orientation process should include an explanation of the termination procedure.

REVIEW EXERCISES

TRUE OR FALSE

1. _____ To undergo a yearly evaluation, an employee should have a job description.

2. _____ An advertisement for new personnel should state the requirements.

3. _____ An interview should always be during working hours.

4. _____ Policies and procedures for termination are necessary.

5. _____ Questions during an interview should be directed at qualifications and experience.

6. _____ A prospective employer can also ask during an interview how many children a candidate has.

7. _____ A background check may be a contingency of employment.

8. _____ Credentialing is a quick process.

9. _____ All employees get the same orientation.

10. _____ Only large organizations will have an organizational framework.

MATCHING

A   Employee Manual

B   Job Description

C   ADA

D   Credentialing

E   I-9

F   W-4

G   OSHA

H   Acceptance Letter

I   Orientation

J   EDI

1. _____ A process that confirms a physician's qualifications.

2. _____ Written expectations of an employee's responsibilities.

3. _____ Prohibits discrimination in hiring based on disabilities.

4. _____ States the position offered, starting date, and salary.

5. _____ An electronic transfer of funds (for payment to a physician).

6. _____ A vehicle through which rules, regulations, and mission are presented.

7. _____ Designates federal income tax withholding information.

8. _____ Proves your identity.

9. _____ Concerned with safety and exposure to hazardous materials.

10. _____ Contains policies and procedures, job descriptions, the company's mission statement, and employer expectations.

CRITICAL THINKING ACTIVITIES

ACTIVITY 1

As a manager, you may be involved in developing a benefits package for the health care facility. Identify 10 benefits you would like to see in the benefits package for your employees.

Benefits Package
1. _____
2. _____
3. _____
4. _____
5. _____
6. _____
7. _____
8. _____
9. _____
10. _____

ACTIVITY 2

Match the following words with each other according to their relationship. Only one answer is valid per question.

1.	_____ Credentialing		A.	_____ CV
2.	_____ Orientation		B.	_____ CEUs
3.	_____ Résumé		C.	_____ Salary
4.	_____ Background check		D.	_____ 401(k) benefit
5.	_____ Privacy		E.	_____ EDI
6.	_____ An offer		F.	_____ Advertisement
7.	_____ Certification		G.	_____ HIPAA
8.	_____ Job description		H.	_____ OSHA training
9.	_____ Employee manual		I.	_____ Raise
10.	_____ Performance review		J.	_____ SBI

ACTIVITY 3

During the interview process, we sometimes forget questions. Potential employees should have particular answers that you as a manager want to know, and you need to remember the questions you need answered during the interview. Create a checklist of questions you want to remember during the interview.

Interview Checklist

☐ _____

☐ _____

☐ _____

☐ _____

☐ _____

☐ _____

☐ _____

☐ _____

☐ _____

☐ _____

☐ _____

☐ _____

☐ _____

☐ _____

☐ _____

☐ _____

☐ _____

☐ _____

☐ _____

CRITICAL THINKING QUESTIONS

1. Describe what type of qualities you would look for in a potential candidate you would want to hire for a health care facility.

2. Debate the pros and cons of hiring a friend or family member if you were the manager. Include personal experience if applicable.

3. Discuss how you would handle the situation where you have a great potential candidate, but the background check came back with one inappropriate warning sign. Then, the candidate explains that this was not what really happened but that it affected his or her license.

4. Explain how you would handle a new employee during orientation when he or she learns about a policy he or she does not approve of and he or she expresses his or her disagreement with you. This happens to be something you do not approve of either, but you must present it to all your employees.

WEB ACTIVITIES

1. Go to the Americans With Disabilities Act (ADA) website at http://www.eeoc.gov/facts/health_care_workers.html to research ADA requirements for a health care facility. The manager must keep ADA requirements confidential from other employees; however, some exceptions exist. Write down five people who are allowed to know about an employee's ADA requirements.

2. Use the Department of Labor's Occupational Outlook Handbook website at http://stats.bls.gov/oco to research the description for a medical assistant. Determine what duties medical assistants can perform in your state. (Save this information for "Think Like a Manager: Create Your Practice.")

THINK LIKE A MANAGER
CREATE YOUR PRACTICE

Using the templates found in Appendix B and the information presented in this unit, complete the following interactive exercises:

1. Write a policy and procedure for the hiring process.

2. Write a policy and procedure for conducting a background check.

3. Write a policy and procedure for terminating employment.

4. Write an employment advertisement to place in the classifieds of the local newspaper for a medical assistant. Include the role, responsibilities, education, and salary.

5. Write a job description for the medical assistant for your practice. Information about this job is located on the Department of Labor's Occupational Outlook Handbook website (http://stats.bls.gov/oco). (See website activities)

6. Write an offer letter for a prospective hire.

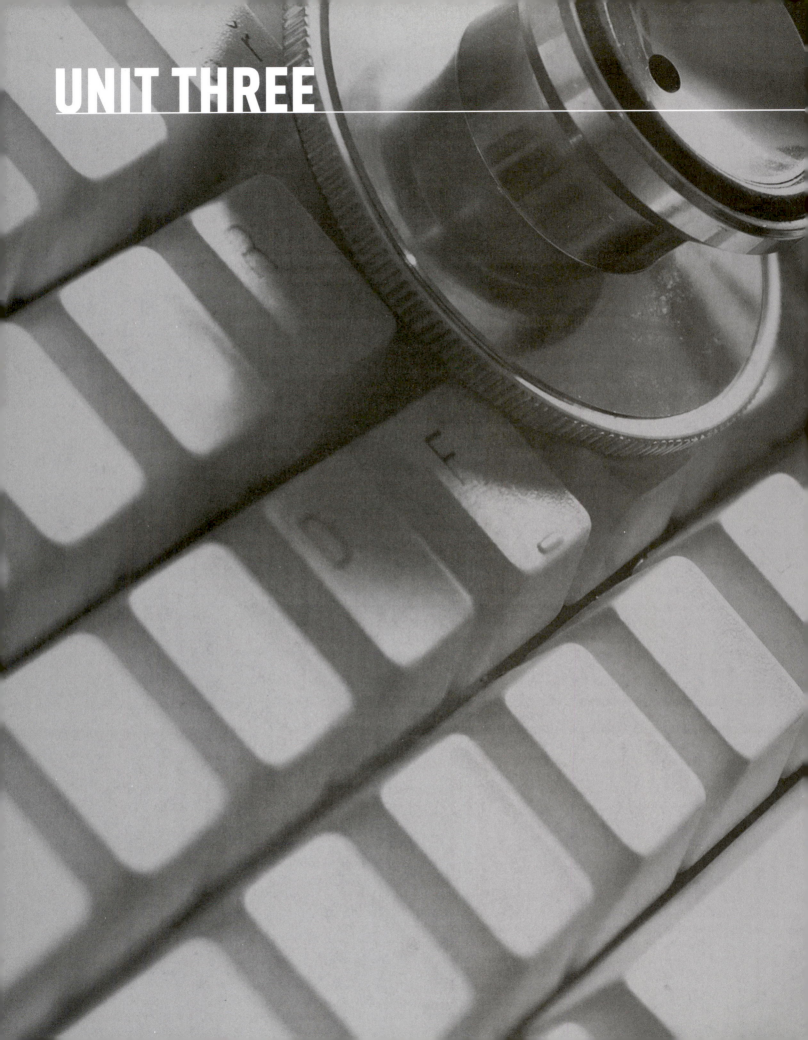

UNIT THREE

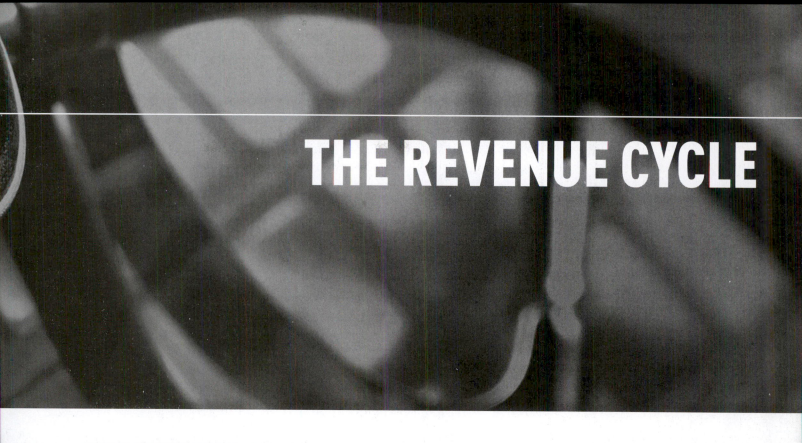

THE REVENUE CYCLE

THE REVENUE CYCLE is essential to the financial success of a health care facility. Reimbursements by payers and patients as well as expenses contribute to the revenue cycle, and maintaining a profit is essential. Each component must be monitored consistently because they all affect one another. Understanding the elements of the revenue cycle as well as performing audits are part of the role of a health care facility's manager.

REVENUE CYCLE

- Manage a medical facility business and its functions.
- Perform bookkeeping procedures, including balancing accounts.
- Manage accounts payable.
- Manage payroll activities.
- Manage accounts receivable.
- Understand basic auditing as a control mechanism.
- Manage patient accounts.
- Perform patient billing.
- Manage collections.
- Understand banking procedures necessary for the facility.
- Track unpaid claims and file and track appeals.
- Facilitate employee meetings and in-service training as part of office communications on procedures of the revenue cycle.
- Manage the components of the revenue cycle.

CHAPTER 5

THE REVENUE CYCLE

FUNDAMENTALS

Chapter 5 will discuss the fundamentals of the revenue cycle. The facility depends on money coming into the practice, and the most important types of accounts receivable are insurance and patient payments. Therefore, it is vital to be proactive in collecting payments from both parties to be successful. This chapter will include reviewing the elements that comprise the revenue cycle as it pertains to the collection of fees for the facility.

OBJECTIVES

Upon completion of this chapter, the student will be able to:

- Identify the elements of the revenue cycle.
- Review each element in the review cycle.
- Apply each element in the review cycle to outpatient and inpatient settings.
- Understand the relationship of the revenue cycle to expenses.

KEY TERMS

- Account aging
- Collections
- Current procedural terminology (CPT)
- Healthcare common procedure coding system (HCPCS)
- International Classification of Diseases
- (ICD-Diagnostic Codes)
- Inpatient
- Medically necessary
- Outpatient
- Remittance advice (RA)
- Explanation of benefits (EOB)
- Third-party payers
- Timely filing

REVENUE CYCLE COMPONENTS

The revenue cycle is a continuum of activities that starts with the new patient needing and making an appointment in the appropriate health care facility and who completes the registration form. The patient receives services that are documented in the patient's medical record. These services, along with a diagnosis for justifying the need for these services, are also documented. The procedures, services, and diagnoses are converted to codes. An insurance form is completed by using these codes and then sent to the patients' insurance carrier for reimbursement. The insurance company processes the claim and sends a payment. The payment is recorded on the patient's ledger and daily log or day sheet. The explanation of benefits (EOB) is examined for correctness, denials, or monies owed. The patient may be responsible for copayments and uncovered services and will be billed.

Revenue Cycle Links

- The patient needs an appointment and seeks services in a health care setting.
- The registration form is completed.
- The patient receives services.
- Services and diagnoses are documented in the patient's chart.
- Services and diagnoses are converted to codes.
- The claim form is completed and sent to the insurance carrier.
- The claim is processed and any payments are sent.
- The payment is recorded on the patient's ledger and daily log or day sheet.
- The explanation of benefits is examined.
- Additional billing is done if warranted.

THE PATIENT VISIT

When a patient needs to see a health care provider, he or she will seek services in a health care setting. A patient may seek services in a variety of settings depending on the nature of his or her health or medical condition. These settings include but are not limited to the physician's office, a specialist, radiology centers, a laboratory, long-term care, hospital **inpatient** (in which patients are admitted), and hospital **outpatient** (where patients are not admitted but seek treatment and leave the same day). When a patient arrives at a health care setting as a new patient, information is obtained by medical personnel, such as the receptionist, as discussed in Chapter 1. Recall that this information includes the reason for the appointment, insurance information, and billing information.

Upon arrival to the facility, all patients have to go through the registration process to be sure their information is accurate. Patients who are there for the first time are considered new patients and need a full registration to be completed prior to the patient visit. Return patients are considered established and require their paperwork and demographics be reviewed and updated prior to their follow-up visit. Obtaining accurate information from both types of patients is pertinent to the billing process because this is the first step to beginning the claim form completion and obtaining revenue for the facility. Avoid errors with the patient registration or else they might be transferred to the claim form and then the claim could be denied.

Reasons for the Appointment

Different specialties and health care settings will have different types of appointments—some routine and some urgent or emergencies. When a patient needs to be seen, he or she does not always know what type of appointment he or she needs. Initially, the patient pays to see his or her own physician and then be referred to the appropriate facility after that. Each insurance is different, and some allow the patient to self-refer and others need a referral from his or her primary care physician, so be cautious when making appointments at different types of facilities. Table 5-1 lists some of the different specialties, appointments that can be routine and those that could be emergencies.

TABLE 5-1: Routine and Emergency appointments by specialty

Specialist	Routine Appointments	Urgent or Emergency Appointments
Radiology	Yearly mammography Follow-up to previous fracture or injury	Suspected internal problems Sudden accident or injury Severe unexplained pain
Laboratory	Periodic follow-up exams, such as blood glucose or hemoglobin tests	Unexplained symptoms Biopsy
Inpatient hospital	Planned routine procedure	Sudden illness or accident
Long-term care/adult setting	Long-term residence for 24-hour care	Need for rehabilitative or respite care
Physician Specialists		
Cardiologist	Follow-up to a previous cardiac condition or surgery	Severe chest pain Complications after surgery or cardiac procedure
Dermatologist	Follow-up appointments to previous skin conditions, such as skin cancer or burns	Burns Skin cancer Severe dermatology reactions
Gastroenterologist	Follow-up to critical conditions, such as bleeding ulcers or cancer	Bleeding Severe abdominal pain
Obstetrics/Gynecologist	Yearly exams Monthly prenatal visits	Sudden vaginal bleeding that is severe in nature Finding a lump in a breast
Orthopedist	Follow-up appointments to previous treatments or conditions	Fracture Sprain or strain injury
Respiratory/Pulmonologist	Follow-up appointments to previous treatments or conditions	Difficulty breathing Acute exacerbation of an existing problem
Urologist	Follow-up appointments to previous treatments or conditions	Blood in urine Severe flank pain Severe pain while urinating
Surgeon	Preoperative appointment Postoperative appointment	Postoperative complication

Insurance and Billing Information

As discussed in Unit 1, the reason for the appointment was determined when the patient called to make an appointment. The completed patient registration form gives accurate information on the insurance company to be billed. This information includes who the patient is, the subscriber or who has the policy, the identification numbers, the patient's employer, and if the patient has a policy with a second insurance company. Copies of all insurance cards are on file. These cards have important addresses and telephone numbers as well as the amount of copayments and if a referral is needed.

When registering patients on the telephone, the facility needs to request that the patient use the insurance card to give information for the registration. Receptionists should know about insurance billing procedures and know what information is needed from the insurance card. All insurance cards are different, and identifying the identification number and the claims address is important to the registration process. Trained staff will be able to guide the patient on the telephone to obtain accurate information and ensure that the registration is accurate in the system. For those patients who already have billing information in the system, this same process should be followed to verify that the information is accurate. Request that the patient view his or her insurance card for appropriate information and then make all corrections on the registration screen.

Following procedures for new and established patients is important for obtaining accurate insurance information because the insurance company pays the claim. Although the process may be different, the end result is the same in creating information for the start of the claim form. This process plays an important role in obtaining money from the insurance as a result of a clean claim, and payment may be received in as little as two weeks.

SERVICES PERFORMED AND DOCUMENTED

Services can take place in the many different health care settings, including the physician's office, the radiology center, the laboratory, the hospital, and long-term care/adult settings (see Figure 5-1). Depending on their circumstances, patients may need orders or a referral to go to these locations. Whatever location the services are provided at, they are all part of the revenue cycle and must follow protocol for billing and coding properly.

After patients have received services in a health care setting, each facility is responsible for documenting the service provided. Medical billing and coding professionals believe that "If the services aren't documented, then it didn't happen." This is another process to the revenue cycle in which the patient's documents allow the billing and coding department to determine fees and

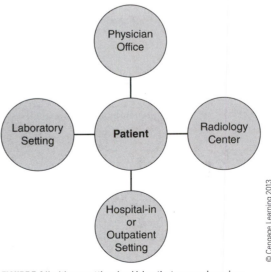

© Cengage Learning 2013

FIGURE 5-1 Healthcare settings in which patients can seek services

send claims for payment. Therefore, without accurately documented services and procedures, the facility will not be reimbursed.

The Physician's Office

The patient receives a service in the physician's office. When patients are in need of treatment, they will call the physician's office first to get further direction. The physician can be a primary care provider or a specialty provider for which the patient is self-referring or has a referral from the primary physician. In addition to an office visit, some patients will also receive procedures, such as an EKG or immunizations.

If the patient contacts your office, your staff must determine whether the patient is going to be able to receive treatment there or whether you should send him or her elsewhere. In most cases, the patient is aware of who he or she is contacting and needs an appointment with you first. After that patient's appointment, you may send him or her to another physician's office for further workup. In scheduling appointments, your staff should always be prepared to question the patient about his or her health or condition to determine his or her need for a visit at your facility or elsewhere.

Services performed are based on the facility. For example, Table 5-2 shows examples of specialties and common procedures.

In addition, diagnostic testing helps to find, confirm, or monitor the patient's condition depending on the health or symptoms of the patient. A physician will order tests as necessary, and the patient will present by appointment or walk in depending on the facility. When presenting for testing, the patient needs to be prepared with orders, insurance information, and a medical history for the registering staff. The facilities that perform diagnostic testing include but are not limited to radiology, laboratory, hospitals, and outpatient clinics.

Radiology

Radiology	Routine procedures performed
	Diagnostic X-rays
	Diagnostic ultrasound
	CAT scans
	MRI

Laboratory

Laboratory setting	Routine procedures performed
	Organ or disease oriented panels, such as obstetrical panels, general health, and lipid
	Urinalysis: the examination of urine, such as for pregnancy, glucose, and bacteria
	Hematology tests (examining the blood)
	Immunology tests: detecting antibodies for infectious diseases
	Microbiology: includes cultures and the identifying of organisms
	Cytopathology: the study of cervical and vaginal screening through pap smears
	Surgical pathology: the study of specimens taken during surgical procedures

TABLE 5-2: Specialties and common procedures

Specialist's Office	Routine Procedures Performed
Cardiologist	Consultations
	EKG
	Stress test
	Blood work
	Echocardiogram
Dermatologist	Consultations
	Biopsy
	Removal of lesion
	Allergy testing
Gastroenterologist	Consultations
	Sigmoidoscopy
	Anoscopy
	Stool exams
Obstetrics/Gynecologist	Pregnancy testing
	Pap tests
	Breast exams
	Prenatal visits
	Follow-up exams to pregnancy
	Follow-up exams to surgery
Orthopedist	Application of cast
	Consultations
	Follow-up exams
	X-rays
Respiratory/Pulmonologist	Breathing tests
	Consultations
	Follow-up to surgery
Urologist	Consultations
	Urinalysis
	Prostate exams
Surgeon	Preop and postop visits

Procedures and services are also performed within inpatient facilities during a patient's stay. Patients are considered inpatient after admission to a facility. Many facilities have patients with inpatient status and a documented medical need must exist for the patient's stay. During the admission, physicians can order diagnostic testing and treatment procedures as required for the patient's care. When the staff performs these procedures or services and clearly documents them with medical necessity, staff can bill insurance companies to receive payment. Staff and management at inpatient facilities must know the requirements when treating patients and follow them precisely. They may include but are not limited to hospitals and long-term care facilities.

Hospital

Hospital setting	Routine procedures not performed, but patients utilize services for acute, emergency, and planned surgeries or deliveries
Emergency room	
Inpatient surgery	
Critical care services	
Observation services	
Labor and delivery	

Long-Term Care

Long-term/adult setting	Admission for housing
	Short-term admission after an illness, such as stroke or heart attack
	Short-term admission for rehabilitative services
	Short-term admission for respite care for families

Although the process is similar, some differences exist when billing in each type of facility, and appropriate guidelines need to be followed to be sure the procedure and services will be reimbursed to the fullest. Some of these differences will be discussed later, as they are essential to good ethics and coding practices. Regardless of the type of facility the patient is in for procedures or services, all services are documented in the patient's chart for all types of health care settings.

ASSIGN CODES

Code assignment is an important aspect in the revenue cycle. The process of code assignment includes diagnostic and procedure coding to ensure medical necessity. When a procedure or service is performed, the ordering provider must justify medical necessity. The provider cannot order anything that is not warranted for the patient's diagnosis or treatment. The method of justifying medical necessity is linking the diagnosis to the procedure on the claim form. For example, an EKG can be done for someone with chest pain but not for someone with an earache. The earache does not justify the need for the EKG; however, it may justify a cerumen removal. This is just one example of many that outlines medical necessity as it relates to coding for the patients. In each case, the patient has a specific need and the provider must identify the need through the patient's interview and the exam as he or she conducts the medical exam on the patient.

As a result of the exam, for all procedures or services, the findings must be identified by the provider to demonstrate the medical necessity. During the patient history and the provider's exam, staff must document as they go. The information obtained during the medical encounter is extremely important and can result in justifying medical necessity for the coder. While documentation can be added anytime during the visit, you should document at the earliest convenience to be sure your information is accurate. In addition, thorough documentation is vital to the process as coders read the documents and accurately code all procedures and services that were performed for maximum reimbursement.

During code assignment, you must know what procedures or services were done and why, which must be apparent through the documentation in the patient's medical record. In some instances, the documentation may be missing despite the direction to code the procedures and services. Coders will be responsible for identifying discrepancies and addressing them appropriately and according to all guidelines. With missing or incorrect information, the coder may not be able to include the procedures or services on the claim submission, resulting in lost revenue. In the end, documentation is vital in all medical facilities. The following sections identify the processes of assignment codes for procedures and diagnoses separately; however, not all scenarios are described.

Procedure

Procedures or services provided by a physician, ambulatory surgical center, hospital observation, laboratory, physical therapy, urgent care, and/or hospital outpatient center are assigned a **CPT** code. The CPT (Current Procedural Terminology) Level I coding system was developed by the AMA (American Medical Association) and uses five-digit numeric or alphanumeric designations to identify the procedure or service provided to the patient (see Figure 5-2). Rather than someone writing out the description of the procedure or service, the CPT coding system assigns a description in the CPT book with a numeric or alphanumeric identifier. The medical coder is able to read the description in the CPT book, identify the description as appropriate for the patient's documentation, and assign the numeric or alphanumeric identifier to submit to the insurance company. This system of codes is copyrighted by the AMA. CPT is one of the coding systems that is compliant with HIPAA regulations and is used by all medical providers and insurance carriers as the accepted coding system, along with HCPCS and ICD-diagnostic codes as described shortly.

Level 11 codes are called **HCPCS** (Healthcare Common Procedural Coding System) codes and include five-digit alphanumeric characters that represent procedures or services provided to the patient (see Figure 5-3). Similar to the CPT codes, the HCPCS coding book has a description

---

BREAST

Incision

19000	Puncture aspiration of cyst of breast
+19001	each additional cyst (List separately in addition to code for primary procedure)
	(Use 19001 in conjunction with 19000)
	(If imaging guidance is performed, see 76095, 76096, 76393, 76942)
19020	Mastotomy with exploration or drainage of abscess, deep
19030	Injection procedure only for mammary ductogram or galactogram
	(For radiological supervision and interpretation, see 76086, 76088)
	(For catheter lavage of mammary ducts for collection of cytology specimens, use Category III codes 0046T, 0047T)

FIGURE 5-2 CPT Code Example

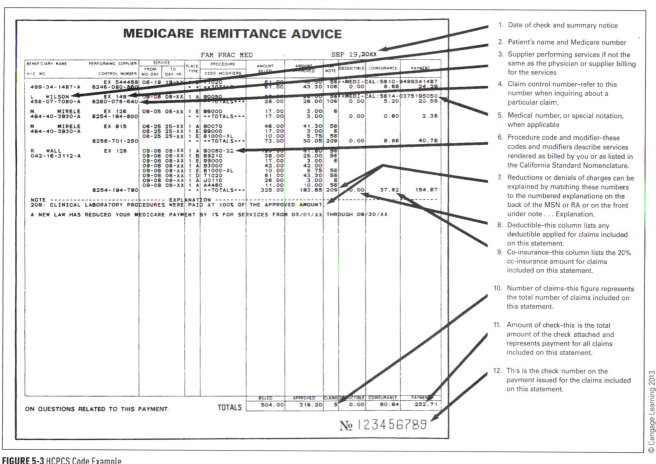

FIGURE 5-3 HCPCS Code Example

that tells the coder about the alphanumeric characters, and the coder must decide which codes to choose according to the patient's medical record. Although the characteristics and coding systems are similar, they are two different code sets and can be used alone or together based on the patient procedure or service provided. In some cases, both code books may have an appropriate code, and the medical biller and coder must decide which code is more appropriate based on the description and the insurance carrier. These codes are used to bill Medicare carriers and some private payers for select procedures, services, and supplies, such as durable medical equipment and injectable medications.

Diagnostic

ICD-Diagnostic Codes (International Classification of Diseases) is a coding system used to report diseases, diagnoses, and reasons for encounters for health care services. The code set is a numeric or alphanumeric three-, four-, or five-digit code with a decimal after the third digit (see Figure 5-4). The ICD-diagnostic code book provides a description of the disease, illness, signs, symptoms, or reason for encounter, and the medical coder must determine the appropriate code(s) based on the patient's medical record. The medical coder and biller must obtain information documented by the provider and use the ICD-diagnostic code book to locate the appropriate codes for the patient's encounter. The ICD-diagnostic coding system fulfills the requirement of **HIPAA** that mandates providers to document and report the reasons for encounters by using a uniform system of code sets. These official guidelines are published by the U.S. Department of Health and Human Services in conjunction with other organizations. The anticipated implementation of ICD-10-CM and ICD-10-PCS is October 2013. This will further fulfill the HIPAA

Chapter heading	**3. ENDOCRINE, NUTRITIONAL AND METABOLIC DISEASES, AND IMMUNITY DISORDERS (240–279)**
Excludes statement	**EXCLUDES** *endocrine and metabolic disturbances specific to the fetus and newborn (775.0–775.9)*
Instructional note	**Note:** All neoplasms, whether functionally active or not, are classified in Chapter 2. Codes in Chapter 3 (i.e., 242.8, 246.0, 251-253, 2555-259) may be used to identify such functional activity associated with any neoplasm, or by ectopic endocrine tissue.
Major topic heading	**DISORDERS OF THYROID GLAND (240–246)**
Category code	✓4th **240 Simple and unspecified goiter** DEF: An enlarged thyroid gland often caused by an inadequate dietary intake of iodine.
Subcategory code	**240.0 Goiter, specified as simple** Any condition classifiable to 240.9, specified as simple

Description statements	**240.9 Goiter, unspecified**
	Enlargement of thyroid Goiter or struma:
	Goiter or struma: hyperplastic
	  NOS nontoxic (diffuse)
	  diffuse colloid parenchymatous
	  endemic sporadic
	EXCLUDES *congenital (dyshormonogenic) goiter (246.1)*

DISEASES OF OTHER ENDOCRINE GLANDS (250–259)

✓4th **250 Diabetes mellitus**
EXCLUDES *gestational diabetes (648.8)*
hyperglycemia NOS (790.6)
neonatal diabetes mellitus (775.1)
nonclinical diabetes (790.29)

> The following fifth-digit subclassification is for use with category 250:
> ▲ **0 type II or unspecified type, not stated as uncontrolled**
>   Fifth-digit 0 is for use for type II patients, *even if the patient requires insulin*
>   ▶ Use additional code, if applicable, for associated long-term (current) insulin use V58.67 ◀
> ▲ **1 type I (juvenile type), not stated as uncontrolled**
> ▲ **2 type II or unspecified type, uncontrolled**
>   Fifth-digit 2 is for use for type II patients, *even if the patient requires insulin*
>   ▶ Use additional code, if applicable, for associated long-term (current) insulin use V58.67 ◀
> ▲ **3 type I (juvenile type), uncontrolled**

Subclassification codes for 5th digit assignment

AHA: 2Q, '02, 13; 2Q, '01, 16; 2Q, '98, 15; 4Q, '97, 32; 2Q, '97, 14; 3Q, '96, 5; 4Q, '93, 19; 2Q, '92, 5; 3Q, '91, 3; 2Q, '90, 22; N-D, '85, 11

DEF: Diabetes mellitus: Inability to metabolize carbohydrates, proteins, and fats with insufficient secretion of insulin. Symptoms may be unremarkable, with long-term complications, involving kidneys, nerves, blood vessels, and eyes.
DEF: Uncontrolled diabetes: A nonspecific term indicating that the current treatment regimen does not keep the blood sugar level of a patient within acceptable levels.

✓5th **250.0 Diabetes mellitus without mention of complication**
Diabetes mellitus without mention of complication or manifestation classifiable to 250.1–250.9
Diabetes (mellitus) NOS
CC Excl: For code 250.01–250.03: 250.00–250.93, 251.0–251.3, 259.8–259.9

AHA: 4Q, '97, 32; 3Q, '91, 3, 12; N-D, '85, 11;
    For Code 250.00;
4Q, '03, 105, 108; 2Q, '03, 16 1Q, '02, 7, 11;
    For Code 250.01:
4Q, '03, 110; 2Q, '03, 6 **For Code 250.02:** 1Q, '03, 5

From ICD-9-CM for Hospitals–Volumes 1, 2 &3, 2005 Professional. Reprinted with permission of Ingenix.

FIGURE 5-4 ICD-9-CM Code Example

requirements for data sets. These codes will be more specific and allow for expansion of new technology. They will have up to 7 digits.

It is the **ICD-diagnostic code** set that justifies the medical necessity of a service and ultimately the payment of that service to the health care provider. When coders and billers identify the reason for a patient's visit, insurance carriers can see the need and then pay the claim. Table 5-3 shows some examples of how ICD-diagnostic codes justify procedures:

TABLE 5-3: Medical necessity for procedures

Service or Procedure	Linking Diagnosis
EKG	Chest pain
Urinalysis	Urinary infection
Blood sugar	Diabetes
Application of cast	Fracture
Prenatal visits	Pregnancy
Removal of skin lesion	Skin lesion
Throat culture	Sore throat

THIRD-PARTY PAYERS

Third-party payers refers to the type of insurance and the company with whom an individual may have an insurance plan. Patients sign a contract with the third-party payer and pay a premium for coverage of medical services and procedures. Each third-party payer has different policies and different coverages, and the patient should know his or her policy and what it covers. In many circumstances, patients are not familiar with their policy and rely on the provider's office to know their coverage. The staff at the facility, including the receptionist and clinical staff, should be familiar with every policy and know when to further investigate for the patient to ensure the procedures and services are covered and the patient does not end up with an unnecessarily large balance. When the insurance rules are followed, most policies will cover procedures and services deemed **medically necessary** when the diagnosis justifies the services and procedure, and the patient will be left with a copayment, deductible, or coinsurance amount. In some instances, when the provider's office does not verify policy guidelines, this can result in lost revenue or high patient balances, which could have been prevented. These insurance companies can be classified as private, commercial, or government. Examples of insurance companies are:

* Medicare

* Medicaid

* Workers' compensation

* Auto insurance

* Disability

* Blue Cross/Blue Shield

* United Health Care

The provider's office should be proactive in obtaining appropriate information as well as checking policy guidelines and coverage for the patient. Ultimately, the patient is responsible for knowing his or her policy, but most facilities will take the time to recognize the policies because they work with them every day. The information on the third-party payer is obtained during the patient's registration and confirmed by the copy of the insurance card on file. Please be sure to copy the front and back of the card upon the patient's arrival, and check the card for information needed during the visit. The start of the insurance process begins with the call to the office and the registration process, and accuracy is important to the revenue cycle.

PAYMENTS RECEIVED

Payments for procedures or services can be from a patient, a patient's primary insurance, or a combination of primary and secondary insurance. Payments from patients are in the form of checks, credit cards, or cash. Checks are endorsed on the back with the facility name, account number, and the statement "deposit only." If accepted, credit card payments must be processed by the servicer before crediting a patient's account. After the credit card payment has been processed, the patient will be given a slip to sign to approve the credit card payment. After producing the slip and obtaining an appropriate signature, the staff should then credit the patient's account, issuing him or her a receipt of payment on the account. All patient payments are also recorded on the patient ledger (see Figure 5-5) and daily log (see Figure 5-6) or day sheet and should be balanced at the end of the day for accuracy.

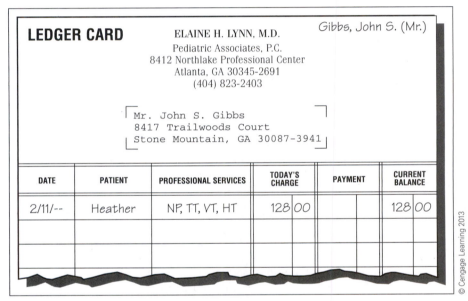

LEDGER CARD

ELAINE H. LYNN, M.D.
Pediatric Associates, P.C.
8412 Northlake Professional Center
Atlanta, GA 30345-2691
(404) 823-2403

Gibbs, John S. (Mr.)

Mr. John S. Gibbs
8417 Trailwoods Court
Stone Mountain, GA 30087-3941

DATE	PATIENT	PROFESSIONAL SERVICES	TODAY'S CHARGE	PAYMENT	CURRENT BALANCE
2/11/--	Heather	NP, TT, VT, HT	128 00		128 00

FIGURE 5-5 Partial Ledger Card

DAILY LOG

ELAINE H. LYNN, M.D.

DATE	PATIENT	PROFESSIONAL SERVICES	TODAY'S CHARGE	PAYMENT	CURRENT BALANCE	PREVIOUS BALANCE	NAME
2/11--	Pat	OV, TOPV	34 00		34 00	0 00	O'Meara
2/11--	Lucinda	OV	35 00		35 00	0 00	Jensen
2/11--	Heather	NP, TT, VT, HT	128 00		128 00	0 00	Gibbs
2/5-2/11--	Matthew	HV	245 00		325 00	80 00	Wiley
TOTALS							

FIGURE 5-6 Partial Daily Log

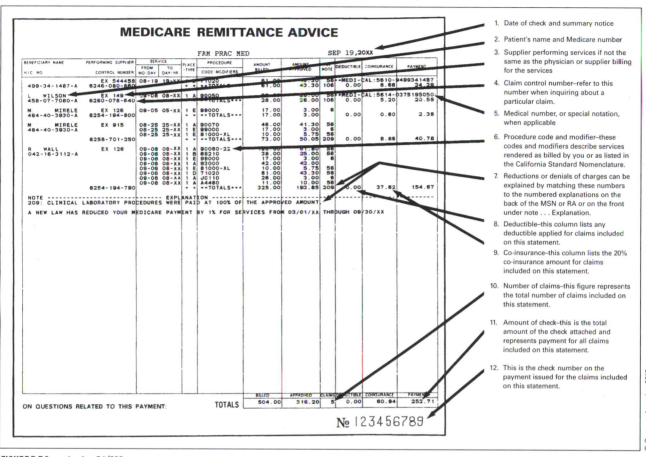

FIGURE 5-7 Example of an RA/EOB

Payments from insurance companies are accompanied by a **remittance advice (RA)** or **explanation of benefits (EOB)** (see Figure 5-7). These documents contain information on the service, date of service, CPT code, charges, allowed amounts, deductible, coinsurance, copayments, and insurance payments. They may also contain information on payments reduced or denied if something was not covered or paid appropriately. It is imperative to examine the RA or EOB thoroughly for comments, denials, or reduction in expected payments.

Reasons that a payment for services might be denied include:

- A service is an uncovered service. This might occur with cosmetic procedures, experimental procedures, or a service limited by the terms of the contract a provider has with the insurance company.

- Not proved to be medically necessary. If the diagnosis does not show a relationship to the services provided, payment may be denied.

- Patient not covered by insurance. This can result from inaccurate information placed on the insurance form or incorrect ID numbers. If the patient is not covered, the balance must be returned to the patient until new information is obtained.

- Timely filing issue. A timely filing issue results when a service is not billed within a certain time period. Different carriers have different requirements, so a health care facility should have up-to-date carrier information on issues such as timely filing limits, especially those carriers with whom they participate with.

If you believe the denial reason is incorrect, a response must be made to the insurance company that identifies the patient and the claim number and includes a letter explaining your situation. In some circumstances, documentation is needed to support your decision to appeal the denial. As stated earlier, each carrier has a different method for appealing a denial, and the carrier must

Doctors Group
Main Street
Alfred NY 12345
March 15, YYYY

Medicare B Review Department
P.O. Box 1001
Anywhere, US 12345

NAME OF PATIENT: _____
MEDICARE HICN*: _____
I do not agree with the determination you made on HICN* _____.

The reason I disagree with this determination is/are: (Check all that apply.)
☐ Service/Claim underpaid/reduced   ☐ Service/Claim overpaid   ☐ Service(s) overutilized
☐ Services not medically necessary   ☐ Duplicate claim submitted   ☐ Other: _____

Services in question are delineated as follows:

Date(s) of Service:	Quantity Billed:	Modifier:	Procedure Code(s):
_____	_____	_____	_____
_____	_____	_____	_____
_____	_____	_____	_____
_____	_____	_____	_____

Additional information to consider, including specific diagnosis, illness and/or condition:
_____
_____

Attachments to consider: (Check all that apply)

☐ Medical Records   ☐ Ambulance Run Sheet   ☐ Copy of Claim   ☐ Certificate of Medical Necessity

☐ Other: _____

_____   _____
Signature of Claimant or Representative   Telephone Number

* HICN = Health Insurance Claim Number

FIGURE 5-8 Sample Appeal Letter

be contacted for direction if necessary. These methods include the online appeal process or the completion of an appeal form specific to that carrier. Figure 5-8 illustrates a sample appeal letter.

PAYMENTS APPLIED

Applying payment to the patient's account is extremely important. The account must be correctly credited with payments from either an insurance carrier or from the patient payment. With proper payment application, someone can determine what is owed by the patient, what was denied by the insurance, and the adjustment of the contractual allowance for contracted insurances. Not all insurance companies are contracted with the provider, so medical billers must be cautious when applying adjustments to the account. In some instances, payments are applied and no other entries are made. However, in most circumstances, insurance payments require posting the payment; transferring the deductible, coinsurance, or copayment; and posting the adjustment to create an appropriate balance on the account. Payments must be applied to the appropriate claim that represents the dates, services, procedures, and billed amounts accurately. Applying payments should be done with caution and not rushed. In the end, all payments, transfers, and adjustments can be viewed on the day sheet or daily log for confirmation. Figure 5-5 showed an example of a partial ledger card. Figure 5-6 showed an example of a daily log or day sheet. Even more important is to determine any additional monies owed to the health care facility. Determining if any monies are due involves:

- Reviewing the RA or EOB for information on payments and denials
- Comparing the information to the patient ledger, which shows what services and procedures the patient had and the fees and any other payments made by the insurance company or the patient
- Reviewing patient balances and transferring them appropriately to the patient
- Making adjustments as required on the RA or the EOB under contractual agreements with insurance companies
- Appealing denials as necessary and with appropriate documentation

Complete Revenue Cycle

1. The patient seeks services and procedures in a health care setting.
2. The new patient completes a patient registration form.
3. Services and procedures are performed.
4. Services and procedures are documented.
5. Services and procedures are assigned a CPT and/or HCPCS code.
6. Diagnoses are assigned an ICD code linking to the services and procedures.
7. The patient's third-party insurance is billed.
8. Payment for services and procedures are made by the insurance company.
9. The explanation of benefits is reviewed.
10. The patient's account is credited with payment.
11. Any additional monies owed are billed.

BALANCES AND DENIALS

After someone completes the process of applying payments, the remaining balance and denials have to be handled properly. The RA or the EOB will identify the process by which to assign the balance appropriately and how to read denials to determine further action for the biller or coder. When the patient account shows a balance at the end of the payment posting process, the balance is either owed by someone or else a denial needs to be appealed. Addressing these situations is handled differently in each scenario and may have different approaches.

When there is a balance left, the biller or coder must determine if this is the patient's responsibility or the insurer's responsibility. When someone views the RA or the EOB, the balance would be determined by reading the deductible, copayment, and coinsurance columns and then applying any credits or adjustments indicated by the amounts in each column of the EOB to the patient. The columns for patient balances can have different column headings depending on the insurance company; sometimes, the columns are added together, so the biller or coder must be cautious when transferring. The balance must be clearly identified for the patient to understand what he or she owes. Getting a statement from the provider can sometimes be confusing if the information is not clearly identified as to what the balance consists of. Another way to confirm the patient balance is to try to locate the patient responsibility amount that is sometimes printed on the RA or the EOB. In getting to know the insurance carriers, the biller or coder will learn how to identify balances that should be transferred; however, if he or she is unsure, he or she should call the insurance carrier for directions. The insurance card can also be of assistance if patient balances are marked on the card; thus, the card can be compared to the RA or the EOB for further clarification. In either case, when transferring balances to the patient, be certain they are accurate.

Although denials leave a balance, they are handled differently from patient balances. Denials can have several different results, such as adjusted denials because they are not covered, transferred denials because they are the patient's responsibility, or appealed denials that need further documentation in order to be paid. Although many denials exist, these are some of the examples that a biller or coder will have to work with. When denials are not covered and are part of the contractual allowance, the balance is adjusted during the payment posting process. However, the denial needs to be viewed carefully for any recourse that may exist. Although a denial may appear to be an adjustment, it may be a result of incorrect information entered during the claim submission process. In this case, the denied service or procedure can be corrected and sent back in. The biller or coder must carefully scrutinize the denials and check all documentation before making an adjustment. Another reason for denial may be something not covered under the patient's policy and thus result in the patient owing the balance. Sometimes, these denials can appear as if they are adjustments on the RA or the EOB; during the payment posting, the columns must be read carefully and the balance for the denied service or procedure must be transferred to the patient, such as a cosmetic surgery. Another typical denial is a claim that can be appealed. In some instances, the insurance carrier views the service or procedure as not typically being covered due to the policy. However, with an appeal and written documentation, the biller or coder can identify the reason for the submission and demonstrate to the insurance carrier the medical necessity of the service or procedure, such as a lesion removal being done in a hospital setting under anesthesia due to the patient being anxious. With an appeal letter, documentation in the patient's chart and a reference to the denial code, the insurance carrier will review the submission and determine payment. After a decision is made, the provider must either make an adjustment or transfer the balance to the patient as directed by the appeal decision, which usually takes some time to render.

Billers and coders will have to pay close attention to balances and denials as they appear on the RA or the EOB. Each balance or denial needs to be handled according to the description and must be appropriately accounted for after payment posting is complete. The balances and denials must be handled immediately upon completion of the payment posting process.

BILLING AND COLLECTIONS

After information is sent to the insurance companies, the collection of funds begins. Two forms of revenue enter the medical facility: insurance payments and patient payments. Each requires a different collection process and must be attended to at all times. For the insurance companies, they are billed directly by using a claim form or CMS-1500. After all CPT, HCPCS, and ICD-diagnostic codes are determined, they are all entered onto a claim form with the patient registration information. This is the beginning of the billing process, as the insurance carriers review the claim form to determine payment to the provider. The majority of insurance carriers require the provider to submit claim forms electronically for payment; however, a few instances exist where claims are printed on claim paper and sent, such as secondary payers who need the primary payer EOB attached. With the electronic claims submission, the billing is cleaner and quicker, which results in a better revenue cycle for the provider's office.

During the billing process, balances are sometimes left for the patient, who can be negligent in paying his or her amount due. In an effort for the facility to maintain cash flow, a collection agency can be used to collect money that has not been paid. After three statements or 90 days, the provider's office can determine whether it wants to get an outside collection service involved or begin its own collection steps with the patient. When a facility uses collection procedures, the state guidelines must be followed precisely. Calling patients at appropriate times and not calling at the place of employment are some of the requirements that some states regulate for the collection process. In billing and collections, be certain that all appropriate staff members are educated on the guidelines and follow them accurately.

EXAMINE THE RA AND THE EOB

To determine if additional payments are due from insurance companies, examine the RA or the EOB attached to the payment from the insurance company. Each insurance carrier has a different layout for its RA or EOB, and knowing how to read the attachment is necessary for the billing and coding staff. There are columns with headings, dates of service, amount charged, CPT and HCPCS codes, allowances, and patient balances, payments, and adjustments that need to be determined. In addition, there are denial reasons for any payment not made on the claim. The reasons may be included with the line item or in a key in a central location. For the RA or the EOB that is difficult to understand, the staff should contact the insurance company to get direction. Understanding the RA or the EOB completely is important to the payment posting and the revenue cycle.

Monies that could still be owed would include:

- Uncovered services
- A difference between the fee for service and the amount covered by the insurance company
- Patient balances
  - Copayment
  - Coinsurance
  - Deductible
- Denied services

RUN ACCOUNTS AGING REPORT

After the payment posting process has been completed, the biller and coder must look at all outstanding balances. The insurance and the patient balances must be viewed, and the next step must be taken in collecting money. You should know if the patient has secondary insurance, which should be billed after the primary insurance has paid. When all insurance payments have been received, the next step is to determine the patient balance and then begin the patient collection process through patient statements. To determine the balances, who owes, and how many days outstanding, the biller or coder must print an accounts aging report. This can be done by insurance balances or by patient balances to help in the process of collecting final balances. The process of collecting payments generally occurs at intervals every 15–30 days. The process includes sending a statement, using a friendly sticker on the statement, calling the patient, and checking on insurance claims. The last action in the collection process would be sending the account to a collection agency. Table 5-4 details this process of collection. Figure 5-9 shows an example of a bill that uses a friendly sticker, and Figure 5-10 shows a sample letter for collection to a patient.

When billing is done each month, printing out an account aging report, which most computer systems can do, will show the age of the bill. Then, follow the actions in Table 5-4 to take appropriate action.

TABLE 5-4: Process of Patient Collection

Current: 1–30 days	30 Days From Date of Service	60 Days From Date of Service	90 Days From Date of Service	120 Days From Date of Service	180 Days From Date of Service
Patient seen in facility for service or procedure. Any payments due or copayments should be made at this time.	Send the bill.	Send a bill with a reminder. This bill can have a personal note on the bill or friendly sticker reminders.	Send a bill but also call the patient. Try to determine reason for nonpayment, such as waiting to hear from insurance. Also, call the insurance company to determine if it has received the bill, is waiting for more information, or has already processed the claim.	Send final notice letter that if there is no payment within a certain time frame, then the account will be sent to collection.	Follow-through with the letter that the account has been sent to a collection agency.

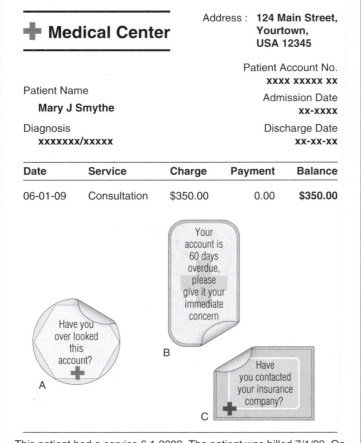

This patient had a service 6.1.2009. The patient was billed 7/1/09. On 8/1/09 the patient is billed again with a reminder sticker. The reminder sticker could be a friendly one (A) or business like one (B) or asking questions such as have you contacted your insurance company (C).

© Cengage Learning 2013

FIGURE 5-9 Billing Using Stickers

Dr. F. Jones
1 Broadway
Yourtown, USA 12345
Telephone 123-456-7890

91/2009
Mary J. Smythe
124 Main Street
Yourtown, USA 12345

Dear Mary,

Your account is now 90 days overdue. We have sent your the bill and reminders, as well as asking you to contact any insurance you have. We have not received any payment as yet. If we do not receive payment at the next billing cycle, your account may be sent to our collection company. Please either send us payment on this account or contact this office as soon as possible so that we may set up a payment plan with you.

Sincerely

Deanne Krum
Office Manager

© Cengage Learning 2013

FIGURE 5-10 Billing Using Letter

COMPLIANCE WITH ALL REGULATIONS

There are many regulations to be aware of in the medical field related to the revenue cycle. These include but are not limited to regulations from the OIG (Office of Inspector General), the CMS (Center for Medicare and Medicaid Services), HIPAA (Health Insurance Portability and Accountability Act), and The Joint Commission. Many agencies will host workshops, seminars, or webinars in accordance with the changes that occur and regulations that are created. Due to the consistently changing regulations, the biller or coder needs to be educated on a regular basis and make changes to the process in the provider's office when necessary. Open communication within the office staff and providers is important to successful updates and accurate information. Keeping abreast of all regulations is important to avoid denials or the appearance of fraud and abuse. Activities that are considered fraudulent are:

- Billing for services not furnished
- Altering diagnoses to justify payment on a procedure or service
- Falsifying medical records
- Using incorrect procedure codes to attain increased payments

EXPENSES AFFECT REVENUE

In accordance with the function of a facility, there are two sides to a revenue cycle: income and expenses. We have discussed income and how the money being collected comes from patients and insurance companies. In order to maintain an efficient revenue cycle, important steps need to be taken to increase income so expenses can be covered. When collecting income, the office staff must keep in mind the amount of expenses to run an office in order to remember to be successful in income collection. With patient care, mistakes can be made in patient registration and insurance billing, which can drastically affect the amount of income coming in. If expenses are considered from the beginning, staff will remember to be proactive in obtaining appropriate information from the patient, submitting clean claims to the insurance, and billing the patients when balances are determined. The parts of the revenue cycle should work correctly and promote a positive cash flow because the other side of the revenue cycle is expenses to be paid. Expenses include:

- Rent or mortgage
- Payroll, including taxes, social security payments, and deductions
- Medical and administrative supplies, which vary by specialty
- Equipment: new, used, and repairs
- Malpractice insurance for all physicians in the practice as well as, possibly, physician assistants and nurse practitioners

The manager is responsible for ensuring that the finances and revenue cycle are efficient, including accounts payable and paying the bills. These areas are discussed in Chapter 6.

SUMMARY

- The revenue cycle begins when the patient makes an appointment at a health care facility.
- The medical personnel, such as the receptionist, gathers information for the visit, such as the reason (symptoms, diagnosis, etc.), insurance information, and billing information.
- The service or procedure is performed and documented in the patient's chart.
- Different specialties have different types of appointments, which staff should be familiar with.
- Medical codes for procedures, services, and diagnoses are assigned that are compliant with all regulations and accurately reflect the chart documentation.
- The insurance company receives the claim from the health care facility, processes the claim, and returns any payment to the health care facility, along with a remittance advice (RA) or an explanation of benefits (EOB).
- Payments are received from either the insurance company or patient, and the appropriate patient account is credited.
- Determinations are made after examining the EOB and other insurance information if additional monies are due from the patient.
- Incorrect payments from insurance companies may prompt an appeal letter.
- At all times, there must be compliance with federal, state, and carrier regulations.
- The efficient application of the parts of the revenue cycle for the finances will ensure the ability to handle the other side of the revenue cycle: expenses.

REVIEW EXERCISES

TRUE OR FALSE

1. _____ An inpatient is one who used a department within a hospital but was not admitted.

2. _____ The revenue cycle is started with the patient completing a registration form.

3. _____ The diagnosis justifies the need for a service.

4. _____ A completed registration form will designate the diagnosis and procedure.

5. _____ CPT codes are for procedures and services.

6. _____ A third party is an insurance company.

7. _____ An EOB and an RA are essentially the same thing.

8. _____ Payment may be denied if not proved to be medically necessary.

9. _____ You cannot appeal a claim that has been denied.

10. _____ An accounts aging record is a bill sent to the patient.

MATCHING

A   CPT
B   ICD
C   HCPCS
D   RA
E   Inpatient
F   Outpatient
    Accounts
    Aging
G   Timely Filing
    Limit
H   Medically
    Necessary
I   Third-Party
    Payer

1. _____ A report that shows how old monies owed are.

2. _____ Admitted to the hospital.

3. _____ Uses a department in a hospital for diagnostic tests.

4. _____ Used for diagnose coding.

5. _____ Used for procedure coding.

6. _____ Level II procedure codes.

7. _____ Same as an explanation of benefits.

8. _____ The amount of time an insurance company gives to file a claim after date of service.

9. _____ When the diagnosis justifies a procedure or service.

10. _____ The insurance company.

CRITICAL THINKING ACTIVITIES

ACTIVITY 1

List the steps to take in the following circumstance.

The RA or the EOB indicates that a service was denied. The reason stated was that there is no such patient with this particular insurance.

Steps for Denial

_____
_____
_____
_____
_____
_____
_____
_____
_____
_____
_____
_____
_____
_____
_____
_____
_____

ACTIVITY 2

What information is gathered by the receptionist, and how does it relate to the elements of the revenue cycle?

_____
_____
_____
_____
_____
_____
_____
_____
_____
_____
_____
_____
_____
_____

ACTIVITY 3

Review this account aging report to determine what type of activity would be taken for each account.

TABLE 5-5: Account Aging Report

Patient Name	Current	30 Days	60 Days	90 Days	120 Days	180 Days
Mary Smith	$700					
Martha Smithe		$500				$250
Michelle Smythe					$5,000	
Michaela Smithee			$675			
Martha Smittey				$550		

PLAN OF ACTION FOR EACH AGE ACCOUNT

Mary Smith _____

_____

Martha Smith _____

_____

Michelle Smythe _____

_____

Michaela Smithee _____

_____

Martha Smittey _____

_____

CRITICAL THINKING QUESTIONS

1. Your facility continuously has timely filing issues with reimbursement. What would you suggest at your next staff meeting?

2. Debate the pros and cons for the revenue cycle if you chose to use an outside billing agency. Consider the outside agency as doing 100% of the billing for the health care facility.

3. Explain the benefits to the revenue cycle if the copayments and patient balances are collected at the time of the encounter. Include the steps that are required if the patient has to be billed.

4. Discuss the time frame in which aging account reports should be run and reviewed by billing staff. Differentiate between the patient and insurance aging. Explain how the revenue cycle is affected by the aging reports.

WEB ACTIVITIES

1. For federal regulations regarding fraud and detection, research the Office of Inspector General (OIG) website at www.oig.hhs.gov. Identify the new regulations for this year that you must consider in the health care facility.

2. For Medicare regulations involving fraud, go to Centers for Medicare & Medicaid Services (CMS) website at www.cms.gov. List five regulations you believe should be discussed in the health care facility.

CHAPTER 6

THE REVENUE CYCLE

MANAGING

Chapter 6 discusses the fundamentals of finances and the revenue cycle by explaining all the factors involved in managing the revenue cycle. There are many policies and procedures that should be created for the successful functioning of all components of the revenue cycle.

These policies and procedures include:

- Determining eligibility for charity care
- Evaluating components of the revenue cycle

OBJECTIVES

Upon completion of this chapter, the student will be able to:

- Understand the role of the registration process to maintain a positive revenue flow.
- Explain the role of contracts to the managing of revenue.
- Establish policies and procedures for the collection of monies.
- Develop benchmarks to evaluate the success of collection.
- Evaluate the relationship of income to expenses.

KEY TERMS

- Accounts aging
- Bad debt
- Benchmarking
- Bundled codes
- Charity care
- Contractual adjustment
- Day sheet
- Denials
- Unbundled codes
- Write-off

EVALUATING THE REGISTRATION PROCESS

In Unit 1, we discussed the diverse role of the receptionist. That very important person has the first contact with a patient, makes appointments, sees that the patient registration form is complete and accurate, and collects any copayments. The revenue process begins with the appointment. There are some good practice activities that when used routinely ensure success. Figure 6-1 demonstrates a method in which staff should reconcile appointment book entries, sign-in sheets, and day sheets. On any given day, the manager would compare the day's appointments with the sign-in list and the **day sheet**, which shows the patient's charges and any payments made. Use this process to go back 30 days and 60 days, comparing the appointment book, sign-in sheet, and day sheet and the current ledgers for payment. When management verifies these items, it is ensuring that all appointments have been billed and paid appropriately, creating a positive cash flow for the revenue cycle.

When you check on payments, note the insurance carrier, the amount paid, and any reduction or denial of payments. Areas to examine more closely are:

- Discrepancies between the appointment book and the sign-in sheet
- Discrepancies between the appointment book and the day sheet
- Discrepancies between the sign-in sheet and the day sheet

Evaluate again in 30 days and 60 days for unpaid or denied claims by insurance.

Today's Date: _____

Total number of patients listed in the appointment book   _____

Total number of patients who signed in on the sign in sheet   _____

Total number of patients who are listed on the day sheet   _____

Discrepancies noted:

Action taken:

Reconciling the above date in 30 or 60 days

Number of patients listed on the day sheet on (date)   _____

Number of patients who had their charges paid   _____

Number of claims outstanding   _____

Notes on outstanding claims:

© Cengage Learning 2013

FIGURE 6-1 Reconciling the Registration Process from the Appointment Book through the Day Sheet

DISCREPANCIES BETWEEN THE APPOINTMENT SHEET, SIGN-IN SHEET, OR DAY SHEET

In some cases, there will be discrepancies found due to new staff or a busy time of day. When there are discrepancies between the appointment books, sign-in sheet, and day sheet, a review of policies and procedures needs to take place. Determine if the sign-in sheet is clearly marked, indicating the need for patients to sign in. Determine if there is a master list of patients for a given day based on the scheduled appointments. Reconcile the two lists each day to determine patients who have not shown for appointments as well as patients who walked in without an appointment. If the patient appears on all three lists, the manager can be certain that the services and procedures will be billed for that appointment. Check that list against the day sheet and look for discrepancies in the numbers and names of patients. A tally of the numbers each day should be recorded for all three documents: the appointment book, the sign-in sheet, and the day sheet.

Checklist for the manager to use daily

- ☐ Sign-in sheet clearly marked
- ☐ Master list of patients for the day matches the sign-in sheet
- ☐ Day sheet matches the master list and sign-in sheet

EVALUATING BILLING PRACTICES

When running a provider's office, the manager must be responsible for keeping the revenue cycle and cash flow at full capacity. By monitoring patient activity, the manager can evaluate the billing procedures and determine if the patient's services and procedures have been billed appropriately according to the documentation and appointment. The first step in evaluating if your billing practices are effective is to review the explanation of benefits (EOB) or remittance advice (RA) from the insurance company. Check if the patient names and charges for services or procedures (CPT codes) are the same as on the patient ledger. After reviewing everything, any actions or payment adjustments must be made.

First step for the manager when checking an EOB

- ☐ Does the patient's name match?
- ☐ Are the services and procedures listed on the EOB or the RA the same as on the patient's chart or ledger?
- ☐ Are the fees listed the same?
- ☐ Is there something that does not match between the EOB or the RA and the patient's ledger?

REVIEWING THE EOB

You must review EOBs or RAs as they come in due to the filing deadline for corrections or appeals with each insurance company. An EOB or an RA is a document that accompanies payments from insurance carriers on claims. Evaluating these documents is often the first step a manager should take to discover areas in the revenue cycle that need improvement. Evaluating EOBs or RAs as well as reviewing claims in 30- and 60-day intervals is a good practice to determine problems in the beginning stages of the revenue cycle. With insurance billing, there is usually a filing limit for each action the biller or coder needs to take. Oftentimes, the biller or coder is busy and does not address the problems with the EOB or the RA immediately, and management must monitor this and ensure the filing limits are being met by the biller or coder. Without appropriate action, the revenue cycle may result in a loss as fees are adjusted for late filing and become uncollectable from the insurance and the patient. Even when payments are processed, the insurance carriers still have filing limits for corrections or appeals, and management must make billers and coders aware of this and oversee the process to be sure they are also meeting those deadlines. When evaluating EOBs or RAs, note reduced payments as well as denials for payment, which would reduce income. The reason for the denial or reduced payment may require submission to the insurance carrier or patient or an adjustment and must be carefully processed.

Some of the reasons for reduced payments or denials include:

- Patient ineligible or no such patient
- No referral or authorization on record
- Not a covered service
- Charges unbundled
- Timely filing
- Duplicate service
- Not part of contractual agreement

Figure 6-2 shows a sample EOB/RA that shows how denials and the reasons appear.

PATIENT RESPONSIBILITY

In many situations, the EOB or the RA identifies an amount that is the patient's responsibility, and the billers and coders must recognize the difference between patient responsibility, an error or denial, and the contractual adjustments so the amounts can be applied appropriately. Management must train billers and coders to be sure they are not accepting the patient responsibility if it is inaccurate. For example, the patient's date of birth could be incorrect and it can easily be corrected; however, on the EOB or the RA, it is listed as the patient responsibility, and the biller or coder may easily transfer the amount to the patient. Further investigation is required by management or billing and coding staff to make the appropriate entries. If the information is incorrect, a correct claim must be submitted, and payment will be made accordingly.

In another situation, the amount could represent a **contractual adjustment**, which represents a write-off after the allowance is determined because the provider is contracted under the insurance. The EOB or the RA may state it is a noncovered benefit and not indicate whose balance it is. Management must train and monitor staff to recognize when contractual adjustments are necessary because you should not adjust something that is owed to the provider. Additionally, it is also against contract policy to bill the patient for that amount. Therefore, careful attention must be used when processing EOBs and RAs, and management must review and advise billing and coding when there are any questions or concerns.

Patient name and ID number	Type of service	Place of service	Procedure code	Amount billed for procedure	Amount carrier will pay for procedure	Deductible and copayments	Total amount payed	Denial code
Mary Monkee No:1234	medical	office	9xxxx	100	0	0	0	U1
Jules Giraf No:2356	consultation	office	9xxxxx	500	0	0	0	V2
Ellie Ellafant No:3456	emergency	office	9xxxx	350	0	0	0	W3
Larry Lyon No:5678	medical	office	9xxxx	250	0	0	0	X4
Zanny Zeebray No:6789	surgery	hospital	3xxxxx	1500	0	0	0	Y5
Carly Kitten No:9357	medical	outpatient	9xxxxx	150	0	0	0	X6

U1   patient ineligible or no such patient

V2   no referral or authorization on record

W3   not a covered service

X4   charges unbundled

Y5   timely filing

X6   duplicate service

FIGURE 6-2 EOB/RA Which Shows How Denials and the Reasons Appear

Mary Monkee No: 1234	medical	office	9xxxx	100	0	0	0	U1

U1   patient ineligible or no such patient

There are a number of common reasons for which a denial from an insurance company would state that the patient is ineligible or no such patient is listed as having that insurance. These reasons could include:

- The patient's spelling of the name could have been spelled incorrectly.

- The ID numbers were mixed up.

- Other demographic information may be incorrect.

- Not identifying who the patient is or who the subscriber is or who has the insurance could cause an error in patient and insurer information.

In a situation where the patient is ineligible and the provider's records are all correct, then the balance will have to go to the patient until additional information is received. Many times, the billing and coding staff think that if the patient is ineligible, then he or she is responsible because they did not check eligibility at the time of the visit. However, this is not the case, as the patient is responsible for giving appropriate information at the time of the appointment regardless of when he or she was in last. In addition, the patient may have changed insurances since the visit and did not call you to update his or her information. You should get the patient involved to understand what coverage he or she has.

You should update records routinely. With insurance changing frequently, it has become routine practice to check demographics and insurance at each visit and then make changes accordingly. Managers should implement guidelines for staff to verify information on each visit and not simply ask if everything is the same. They should request the type of insurance and identification number on each visit to maintain a successful revenue cycle for the practice.

COMMON DENIAL REASONS

With each denial from the insurance carrier, steps can be taken in order to obtain appropriate payment. Management must identify the common denials and clearly outline steps to take in processing the EOB or the RA for the biller or coder. Although every insurance carrier has its own rules, most of the concepts are similar, as are how to recognize and work with the denial. For example, a noncovered procedure can be listed as an uncovered procedure for a different insurance carrier. This can be confusing to billing and coding staff, as some carriers require this denial to be an adjustment and others bill it to the patient depending on the policy. Guiding staff through this process is pertinent to management so they can avoid unnecessary adjustments by the billing and coding staff. Management must monitor adjustments on the end-of-month reports closely and confront billing and coding staff if necessary. The most common denials in the industry will be discussed in the following sections, but they are not limited to these examples.

List of Common Denials

- Wrong spelling of name

- ID number incorrect

- Mixing up the patient and the subscriber

- Wrong insurance carrier

- Mixing up the primary or secondary insurance

NO REFERRAL OR AUTHORIZATION

Jules Giraf No: 2356	Consultation	Office	9xxxxx	500	0	0	0	V2

© Cengage Learning 2013

V2   no referral or authorization on record

Denials on EOBs or RAs occurring as not paid because there was no written referral or authorization indicate the need to review contracts with insurance carriers. Each insurance carrier has different guidelines on referrals and authorization, such as backdating guidelines. Some insurance carriers allow backdating but within a certain time frame, while others do not allow backdating. Personnel, including clinical and administrative staff, need to know how to determine if a procedure or service needs to have a referral or authorization. When referrals or authorizations are necessary, the appropriate staff needs to obtain them in a timely manner and management should maintain guidelines on requesting them.

Appropriate billing of the patient without a referral or authorization is another issue and also differs with each insurance carrier. Signing insurance waivers is one method of obtaining payment from the patient upon denial of no referral or authorization; however, some insurance carriers do not recognize waivers and expect the provider's office to adjust the balance. Management must educate all staff on the different regulations and clearly demonstrate the need to have referrals or authorizations ahead of time with particular insurance carriers to be sure that anyone involved in the patient's visit is aware. They should also review with all personnel when patients should sign an advanced beneficiary notice (ABN) prior to services or procedures when amounts are higher and the patient's insurance may not cover them. This allows the patient to be aware of the potential for a balance. Also, Medicare secondary payer (MSP) is an issue that should be reviewed by the manager with personnel. Finally, being aware of national coverage determination (NCD) policies from Medicare for your health care setting is of fundamental importance. All these policies play an important role in the revenue cycle, and direction from management will create a positive cash flow.

NOT A COVERED SERVICE

Ellie Ellafant No: 3456	Emergency	Office	9xxxx	350	0	0	0	W3

© Cengage Learning 2013

W3   not a covered service

When the reason for denial is stated as not a covered service, you must go back again to the insurance carrier's rules and policies, review contracts for included and excluded services, and check that the codes on the EOB or the RA are indeed the ones performed and submitted. Other reasons that denials may state the reason as not a covered service can be traced to CPT and ICD-diagnostic code errors. For example, the ICD-9 codes do not prove the medical necessity of the procedure or service or the codes are not specific enough per established guidelines. ICD-10 codes will have more specificity when they are implemented in the future.

Management needs to be proactive with the billing and coding staff in knowing the potential for having different outcomes for not covered services or procedures. Many times, the amount not covered appears to be unaccounted for in the ledger and may be incorrectly adjusted off without further investigation. Management needs to be aware and make staff aware of the differences and the risk of making an incorrect adjustment, as unnecessary adjustments can have a negative effect on the revenue cycle.

CHARGES UNBUNDLED

Larry Lyon No: 5678	Medical	Office	9xxxx	250	0	0	0	X4

X4   charges unbundled

In billing, there are such services as surgeries, laboratory tests, and other diagnostic tests that are **bundled codes** together in one code, meaning there is one fee and payment for multiple services or procedures. For example, during surgery, the suturing is included in the surgery as part of the surgical package and cannot be billed separately. If the services or procedures within that bundle are separated and billed separately as individual CPT or HCPCS codes, that would lead to the denial reason as **unbundled codes**. Educating staff on the idea of a bundled service or procedure and a separate service or procedure is pertinent to understand what codes are billed and what adjustments need to be made.

When billing and coding staff refer to bundled codes, they are usually dealing with a true bundled procedure; however, some circumstances have patient services or procedures that are separate and are not considered bundled. If a separate service or procedure is performed and is different from the bundled service or procedure, it can be billed separately with a modifier and usually receives a separate reduced payment. For example, if the suturing during surgery was done on another part of the skin other than the surgical incision, then it is not included and can be billed separately with a modifier. With billing and coding staff, the manager must clarify these situations and ensure that they do not adjust or leave out separate procedures when appropriate because this can decrease the revenue cycle.

Figure 6-3 demonstrates a service that is considered bundled and what would be considered **unbundled**.

Bundled codes:

The physician ordered an electrolyte panel on his patient.

CPT code for this panel is 80051

Unbundled codes:

Carbon dioxide CPT code: 82374

Chloride CPT code 82435

Potassium CPT code 84132

Sodium CPT code 84295

FIGURE 6-3 The Bundling and Unbundling of Services

TIMELY FILING

Zanny Zeebray No: 6789	Surgery	Hospital	3xxxxx	1500	0	0	0	Y5

Y5   timely filing

Within the insurance industry, many insurance carriers have a set filing limit for providers to submit claims. Each insurance company has its own guidelines, and they are listed in the insurance contracts signed by providers. The office manager is responsible for educating providers and billing staff on the risk of filing claims timely because claims beyond the filing limit result in loss revenue and cannot be recovered. Providers and billing staff should be aware and always submit within the filing limit to prevent the unnecessary adjustments. As a result, denials that state the reason as timely filing indicates the claim was not filed in a timely fashion and policies need to be reviewed to determine why. Denials for timely filing reasons indicate they need to know insurance carrier and state filing requirements. The billing process also needs to be reviewed. Let us look at a hypothetical situation:

> An insurance company wants a claim submitted within 30 days of the date of service. A physician performs a consultation on a patient on June 1, 2011, and sends the written report to the primary care physician, who reviews the findings with the patient and the patient's family. Care is then assumed by the consulting physician. These events occurred over a 45-day period. The consulting physician then submits the claim for the consultation, and that claim is now past the 30 days requirement and therefore outside the timely filing range.

When situations such as this occurs, the physician as well as the billing staff need to be educated about what timely filing is and the importance of submitting bills within the range of each insurance carrier. If the provider and billing staff understand the timely filing deadlines, they can be proactive in obtaining the necessary information in order to submit the claim on time. In knowing the risk of having to lose the revenue, the provider and billing staff will be more educated in the importance of submission. Figure 6-4 demonstrates how to create a tracking system for each carrier and the timely filing limits.

Carrier	30 days	45 days	60 days	90 days	other
Carrier Z	✔				
Carrier Y		✔			
Carrier X			✔		
Carrier W					
Carrier V					✔
Carrier U				✔	

FIGURE 6-4 Tracking System for Each Carrier and Their Timely Filing Limits

DUPLICATE CHARGES

Carly Kitten No: 9357	Medical	Outpatient	9xxxxx	150	0	0	0	X6

X6   duplicate service

Circumstances arise where the claim will be denied as duplicate and further investigation is necessary. Billing and coding staff may view duplicate denials as an adjustment because it was processed before, but some duplicate denials are not accurate and need corrected claims. Management should educate staff not to adjust duplicate denials until everything has been reviewed and they are absolutely sure the claim is a duplicate that will not be paid twice; otherwise, this could result in lost revenue. For example, if a patient has a repeat procedure on the same day, this can be paid with a modifier 76, and if the modifier was not added, then the denial will be a duplicate denial. The biller or coder can send a correction with the modifier to receive payment. In addition, when a denial is considered a duplicate charge on an EOB, managers need to evaluate the billing process for the reason charges are being billed more than once. They must investigate whether this was a situation for a duplicate charge. The whole cycle of revenue needs to be evaluated, starting from the registration process to the billing process. When reviewing the process for why duplicate charges are being submitted, some to the questions to ask include:

- Are multiple people performing billing routines?
- Is there a system in place that defines who bills for a service?
- What type of billing logs are in place?
- Is there a computer system in use, and does it flag duplicate services being billed?

If duplicate denials are not considered and investigated, the billing and coding staff eventually performs an adjustment, removing the balance from the aging. If the adjustment is done, the amount is no longer there for anyone to question whether payment should be made by adding a modifier or documentation of a duplicate service or procedure. These unnecessary adjustments can have a negative impact on income and the revenue cycle, and management must educate billing and coding staff to do a thorough search before making any duplicate adjustments.

PAYMENT ADJUSTMENTS

Adjustments can be detrimental to the health care facility if performed unnecessarily; complete consideration must be given before performing the task. After reviewing an EOB/RA for payments and denials, the manager also needs to review the part of the EOB/RA that indicates any adjustments in payment. Each carrier may use different codes to identify the reason for the adjustment, such as contractual or unbundled, and management must confirm that the billing and coding staff are familiar with the differences in each insurance carrier. Medicare publishes a guide on understanding remittance advice for providers, physicians, suppliers, and billers. You can access this guide by going to https://www.cms.gov/MLNProducts/downloads/RA_Guide_Full_03-22-06.pdf. When an adjustment is performed on the patient's ledger, the amount adjusted is removed from the books, and determining an error is difficult if the amount does not appear on aging reports or day sheets as outstanding. The amount adjusted becomes uncollectable to the office, and management must explain the importance of losing track of money owed if it is adjusted incorrectly by the billing and coding staff. In addition, management should review adjustment totals as they appear on the day sheet and end-of-month report to be sure the adjustment amounts are not exceedingly large for the report. The percentage of adjustments to payments should be known by management and must be monitored at least monthly to maintain a positive revenue cycle within the practice.

COLLECTION PRACTICES

When patients are delinquent in paying their bills to the practice, after a certain amount of time (which is determined by management) the patient can be sent to collections as an option to help increase revenue. Three months of nonpayment is a sign that the patient does not intend to pay his or her balance. During the billing process, the billing staff must identify the delinquency to the patient and inform him or her of the potential for further action with the collection agency. Management must ensure that proper collection processes are used and that staff is fully educated on the procedure, including the delinquent amounts, the time frame in which collection proceedings begin, and the letters and calls that can be placed before using the collection agency. There are certain guidelines for each state on what can be done to pursue the delinquent amount, and management must oversee this process and confirm that procedures are being followed for every patient with a delinquent balance. The manager needs to make a regular practice of reviewing collection practices and addressing billing staff when there are discrepancies or complaints from the patients. The collection process includes reviewing existing contracts for payment fees as well as evaluating whether write-offs, bad debts, and charity care are following best practices—also referred to as *benchmarks*.

Collection practices include:

- Evaluating contracts with third-party payers
- Evaluating accounts that have been written off as bad debts
- Evaluating accounts that are classified as charity care
- Using benchmarks as guides

REVIEWING CONTRACTS

The insurance company and the provider will sign a legal contract that covers fee schedules, covered services and procedures, and claim submission rules and regulations that both parties must adhere to. When you evaluate the components of the revenue cycle, if a pattern of denials by one carrier becomes evident, this is an indication that a review of the contract between that provider and the insurance carrier is necessary. This may be an indication that the provider is submitting the claim incorrectly or the contract is not appropriate for the provider as to what services or procedures are covered under the contract. Another situation that should result in review of the contract is payment in full by the insurance carrier. If the payment meets 100% of the billed amount, that is an indication that the provider is billing below the insurance carrier fee schedule, and they may want to review the contract for the current fee schedule to see if changes are necessary. In addition, if a need for changing the fees is necessary, the office manager will make a permanent change to the provider's fee schedule that will reflect the billed amount to every insurance carrier as well as patients. Fees cannot be adjusted to fit the insurance carrier's fee schedule; they must be changed permanently for everyone. Once a contract is negotiated and a fee schedule established, they should be reviewed annually for changes. The medical office manager should review all negotiated contracts on an annual basis and make adjustments accordingly. Figure 6-5 shows a log that the manager can create that lists the carriers the health care facility contracts with, the dates the contracts were originally signed, and the dates they are reviewed and updated. The termination date can also be a part of the log.

Carrier	Date contract initially signed	Date updated	Changes	Dates updated	Changes	Terminated
Carrier Z	3/2006	3/2007	Yes	3/200x		
Carrier y	1/2006	1/2007	No	1/200x		
Carrier X	12/2005	12/2006	No	12/200x		
Carrier W	10/2005	10/2006	Yes	10/200x		

© Cengage Learning 2013

FIGURE 6-5 A Log Which Lists Carriers the Healthcare Facility Has a Contract With

WRITE-OFFS, BAD DEBT, AND CHARITY CARE

In many situations, required adjustments are made to the patient's account to represent a reduction in the balance. When a patient balance is delinquent or will not be paid, there are circumstances in which the account must be adjusted to remove the balance from the record. If the biller or coder makes an unnecessary adjustment to the patient account, it will result in loss of revenue, and staff must therefore be educated on the process by the manager before attempting to adjust patient balances. Knowing the difference between write-offs, bad debt, and charity care is the first step in knowing how to handle these situations for improving the collection process and revenue cycle. The office manager should be involved in the training and alert when viewing end-of-month summaries for any large adjustments that are not appropriate.

Bad debts are typically from patients who have not paid their bills or have not or cannot pay, even with the use of a collection agency. With a bad debt, patients need to be billed appropriately with letters requesting payment and at least three statements mailed. After an aggressive and appropriate collection process is followed, the patient's account needs to be cleared from the aging report by using a bad debt adjustment. With this type of adjustment, the patient is still liable to pay the balance if he or she returns for another appointment, and management should be notified. The account will be flagged, and the office staff can still request payment from the patient until the time limit is reached according to state regulations. If a patient does attempt to make payment after a bad debt adjustment, the office staff will reverse the adjustment and accept payment accordingly.

Write-offs are debts that cannot be paid, as in the case of deceased patients with no estates. When a balance needs to be removed from a patient's account permanently, the appropriate write-off is done as an adjustment and is typically not reversed. When the patient is not going to pay the balance and it needs to be removed from the aging report, the write-off is done to reflect that no balance is owed. If these balances were left, they would appear to be money owed, when in fact that the money will not be collected. Using an adjustment to remove the balance will allow the provider's office to be clearer on its expected income and plan expenses accordingly, thus maintaining a better revenue cycle.

Charity care refers to patients with no insurance and who fall below a certain income level. When patients suggest they may be eligible for charity care, they are usually asked to submit an application with certain criteria to determine their eligibility. If they are eligible according to the state regulations and local hospitals, they are not responsible for their balance at the provider's office. If the patient has a balance and you determine he or she is eligible for charity care, the adjustment is made to remove the balance so it does not appear on the aging account report. Charity care adjustments are important when the money is not going to be collected by the office as income. For health care settings that do see patients that fall into this charity care category, you should know what each state has as a documentation process that certifies eligibility as a charity case patient. Figure 6-6 shows an example of a documentation checklist from the New York State Department of Health.

DOCUMENTATION CHECKLIST

For Health Insurance

All documentation must be included for the application to be considered complete.

Applicant Name _____   Application Date _____

PROOF OF IDENTITY/DATE OF BIRTH AND RESIDENCE: You must show ONE of the documents listed in both categories to see if you are eligible for health insurance. Discuss this with the person helping you with your application. Photocopies are acceptable.

☐ IDENTITY/DATE OF BIRTH
(not required for recertification)

- ☐ Driver's license/Official Photo identification
- ☐ Passport*
- ☐ Birth certificate*
- ☐ Baptismal/other religious certificate*
- ☐ Official School records
- ☐ Adoption records
- ☐ Official Hospital/doctor birth records*
- ☐ Naturalization certificate*
- ☐ Marriage records

*May also be used to document citizenship or immigration status.

☐ RESIDENCY/HOME ADDRESS
(this must match the home address in Section A, and the proof must be dated within 6 months of the application)

- ☐ ID Card with address
- ☐ Postmarked envelope, postcard, or magazine label with name and date
- ☐ Driver's license issued within past 6 months
- ☐ Utility bill (gas, electric, cable), bank statement, or correspondence from a government agency which contains name and home address (not a P.O. Box)
- ☐ Letter/lease/rent receipt with home address from landlord
- ☐ Property tax records or mortgage statement

PROOF OF CURRENT INCOME: You must provide a letter, written statement, or copy of check or stubs, from the employer, person or agency providing the income. Submit all that apply. Provide the most recent proof of income before taxes. The proof must be dated, include the employees name and show gross income for the pay period.

☐ Wages and Salary

- ☐ Paycheck stubs *(4 consecutive weeks)*
- ☐ Letter from employer on company letterhead, signed and dated
- ☐ Income tax return**
- ☐ Business records

☐ Self-Employment

- ☐ Signed and dated income tax return and all Schedules**
- ☐ Records of earnings and expenses

☐ Unemployment Benefits

- ☐ Award letter/certificate
- ☐ Benefit check
- ☐ Correspondence from NYS Dept. of Labor

Private Pensions/Annuities

- ☐ Statement from pension/annuity

☐ Social Security

- ☐ Award letter/certificate
- ☐ Benefit check
- ☐ Correspondence from Social Security Administration

☐ Child Support/Alimony

- ☐ Letter from person providing support
- ☐ Letter from court
- ☐ Child support/alimony check stub

☐ Worker's Compensation

- ☐ Award letter
- ☐ Check stub

☐ Veteran's Benefits

- ☐ Award letter
- ☐ Benefit check stub
- ☐ Correspondence from Veteran's Administration

☐ Military Pay

- ☐ Award letter
- ☐ Check stub

☐ Interest/Dividends/Royalties

- ☐ Statement from bank, credit union or financial institution
- ☐ Letter from broker
- ☐ Letter from agent

☐ Income from Rent or Room/Board

- ☐ Letter from roomer, boarder, tenant
- ☐ Check stub

☐ Support from Other Family Members

- ☐ Signed statement or letter from family member

**Income tax returns for other than self-employed may be used for applications prior to April of the following year. If later, you must include another form of documentation.

DOH-4220B (page 1 of 2)   NYS DOH

FIGURE 6-6 Documentation List for Eligibility for Charity Care from the NYS Department of Health

DOCUMENTATION CHECKLIST

For Health Insurance

DEPENDENT CARE COSTS:

☐ Written statement from day care center or other child/adult care provider   ☐ Canceled checks or receipts

PROOF OF HEALTH INSURANCE:

☐ Insurance policy   ☐ Certificate of Insurance   ☐ Insurance card

☐ Termination Letter   ☐ Other _____

FOR MEDICAID, CHILD HEALTH PLUS A AND FAMILY HEALTH PLUS ONLY

☐ **Social Security Number** (not required for recertification)

   ☐ Social security card

   ☐ Application for Social Security # (SS-5)

   ☐ Correspondence from Social Security

   ☐ Tax Return

☐ **Resources**
(persons age 19 and over, only if checked by interviewer)

   ☐ Bank Statement

   ☐ Life Insurance policy

   ☐ Deed or Appraisal for Real Estate

   ☐ Copies of stocks, bonds securities

   ☐ Motor Vehicles - Estimate from dealer, "blue book" value

   ☐ Burial Agreement

☐ **Citizenship and Alien Status** (not required for recertification)

   ☐ U.S. Birth Certificate

   ☐ U.S. Baptismal record, recorded within 3 months of birth

   ☐ U.S. or other Passport

   ☐ Naturalization certificate

   ☐ INS form I-551 (Green Card)

   ☐ INS form I-94

   ☐ Official Hospital/doctor birth records

   ☐ INS form I-220B

   ☐ INS I-210 letter

   ☐ INS form I-181

   ☐ Other INS documentation, or correspondence to or from the INS, that shows that the alien is PRUCOL; that is, the alien is living in the U.S. with the knowledge and permission or acquiescence of the INS, and the INS does not contemplate enforcing the alien's departure from the U.S.

PREGNANT WOMEN ONLY

☐ **Proof of Pregnancy**

   ☐ Presumptive Eligibility Screening Worksheet completed by qualified provider

   ☐ Statement from medical professional with expected date of delivery

   ☐ WIC Medical Referral Form

CHILD HEALTH PLUS B ONLY

Noncitizen children who belong to one of the categories in Section D:

☐ INS form I-551   ☐ INS form I-94   ☐ Other INS Documentation (See above)

MEDICAID/CHILD HEALTH PLUS A ONLY

For determination of eligibility for medical expenses from the past three months:

   ☐ Proof of income for the month(s) in which the expense was incurred

   ☐ Proof of residency/home address for the month(s) in which the expense was incurred

**Your enrollment cannot be completed until all checked items are received. Please return these items by _____ .
If you need help getting any of these items, let us know.**

DOH-4220B (page 2 of 2)   NYS DOH

FIGURE 6-6 continued

Some of the reasons payments are not made on charity care patients may be that the application is not complete and that information cannot be verified.

REPORTS AND BENCHMARKING

When determining the success of your practice, the manager should develop good practice standards and then evaluate these standards with weekly and monthly reports. Industry standards, also called **benchmarks**, are tools to assess the effectiveness of practices in a health care facility. Benchmarks and reports go hand in hand as the manager compares the industry standards with his or her own practice reports. The facility type, equipment, expenses, and staff can be compared to current practices to determine whether they are in line with others practices—failing or succeeding. Without using a benchmark to gauge the practice, your expectations could be higher or lower depending on your income and expense. It is difficult to know whether you are successful without knowing how other providers' offices are doing. Using benchmarks allows the provider's office and office manager to identify strengths and weaknesses in the office and make changes accordingly. When the reporting and benchmarking are performed on a consistent basis, the provider's office has more chance of success as it identifies loopholes and finds ways to overcome them.

RUNNING REPORTS

To manage the collection process and revenue cycle effectively, you should run reports on a daily, weekly, and monthly basis. Reports that are run help to identify money outstanding by the insurance and the patient as well as adjustments and payments that have been collected and services and procedures being billed. With each report, the manager or biller can help to identify anything that stands out and does not look appropriate. For example, if there is a high bad debt adjustment and the patient statements were not processed, the manager or biller will look into that adjustment and ensure that it was not a mistake. In addition, if there is a high outstanding balance to Medicaid and the claims are over 60 days old, it could be an indication that Medicaid is not receiving claims and there is a problem. With different reporting options done on a consistent basis, management and billers are able to maintain a better revenue cycle by ensuring income is being received and adjustments are minimal. These reports are examined, and the type of action is determined. The types of reports that should be run on a regular basis are:

- **Accounts aging reports by patient:** This report examines how long monies have been owed. Different activities are performed for accounts that are 30, 60, 90, 120, and more than 180 days old. Generally, at 30 and 60 days, a bill is sent. At 90 days, a note can be attached and phone call can be made. By 120 days, the insurance company should be contacted if payment expected from a payer has not happened. Figure 6-7 shows an account aging report.

- **Accounts aging reports by payer:** This reports looks at the third-party payers that have not paid claims. The report also looks at claims after 30, 60, 90, 120 and 180 days. Carriers need to be contacted when claims are held more than 60 days to see if the claim was received, if additional information is needed, or if the claim was paid but not received or recorded.

- **Denial reasons by payer:** This identifies the money still owed by the payer and what changes need to be made based on the denial reason. Some denials are transferred to the patient, while others have to be handled with the insurance carrier (see Table 6-1).

VERIFYING AND CORRECTING DENIALS

When the insurance carrier denies a procedure or service, the first step is to recognize the denial reason and determine if there is recourse for the billing and coding staff. In some circumstances, denials can be fixed if the documentation supports the changes. Many times, denials appear to be

Insurance Aging

Friday, January 02, 20XX

MEDICAID

Clyde E. Williams (WILLIA0010)   Date of Birth: 03/17/1933   Insured: Self
Insurance: Secondary   Policy: 5133031815   ID: 5133031815

Billing	Date	Code/CPT	Billed	Amount	Current	31 - 60	61 - 90	91 - 120	> 120	Total
Patient Total				95.00	95.00	0.00	0.00	0.00	0.00	95.00
Insurance Total				111.40	111.40	0.00	0.00	0.00	0.00	111.40

MUTUAL - Mutual of Omaha   Mutual of Omaha Plaza, Omaha, NB 68175 (555) 327-8870

James K. Froist (FROIST0000)   Date of Birth: 07/11/1972   Insured: Self
Insurance: Primary   ID:CMZX1C-193591-97

Billing	Date	Code/CPT	Billed	Amount	Current	31 - 60	61 - 90	91 - 120	> 120	Total
5170233	12/05/20XX	99204/99204	01/03/20XX	175.00	175.00					175.00
5170233	12/05/20XX	87070/87070	01/03/20XX	35.00	35.00					35.00
5170233	12/05/20XX	36415/36415	01/03/20XX	20.00	20.00					20.00
5170233	12/05/20XX	81002/81002	01/03/20XX	21.00	21.00					21.00
517305	12/11/20XX	99213/99213	01/03/20XX	95.00	95.00					95.00
Patient Total				346.00	346.00	0.00	0.00	0.00	0.00	346.00
Insurance Total				346.00	346.00	0.00	0.00	0.00	0.00	346.00

PAC POS - Pacificare POS P. O. Box 6099, Cypress, CA 90630 (555) 316-9776

Dorothy J. Blan (BLAN0000)   Date of Birth: 02/23/1950   Insured: Self
Insurance: Primary   Policy: 90158778   ID: 463808651 01

Billing	Date	Code/CPT	Billed	Amount	Current	31 - 60	61 - 90	91 - 120	> 120	Total
5170434	12/20/20XX	99214/99214	01/03/20XX	150.00	150.00					150.00
5170434	12/20/20XX	93000/93000	01/03/20XX	85.00	85.00					85.00
5170434	12/20/20XX	36415/36415	01/03/20XX	20.00	20.00					20.00
5170434	12/20/20XX	81002/81002	01/03/20XX	21.00	21.00					21.00
5170434	12/20/20XX	Patient co-pay	01/03/20XX	-10.00	-10.00					-10.00
Patient Total				266.00	266.00	0.00	0.00	0.00	0.00	266.00

Alice Oganesyan (OGANES0000)   Date of Birth: 06/17/1960   Insured: Self
Insurance: Primary   Policy: 00010085   ID: 564972684

Billing	Date	Code/CPT	Billed	Amount	Current	31 - 60	61 - 90	91 - 120	> 120	Total
5166555	06/04/20XX	99213/99213	06/13/20XX 08/29/20XX	95.00					95.00	95.00
5166555	06/04/20XX	Patient co-pay		-10.00					-10.00	-10.00
5170283	12/09/20XX	99213/99213		95.00	95.00					95.00
5170283	12/09/20XX	Patient co-pay		-10.00	-10.00					-10.00
Patient Total				170.00	85.00	0.00	0.00	0.00	85.00	170.00

Mona Vargas (VARGAS0001)   Date of Birth: 07/23/1973   Insured: Self
Insurance: Primary   Policy: 00010659   ID: 584-69-5112 01

Billing	Date	Code/CPT	Billed	Amount	Current	31 - 60	61 - 90	91 - 120	> 120	Total
5167164	05/16/20XX	99213/99213	07/12/20XX	95.00					95.00	95.00
5167164	08/07/20XX	IA		-25.69					-25.69	-25.69
5167164	05/16/20XX	Patient co-pay		-15.00					-15.00	-15.00
Patient Total				54.31	0.00	0.00	0.00	0.00	54.31	54.31
Insurance Total				490.31	351.00	0.00	0.00	0.00	139.31	490.31

PRU - Prudential HMO

Patty J. Smith (SMITH0002)   Date of Birth: 09/12/1946   Insured: Robert Smith, Sr. (SMITH0000)
Insurance: Primary   Policy: 23236   ID: 54650875702

Billing	Date	Code/CPT	Billed	Amount	Current	31 - 60	61 - 90	91 - 120	> 120	Total
5166497	04/30/20XX	99213/99213	06/13/20XX	95.00					95.00	95.00
5166497	04/30/20XX	Patient co-pay		-10.00					-10.00	-10.00
5167710	07/09/20XX	99214/99214	07/12/20XX	150.00					150.00	150.00
5167710	07/09/20XX	Patient co-pay		-10.00					-10.00	-10.00
Patient Total				225.00	0.00	0.00	0.00	0.00	225.00	225.00
Insurance Total				225.00	0.00	0.00	0.00	0.00	225.00	225.00

Provider Totals

				Amount	Current	31 - 60	61 - 90	91 - 120	> 120	Total
Fran Practon, M.D.				45979.01	29743.84	2851.42	1114.13	600.94	11668.68	45979.01
Gerald Practon, M.D.				17885.34	7476.27	1413.79	414.85	805.00	7776.43	17855.34
Report Totals				63864.35	37219.11	4265.21	1528.98	1405.94	19445.11	63864.35
Percent of Total					58.28%	6.68%	2.39%	2.20%	30.45%	100.00%

© Cengage Learning 2013

FIGURE 6-7 An Accounts Aging Report

adjustments to the billing and coding staff when they first begin posting to the patient's ledger. Management should educate their billing and coding staff to question all denials and see them as a red flag requiring further research. For example, a denial missing a modifier can appear to be a noncovered procedure or service; trained billing and coding staff can recognize the need for a modifier and make appropriate changes and resubmissions. Recognizing the need for changing the denial avoids unnecessary adjustments and contributes to the revenue cycle.

TABLE 6-1: A report that looks at denial reasons by payer

Insurance Carrier	Patient Ineligible	No Referral of Authorization	Not a Covered Service	Charges Unbundled	Timely Filing	Duplicate Charges
Medicare						
Blue Shield						
Aetna						
Oxford						
Healthcare Plus						

Table 6-1 offers examples that may cause a claim to be denied and solutions that may help with correcting the denial.

If the reason for a denial is that the patient is ineligible, the following actions should be taken:

- Check the spelling of the name on the insurance card and the name on the claim submitted.
- Check that the ID numbers are correct.
- Check that the name of the patient and the name of the subscriber have not been mixed up; they may be different people.
- Check the date of birth to make sure it matches the claim and the insurance card.

If the reason for the denial indicates that there was no referral or preauthorization, these actions should be taken:

- Review the patient's chart for communication with the insurance company and notation of a referral or authorization given.
- If there was preauthorization obtained, was there a preauthorization number assigned; if there was, was that number placed on the claim in the appropriate block?
- Look at the insurance card for the patient for information about authorizations.
- If no authorization was obtained, contact the insurance carrier to obtain a backdated referral or authorization if permitted by the carrier.
- Check the patient's medical file to see if there is a waiver on file, stating that he or she is aware of no referral or preauthorization.
- Resubmit with referral or authorization, make any adjustments as needed, or bill the patient as appropriate according to insurance carrier guidelines.

If the reason for the denial is that the service is not a covered service, then you can take these actions:

- Check that the procedure codes submitted were the correct codes.
- Check that the diagnosis code was correct and that it was correctly linked to the procedure justifying the medical necessity.
- If the claim was a Medicare claim, was an ABN completed prior to the service?

If the reason for the denial is that the service was unbundled, then you should:

- Check the codes in the CPT manual. If the individual CPT codes could have been combined into one inclusive code, then that inclusive code needs to be resubmitted.

- If the code was for a separate procedure from the bundled service, then add the appropriate modifier stating an additional procedure or service was performed.
- If the claim was sent correctly and the codes were done separately, resubmit with a special report documenting the separate procedure or service.
- When the code is determined to be bundled with another procedure or service code that was already billed and paid, make an adjustment against the bundled procedure code to the patient's ledger to avoid the procedure or service being resubmitted incorrectly and then create an accounts receivable that reflects the correct amount due according to the revenue cycle.

If the reason for the denial is a timely filing issue, then you should:

- Check the carrier requirements, and if it is a claim that was filed past the time frame, then send an appeal to the carrier indicating why the claim was filed past the timely filing limits.
- Check the claim status reports for the date of service and thereafter. If the claim was proven to be submitted within the filing limit, then send an appeal with the proof of timely filing to the insurance carrier.
- If it is determined that the claim is beyond the filing limit and there is no recourse to recover the money, then make an adjustment to the patient's ledger to avoid the procedure or service being resubmitted incorrectly and then create an accounts receivable that reflects the correct amount due according to the revenue cycle.

If the reason for the denial states that these are duplicate charges, then the actions you should take are:

- Check the dates of service listed on the EOB/RA to see if these dates were previously submitted and paid.
- Check to see if there were any outstanding claims not paid.
- Check to see if an appeal, corrected claim, or resubmission was done in the time between the claim submission and receiving the EOB/RA.
- Read medical documentation to be sure the procedure or service was not repeated or performed bilaterally on the same date of service, which requires payment twice in one day.
- A call to the insurance carrier could also help clarify what claims were not submitted based on the patient's ledger card.
- If it is determined that the claim is a duplicate and there is no recourse to recover the money, then make an adjustment to the patient's ledger to avoid the procedure or service being resubmitted incorrectly and then create an accounts receivable that reflects the correct amount due according to the revenue cycle.

BENCHMARKING

Benchmarking is a process whereby standards are established to evaluate different practices in health care. A percentage is usually established that represents good practice results for that health care setting. There is no single benchmarking standard. Instead, many factors are established that result in the best practice standard. In the area of the revenue cycle, benchmarking is used to promote a positive cash flow and lower monies owed to the health care provider. Management should rely on benchmarking as a guide to determine the success for the provider's office. With benchmarking references in a medical facility, the success of the facility will increase as the benchmarking indicates the need for change. Although benchmarking may be time consuming, without referencing the industry standards, it is difficult to determine where you should be at as a practice manager of a provider's office. Making changes appropriately and timely are important, and benchmarking is one method used to identify the need as it relates to a positive income and revenue cycle.

Benchmarking standards should include:

- Paid claims versus denied claims
- Expenses versus income
- Amounts billed versus amounts collected
- Correct codes billed versus incorrect

For example, if the amount of monies received is $75,000 and the amount of the total charges is $100,000, then another way of looking at this is:

$75,000 = 75% of the total charges received

$100,000

Let us look at an example:

Figures 6-8A and 6-8B demonstrate a positive cash flow scenario and a negative cash flow scenario, respectively. If the income in a given month is $20,000 and expenses are at $14,850, then there is a positive cash flow.

If the amount of income per month is $13,000 and the amount of expenses is $14,850, then this health care facility does not have a positive cash flow.

Expenses vs Income

Month of June

Expenses		Income
Mortgage	$2500	Insurance payments $15,000
Taxes	$700	
Telephone	$300	Patient payments $5000
Electric	$350	
Salaries	$10,000	
Supplies	$1000	

Income: $20,000

Expenses $14,850   positive cash flow of $5150 for the month of June

A. Example of a positive cash flow

Month of June

Expenses		Income
Mortgage	$2500	Insurance payments $10,000
Taxes	$700	
Telephone	$300	Patient payments $3000
Electric	$350	
Salaries	$10,000	
Supplies	$1000	

B. Example of a negative cash flow

Income: $13,000

Expenses $14,850   negative cash flow of $1850 for the month of June.

FIGURE 6-8A, B Example of a Positive Cash Flow Scenario and a Negative Cash Flow Scenario

INCOME AND EXPENSES

As you can see, equally important in the continuous monitoring and evaluating of the components of the revenue cycle is to also evaluate the total expenses of maintaining the health care facility. To have a positive cash flow, expenses should not be greater than the income received at the facility. In the process of maintaining increased income and low expenses, you should identify opportunities for cutting back on expenses, as long as the process does not overcome the savings. Paying a staff member to research can be as much as the savings, and the manager must realize the potential for this occurring. In addition, lower prices sometimes result in cheaper products that do not last as long and in the end cost more money. Monitoring expenses is a difficult task, and the office staff must come together and assist in this process, as ordering is monitored and kept at a minimum. For example, ordering cases of paper because of printing errors that could have been avoided. Income comes into the practice through insurance payments and patient payments. At the time of the visit, cash will be given by some patients and should be recorded in the patient's account immediately to be sure the patient is credited for the payment. In some circumstances, patients may send cash in the mail, but it is not likely. If they do send cash, the payment should be applied to their account appropriately and deposited with the daily cash and checks. Checks will come either direct deposit through an EFT (electronic fund transfer) or through the mail from patients and insurance carriers. The online bank and the mail must be checked daily, and discrepancies should be identified and cleared up immediately. Credit card payments from patients are also usually electronically deposited and can appear within 1–2 days after processing. Credit card payments can be processed at the time of the visit or through the mail or telephone call. Keeping track of the different payments can be challenging, and a day sheet with all the totals must be run to identify expected deposits and compare the totals. Deposits should be made daily or as often as necessary to ensure consistent cash flow.

MAKING DEPOSITS

In most providers' offices, management should require that deposits be made daily to prevent stealing, keep patient's accounts current, identify outstanding income easier, and maintain a positive cash flow. Cash should be totaled for the deposit slip. This cash should equal the amount on the daily ledger or day sheet. In addition, checks from patients and insurance carriers should be listed separately on the deposit slip. On each entry is room for a check number and sometimes a name. Using the name is sometimes easier for locating the posting of the payment if needed in the future. The manager can determine the best method of recording checks on the deposit slip as it fits his or her practice and the deposit slip space availability. Deposits should also match the ledger, and a carbon copy of the deposit slip should be kept for future reference of payments that were incorrectly recorded. Figure 6-9 shows an example.

EXPENSES TO INCLUDE

Although most expenses are the same for medical facilities, there can be a variance within different specialties. Most supplies are the same when dealing with administrative supplies, but medical supplies are different for different specialties. When determining expenses in a provider's office, the office manager should keep in mind the type of specialty and design purchases around the need for the office. Some expenses can be one-time purchases, whereas others are ongoing and must be compared carefully (see Figure 6-10). While researching pricing for the office expenses, consider asking other facilities where they purchase their supplies and equipment to get a better idea of cost and quality.

List all items separately		
Total Enter on front side		

DEPOSIT SLIP

CURRENCY		
COIN		
CHECKS		
TOTAL FROM OTHER SIDE		
TOTAL		

Sorena City Bank

2204 Lancaster Highway

Berwyn, PA 19312

© Cengage Learning 2013

FIGURE 6-9 Sample Deposit Slip

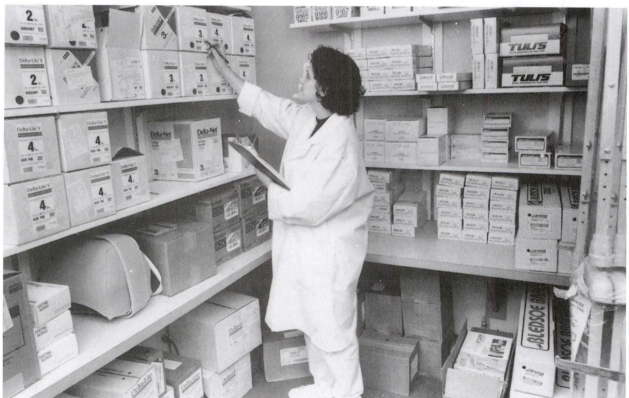

© Cengage Learning 2013

FIGURE 6-10 Taking Inventory

TABLE 6-2: Types of supplies

Speciality	Type of Supplies
Orthopedist	Chet Payne
Obstetrician	Prenatal supplies
Surgeon	Surgical trays, suture removal
Cardiology	Exercise stress testing, echocardiogram supplies

The most common expenses include:

- Rent or mortgage of facility
- Utilities, such as telephone, electric, and Internet lines
- Payroll, such as salaries of employees, including taxes, social security, and benefits paid by the health care facility
- Medical expenses, including supplies, disposables, new and used equipment, and repairs or servicing of equipment
- Costs of procedures performed in the facility

Some costs have little control, such as mortgage and utilities. Other costs, such as medical supply costs, can be compared between different companies. While many supplies are similar, different specialties have some different equipment or supplies. Making a comparison chart of prices is a great approach to comparing and saving; however, be sure the cost of the employee is not more than the savings on the expenses.

Table 6-2 shows some of the different types of supplies.

Periodically checking the costs of all supplies with different supply companies can be effective in controlling costs. In some instances, companies may negotiate rates for larger quantities purchased, although these are often not advertised. Management should ask what the best price is for the quantity purchased. Another way to watch for savings is to find sales or promotions. The manager should encourage ordering staff to become part of the network and receive e-mails when there are specials being run to take advantage of the savings.

For example, when comparing the costs for performing medical procedures, the following companies quoted these prices (see Table 6-3 sample of quotes on supplies):

TABLE 6-3: Sample of quotes on supplies

Items needed	EKG paper	X-ray film	Culture supplies	Spirometry materials
ABC Company	$125 for package of 100	$250 for 50	$50 for 50	$75 for 100 packages
XYZ Company	$150 for package of 100	$250 for 75	$50 for 100	$75 for 50 packages
Yourre Company	$300 for package of 250	$300 for 100	$100 for 75	$150 for 100 packages
Owr Company	$300 for package of 200	$300 for 150	$100 for 100 items	$150 for 200 packages

As the manager, when comparing these costs, you should look for quality besides cost. Saving on expenses is important; however, when you purchase a cheaper product because of the price, you sometimes sacrifice quality and the product does not last as long. When checking for pricing, you must be aware of the quality or request a sample until you are sure the product will withstand its use in the office. This can sometimes be a long process but is definitely worth it for the items that are used long term by the provider's office. Researching quality and price is important if the end result is saving on expenses.

Checklist for managers to use for supplies:

- ☐ Make a list of the supplies used for procedures.
- ☐ Determine current costs from your suppliers.
- ☐ Research other companies for their prices on the same items.
- ☐ Ask if ordering in quantity reduces the price.
- ☐ Get the quote in writing.
- ☐ Determine the company to use.
- ☐ Keep a list of supplies and companies.
- ☐ Check prices on the invoice against quotes.

DETERMINING FEE SCHEDULE

The office manager is responsible for monitoring the fee schedule for the services and procedures provided in the facility. They must create a permanent fee schedule to coincide with the CPT and HCPCS codes that are used when billing the insurance company and the patients. Once the fee schedule has been set by management and the provider, future changes have to be permanent and apply to all parties that are being billed. Prices cannot change based on the insurance carrier or lack of insurance. In addition, the fee schedule should coincide with the industry standards and be within the range of the Medicare fee schedule. For example, if the Medicare fee for an EKG is $50, it is unreasonable for the facility to charge $500, which is 10 times the Medicare fee. On the other hand, the manager must ensure that the fee is not too low compared to the expenses involved. Even if the fee schedule is set high enough, not all insurance carriers honor the fee that the provider submits and the amount of reimbursement must be checked with each insurance carrier. For example, in the specialist office, the manager needs to compare the cost of doing the procedure with the cost of reimbursement. If the cost is greater than the insurance carrier reimburses, then the manager and the physicians need to decide if this service or procedure should continue to be performed in the health care facility.

Let us look at this hypothetical scenario: An orthopedic practice performs X-rays on all accident patients. The cost of performing the X-ray, including personnel, is $200 per X-ray. The insurance carrier reimburses $135. If the practice performs five X-rays per day five days a week, the cost is $5,000 per week. The insurance carrier reimburses $3,375 per week. The manager needs to discuss this procedure with physicians to determine the cost-effectiveness of continuing this procedure.

In this situation, the expenses of the procedure cost more than the procedure, and continuing to lose money is not conducive to maintaining income or a positive revenue cycle. For the provider's office to be successful, it would have to discontinue the procedure or find supplies or personnel that are less expensive to support its decision. Either way, the fee schedule needs to be monitored and compared to the industry standards and the insurance carriers on a consistent basis.

PAYROLL

Payroll needs to be addressed with each employee. An employee being hired must complete appropriate paperwork for payroll to begin. Each state has different guidelines in addition to the federal guidelines, and management must follow all the guidelines accurately. Most large facilities have human resource departments or payroll companies that perform payroll functions. As a manager, you must understand the components of payroll in order to explain the paperwork and assist new employees as they complete all requirements. If changes occur for the employee during the course of his or her employment, he or she will be asked to complete new paperwork with the changes.

When an employee is hired, he or she is offered a salary—either hourly or salaried.

From that base salary, federal and state taxes are taken out as well as social security deductions, Medicare deductions, state disability deductions, and benefit deductions. The amount of each deduction is based on the number of deductions claimed on the employee's W-4 form, which was completed when hired. As the manager, you may have a duplicate payroll register that summarizes this. As the manager, you should also keep track of paid holiday's vacations, PTO time, or sick time (see Figure 6-11).

In addition to the payroll register, keep track of employee time off by using a system such as a yearly calendar in each file, which shows time off each month for vacation, sick time, etc. (see Figure 6-12).

PAYROLL REGISTER FOR PERIOD ENDING: August 31, 20--

EMPLOYEE NAME				EARNINGS			DEDUCTIONS							
	No. of Exempts	Hours Worked	Hourly Rate	Reg. Pay	Over-time	Gross Pay	FICA	Fed Inc. Tax	State Inc. Tax	SDI	Medicare	TOTAL DEDUC.	Check No.	NET PAY
Mary Jo Davis	1-S	90	13.	1170	39.	1930.50	73.35	145.	36.51	—	17.15	272.01	554	1658.49
Beverly Woo	0-S		Salary	1200		1200.	75.64	145.	39.30	—	17.40	277.34	555	922.66
Harold Bohrn	2-M	88	12.	1056		1056.	65.47	84.	23.46	—	15.31	188.24	556	867.76
Joan Gonzalez	1-M		Salary	1000		1000.	62.00	92.	23.85	—	14.50	192.35	557	807.65

FIGURE 6-11 Payroll Register

Employee name: Anna Thimely						
Date of Hire: 12/1/2011				Date of Termination:		
Month of: January 2012						
Monday	Tuesday	Wednesday	Thursday	Friday	Saturday	Sunday
	S	S				
V	V	V	V	V		

H: Holiday

V: Vacation

S: Sick time

PTO: Personal time off

FIGURE 6-12 Example of Tracking Employee Time Off

Each month would be marked for each employee.

SUMMARY

- The manager's role in the revenue cycle includes the monitoring of each component, including income and expenses, and identifying and resolving any issues.

- The manager performs evaluations daily and at 30- and 60-day periods to identify and take action on discrepancies in patient balances, insurance claims, and payments.

- The manager evaluates EOBs and RAs for denial reasons and takes action to prevent future denials by establishing policies and procedures according to regulations and guidelines.

- The manager reviews aging reports to determine the action that needs to be taken on claims at intervals of 30, 60, 90, 120, and 180 days. Policies and procedures are established for uniformity of action by all people involved in this process.

- Management evaluates costs of materials, supplies, and procedures for cost-effectiveness and to maintain a positive revenue cycle.

REVIEW EXERCISES

TRUE OR FALSE

1. _____ Good practice for managers is to reconcile the appointment book.

2. _____ The manager should check the sign-in sheet against the master list daily.

3. _____ EOBs do not need to be reviewed regularly.

4. _____ The denial reason of patient ineligible means the patient is not your patient.

5. _____ A bundled code is one service for one group of codes and one fee.

6. _____ A duplicate service means the patient had the service twice on the same day.

7. _____ Bad debt results when a patient cannot pay the bill.

8. _____ A patient is eligible for charity care if income is below a set level.

9. _____ A patient must complete an application for charity care.

10. _____ An accounts aging report is a report run on only patient accounts.

MATCHING

A   Accounts Aging

B   Bench-marking

C   Bundled Codes

D   Day Sheet

E   Unbundled Codes

F   Bad Debt

G   Write-Off

H   Charity Care

I   RA

J   Denial

1. _____ One fee for one group of codes.

2. _____ Breaking apart of a grouping of codes and charging individual fees.

3. _____ When an insurance company does not pay a service submitted.

4. _____ Patients who are deceased with no estate to pay bills.

5. _____ Patients with no insurance and whose income is below a set level.

6. _____ Considered to be an industry standard.

7. _____ A report of how long monies are owed.

8. _____ A record of each day's charges and receipts.

9. _____ Patients who do not pay their bills.

10. _____ A statement of services, charges, and payments by an insurance carrier.

CRITICAL THINKING ACTIVITIES

ACTIVITY 1

Review this aging report to decide what action you would take for each patient who owes money at each level. Using number 1 as the first contact and 5 as the last contact, number each in order of what you would consider the first phone call to make in trying to reach the patient.

Patient Name	30 Days	60 Days	90 Days	120 Days	Over 180 Days
Aalyce Aeye		$795 _____			
Becky Bee	$1,200 _____				
Carly Cee					$315 _____
Debby Dee				$925 _____	
Elli Eeyee			$1,050 _____		

ACTIVITY 2

You are the manager of a large practice. Your daily routine includes:

- Checking the daily schedule
- Checking the sign-in sheet
- Reviewing the day sheet, the number of patients, charges, and payments

Your job includes finding any discrepancies and deciding on a course of action.

Review this appointment book, sign-in sheet, and day sheet and then note any problems. Use the checklist for a manager from this chapter to help you find discrepancies.

Checklist for the manager to use daily:

☐ Master list of patient's appointments for
    the day matches   Number of patients _____

Appointment Schedule

8:00 Mary Smith
8:15 Joan Brown
8:30 Jack White
8:45 ↓
9:00 John Black
9:15 Heidi Jones
9:30 Shannon Small
9:45 ↓
10:00 Rose Flowers
10:15 Alex McBrown

10:30 Allison Whiteson
10:45 Betty Blooper
11:00 ↓
11:15 Harry Harrison
11:30 Henry Hudsonville
12:00 Jon James
12:15 James Yellow
12:30 Dave Sideson
1–4 At Hospital

ACTIVITY 3

Checklist for the manager to use daily:

☐ Sign-in sheet clearly marked.   Number of patients _____

Sign-In Sheet

Name	Time In
Mary Smith	8:00
Joan Brown	8:15
Jack White	8:30
John Black	8:30
Mary Blanco	8:45
Heidi Jones	9:00
Shannon Small	9:20
Rose Flowers	9:45
Allison Whiteson	10:30
Betty Blooper	10:45
Henry Hudsonville	11:30
Jon James	11:30
Dave Sideson	12:00
Harry Harrison	12:15

ACTIVITY 4

Checklist for the manager to use daily:

☐ Day sheet matches the master list and sign-in sheet.   Number of patients _____

Day Sheet With Charges and Payments (modified for exercise)

Charges	Payments	Name
$100	$100	Smith, Mary
$100	$100	Brown, Joan
$100	$100	White Jack
$100	$100	Black, John
$100	$100	Jones, Heidi
$100	$100	Small, Shannon
$100	$100	McBrown, Alex
$100	$100	Whiteson, Allison
$100	$100	Blooper, Betty
$100	$100	County, George
$100	$100	Harrison, Harry
$100	$100	Hudsonville, Henry
$100	$100	James, John
$100	$100	Yellow, James
$100	$100	Sideson, Dave
$100	$100	Jones, John
Totals: $1,600	Totals $1,600	Total patients: 16

Then, decide on a course of action for any problems.

Course of Action for Discrepancies

_____

_____

_____

_____

_____

CRITICAL THINKING QUESTIONS

1. Review the specialties in Appendix D. Make a list of procedures or services that could generate income.

2. Once that list is done, what elements of the revenue cycle are important to ensuring payment for these procedures or services?

3. Discuss the result of a missing referral or authorization on the revenue cycle. Include a discussion about obtaining retroactive referrals or authorizations as an option.

4. Explain a day sheet as it pertains to the revenue cycle as well as a reason why it would be run more than once a day.

WEB ACTIVITIES

1. Go to https://www.cms.gov/MLNProducts/downloads/RA_Guide_Full_03-22-06.pdf to complete the codes for these situations in which Medicare indicates any financial liability:

Contractual Obligations	
Correction and Reversal	
Patient Responsibility	

2. For your specialty, make a list of services and procedures that would be performed. Go to supply companies online and in your area to research costs for these supplies. Refer to Appendix D for assistance.

3. Research on the Internet for templates that can be used as overdue notices. Search for the format and appropriate template you would choose for your health care facility.

4. Search the Medicare website in your area. Find the fee schedule for any physician's office. Look up 10 codes to see what the different prices are for facility and nonfacility fees.

THINK LIKE A MANAGER

CREATE YOUR PRACTICE

Using the templates found in Appendix B and the information presented in this unit, complete the following interactive exercises:

1. Write a policy and procedure for determining eligibility for charity care.

2. Write a policy and procedure for taking action based on the aging report.

3. Write a policy and procedure for whose responsibility it is for collection activities.

4. You want to teach your new employees about accounts aging reports and collection activities. Plan a teaching session:

    - Create an outline of content to be discussed.

    - Create a sign-in sheet.

    - Review the policies and procedures you created for your practice.

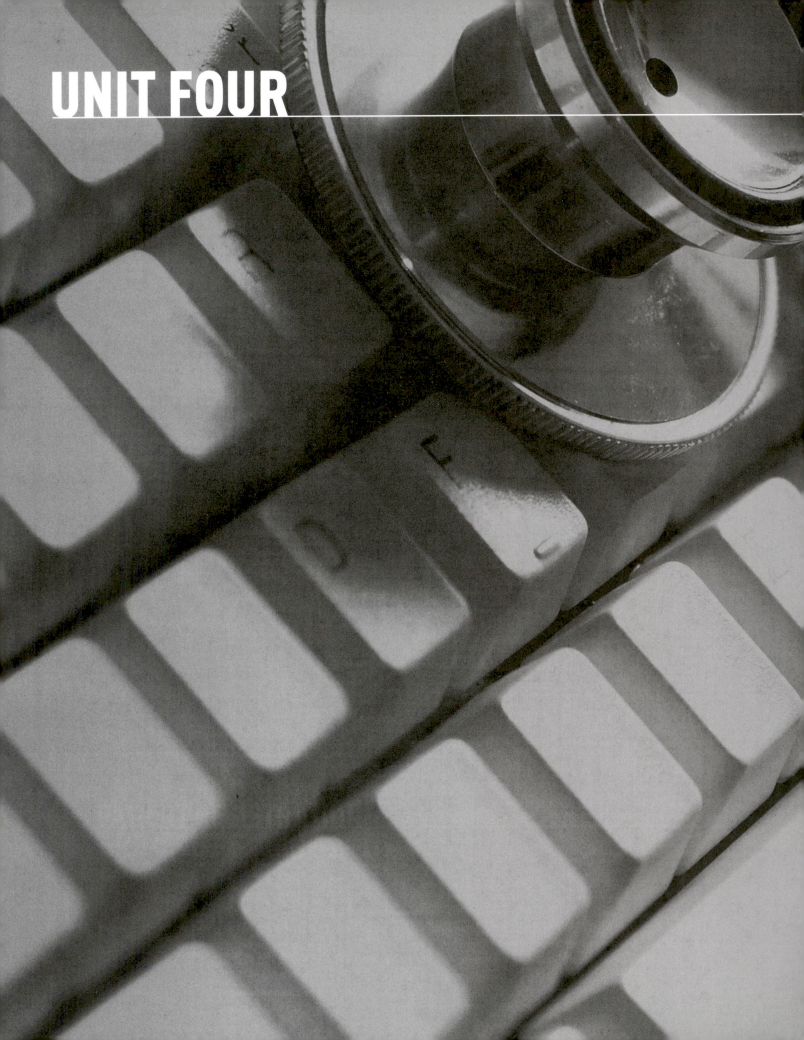

UNIT FOUR

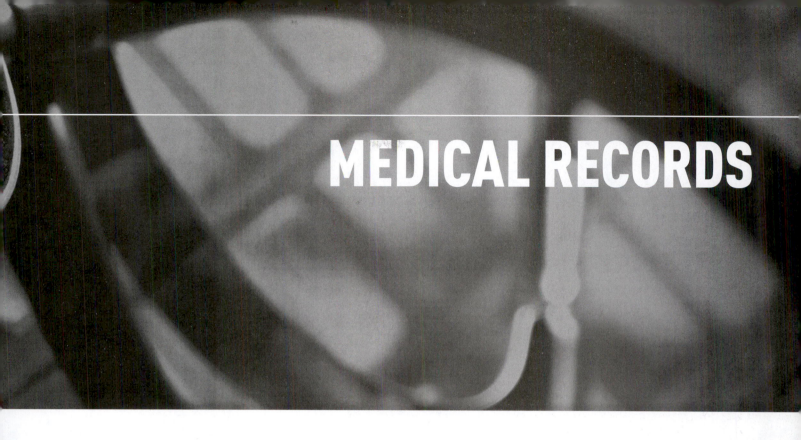

MEDICAL RECORDS

MEDICAL RECORDS ARE vital to all health care settings. They assure continuity of care with health care providers, support compliance with regulatory agencies, and provide a source of statistics. Policies and procedures for documenting, maintaining, and organizing the medical facility must be adhered to by all employees, including management. Training is an ongoing process as updates are received. Management is responsible for performing audits consistently to detect issues and determine further actions based on the results.

MEDICAL RECORDS

- Manage accuracy in documentation of a patient's medical record.

- Determine documentation types as needed for the health care facility.

- Conduct audits on patient records on a monthly basis to ensure consistency.

- Evaluate employees and inform them of any inaccuracies.

- Maintain policies and procedures on documentation guidelines.

- Obtain updates on medical record policies and procedures on a regular basis.

- Educate employees about policies and procedures in place.

- Conduct new training when policies and procedures change.

- Manage medical record completeness to coincide with billing and coding.

- Track errors and inconsistencies and provide in-service training as necessary.

CHAPTER 7

MEDICAL RECORDS

FUNDAMENTALS

Chapter 7 will discuss the fundamentals of medical records, concentrating on the outpatient record and including the name of each section, along with the content included, in each portion. In addition, documentation requirements as well as sources of the information will be covered. Pertinent laws and regulations will also be identified as to their importance in patient care and the facility's obligation in completing a thorough and accurate document.

OBJECTIVES

Upon completion of this chapter, the student will be able to:

- State at least three purposes for keeping a medical record.
- List the components of a medical record.
- Identify the purpose of each component.
- Recognize laws that affect the medical record.

KEY TERMS

- American Medical Association (AMA)
- Date of birth (DOB)
- Centers for Medicare and Medicaid Services (CMS)
- Chief complaint, History, Exam, Details, Drugs, Assessment, and Return (CHEDDAR)
- Continuity of care
- Current Procedural terminology (CPT)
- Healthcare Common Procedural Coding System (HCPCS)
- Insurance carrier
- International Classification of Diseases – Clinical Modification (ICD-diagnostic codes)
- Internet-Only Manual (IOM)
- National coverage determination (NCD)
- Notice of privacy
- Problem-oriented medical record (POMR)
- Subjective, Objective, Assessment, and Plan (SOAP)
- Subscriber

THE PURPOSE OF MEDICAL RECORDS

In any medical environment, the medical record is vital for accurate patient care. When patients have an appointment, medical providers might forget what each patient encounter involved, which can result in improper treatment. The medical record is developed by all participants involved in the patient's encounter to provide a consistent and thorough documentation of the events that occurred. Documentation is completed by administrative and clinical staff involved in the patient care and serves as a guide to demonstrate all aspects of the demographics, procedures, services, history, examination, diagnoses, and much more. Promoting quality care for patients is important, and medical records serve a number of purposes, including:

- Continuity of care
- Compliance with coding and reimbursement policies
- Source of statistics

CONTINUITY OF CARE

In a continuum of care, a patient has a medical record—either in paper or electronic form—at his or her family physician or primary care physician offices. Medical documentation is important to patient care, and maintaining a thorough and accurate medical record helps the health care facility provide quality treatment to its patients. In order to maintain an up-to-date, thorough medical record, providers share medical documentation among each other that represents the patient's history of treatment in other facilities as well as their own. Every time a patient is sent for a service at another health care facility, such as a laboratory, a radiology center, or a physician for a consultation, a report is generated and placed in a medical record in that setting and a report is also sent back to the family or primary physician's office and placed in the patient's medical record. This allows the patient's primary physician and other providers to have a chronological record of symptoms, diseases, and other disorders, along with diagnostic tests and outcomes or diagnoses. This is important for safe treatment as well as providing optimum care for the patient. It serves as a reference from the past to the present. Figure 7-1 shows a continuity of care "wheel" in which the patient and the medical record are the center and all services link back to the medical record of that patient.

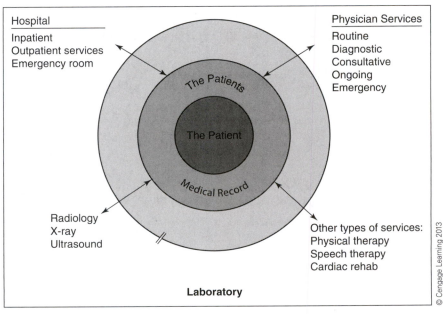

FIGURE 7-1 Continuity of Care Wheel

COMPLIANCE WITH CODING

The medical record is of the utmost importance to coding and reimbursement. If something is not documented in the patient's medical record, then the medical coder is unable to determine the services or procedures provided to the patient. Information in the medical record is what coding is based on, and if something is missing, then the coder will not be able to submit for reimbursement, thus losing the facility revenue. The coder depends on the information within the medical record to be accurate and complete in order to justify medical necessity to the services and procedures provided to the patient. Procedures and services need to be detailed and specific to the nature of treatment provided to the patient in order for the coders to achieve the highest level of services and procedures. Diagnoses need to be accurate so the medical coder can code to the highest level of specificity for each diagnoses the patient has documented. Correct diagnoses and procedures are also important for compliance with insurance carriers' coverage determination policies, as each **insurance carrier** who reimburses the provider has different requirements. The coder must understand the differences to be able to code services, procedures, and diagnoses accurately and according to the medical record.

SOURCE OF STATISTICS

Research is important for the development of new cures, procedures, and medications. The information gathered during research can also be used to predict the need for services in a given area. One way to gather information for statistical purposes is to convert procedures and diagnoses from the patient's medical record into codes and then input them into the computer, becoming a source of statistics for various studies. These studies can help determine clusters of diseases, such as in the flu season, the severity of an allergy season, or to determine and prove the need to receive approval for a health care facility in an area, such as a cancer center. Another benefit to using statistical information for services, procedures, and diagnoses is to identify what types of treatments are able to help with severely ill patients or chronic diseases. Ongoing studies make it easier for health care facilities to identify improved treatment options based on the diagnostic testing, results, and treatments used for certain diagnoses in each area. When documentation in a medical record is thorough and accurate, it can be a tremendous resource to developing statistical information for the future of medicine.

PARTS OF THE MEDICAL RECORD

Consistency is necessary for the patient's medical record to maintain accurate information regarding the patient's medical background in the facility. You can think of the medical record as being divided into an administrative section and a medical or clinical section. The start of a medical record begins when the patient makes the first appointment to the office with a complaint or request for a medical encounter and also provides demographic information. All the information obtained during the appointment scheduling is entered into the medical record, and the administrative and clinical sections are generated as a result. Despite the different sections in the medical record, each area must be documented appropriately to reflect the patient's appointments and to maintain accurate information regarding the patient at all times. Maintaining identifying patient information on all documents in the medical record will allow the facility to ensure proper treatment and continuity of care.

The administrative sections of the medical record are just as important as the medical or clinical sections. Without identifying demographic information, such as the patient's name and **date of birth (DOB)**, documentation can be misplaced and result in poor treatment of the patient. In addition, without proper payment from the insurance carrier, the facility would lose revenue and may provide poor quality treatment or have to close as a result. Maintaining demographics is important to the function of the office and should be checked with each appointment to the facility. If different from the appointment record, the medical record should be updated when the patient identifies changes. Administrative and clinical staff should take part in ensuring that the administrative section of the medical record is updated. If something appears different, the clinical staff should also take the initiative to make changes as appropriate. The administrative section of the medical record will contain demographic information and financial information, such as:

- Patient registration
- An acknowledgment of receipt of the facility's notice of privacy
- Copies of the front and back of the insurance card(s)
- Correspondence

When you document in the medical or clinical sections of the medical record, the documentation is primarily completed by clinical staff, with some minimal administrative entries, such as the documentation of missed appointments. Maintaining accurate medical information is vital to the treatment of the patient, and clinical staff is trained on what information is needed and how it should be documented. The beginning of the clinical section is generated as a result of the information provided during the appointment scheduling, and this could be a result of the administrative staff; however, the clinical staff must verify with the patient the reason for the encounter. The clinical staff must obtain a patient history, perform an exam, and design a plan of treatment based on the patient's medical status. Identifying clinical information and knowing what to obtain is pertinent and requires training to be able to document all necessary information in the patient's medical or clinical sections of the medical record. The medical and clinical will contain sections for:

- Progress notes
- Documentation record formats
- Medication record
- Diagnostic tests
- Hospital records (when applicable)

Within the administrative, medical, and clinical sections of the medical record, each of these documents should always contain the patient's full name, DOB, and medical record ID number. All services and procedures should have a complete date of service (mm/dd/yyyy), and the entry should be signed by the person who documented the medical record. In addition, the place where the medical services or procedures took place should be clearly documented, with the name of the facility and the physician's name appearing on all inpatient reports and outpatient services. You should ensure that medical documents are not filed in the wrong chart to avoid any type of medical malpractice or legal issues. With thorough and accurate documentation, identifying the patient and following his or her plan of treatment will improve the quality of care provided to the patient.

PATIENT REGISTRATION

A patient registration form—used in physician offices and other outpatient settings—is an important document for determining insurance coverage, billing information, and a patient's identification. The information on this form will include the patient's full legal name, address, telephone number, date of birth, gender, place of employment, and marital status. The registration form also includes information about the **subscriber** (the person who has the insurance coverage), if different from the patient. The subscriber's address and telephone number should be on the patient registration form, especially if the address is different from the patient's. In addition, the subscriber's place of employment is also on this form to identify who issues the insurance policy. Insurance information on the registration form includes the name, address, and telephone number of the insurance carrier as well as the ID number and policy number, if one is included. The information written on the registration form by the patient or guardian should be confirmed by matching it with the insurance card, which should also be copied and kept in the patient's record. Other parts of the registration form include signatures necessary for the release of information to other health care providers for insurance purposes, permission to bill the insurance carrier, and permission to treat the patient. Many registration forms include a section for the patient to include his or her previous medical history, illnesses, allergies, surgeries, and medications as well as a referring or primary care physician. Refer back to Figure 1-3, which shows a patient registration form.

Patient Registration:

Patient's legal name

Address

Telephone number

Date of birth

Gender

Marital status

Employment information

Subscriber information

Insurance carrier information

Signatures

Laws and Regulations for the Patient Registration Form

Requiring the patient or guardian signature on the patient registration form provides the necessary information to bill an insurance carrier as well as allow this form to serve as a legal document for the health care facility to perform treatment. The signature of the patient or guardian gives authorization for the insurance carrier to pay the provider directly as well as for the provider to release medical information to the insurance carrier that pertains to the patient's visit. HIPAA regulations allow information to be exchanged for the treatment and payment to the health care provider. The signature on the registration form gives consent for these activities to take place, and administrative and clinical staff must obtain the appropriate information and signatures from the patient or guardian before treatment is administered.

ACKNOWLEDGMENT OF NOTICE OF PRIVACY

A **notice of privacy** is a requirement of HIPAA regulations. The HIPAA policy information is given to patients the first time they seek health services at a health care facility. There are a number of different components, including who has access to the patient's medical information and how medical information from the facility is shared, stored, and destroyed. It also informs patients that they have the right to access their medical information, request copies, and even amend medical information if necessary. When patients receive this notice, they are asked to sign an acknowledgment of its receipt. This means they acknowledge they have received the notice of privacy and they understand that in addition to the aforementioned information, the physician or facility will release information for treatment, payment, and activities for the operation of the facility. The patient's signature acknowledging the facility's HIPAA policy is kept in the patient's chart.

A notice of privacy includes information for a patient on:

Accessing your medical record

Requesting a copy of your medical record

Amending the medical record

INSURANCE CARDS

Every insurance carrier is different in the way it provides its information to its subscribers and dependents. When making an appointment, the patient should access his or her insurance card to complete the telephone registration, and the insurance card should be presented at the time of the first appointment. Billing should ensure that the medical record contains a copy of the front and back of each patient's insurance card(s). The insurance card provides information about the insurance carrier as well as copayment amounts for the primary care physician, emergency departments, and specialists. The front of the insurance card may also list the subscriber's name and sometimes the subscriber's DOB, which is needed for billing purposes. In addition, the back of the insurance card will provide an address for submitting claims and may provide important telephone numbers for contacting the insurance carrier. At the first visit to a health care facility, patients should be asked to bring their insurance cards for proof of insurance and identifying insurance information needed for patient registration and billing. Patients need to be asked if they are covered by more than one insurance policy. If this is the case, one insurance company will be the primary insurance (or first billed policy) and the other is considered secondary insurance. Both insurance cards need to be copied—front and back—to provide all pertinent information needed by billing for claim submission. You should ask the patient at each subsequent appointment if there are any changes to insurance information. Be sure to check the name of the insurance carrier as well as the ID numbers, as the patient may not realize the information has changed. With each new insurance card the patient receives, ask to see a copy, and if there are changes, copy the fronts and backs of the new cards and then update the financial record of the patient and all aspects of the medical record that contain insurance carrier information.

The front of an insurance card contains:

The name of the insurance carrier

The name of the subscriber

The name of the patient

Copayment amounts

The back of an insurance card contains:

The address to send claims

Phone numbers to call

CORRESPONDENCE

Correspondence in a medical record can come from many sources and includes medical and non-medical documentation. It can come from an insurance carrier, such as requiring further clarification of a claim. Correspondence may be from other health care providers concerning the care of that patient or it can even be from the patient. When filing correspondence in a patient's medical record, be sure to include the appropriate information to identify the patient, including medical and nonmedical correspondence. The document should include the patient's legal name, DOB, physician, and any other identifying information needed for that particular document. If any of the information is missing, be sure to add necessary information prior to filing. Nonmedical correspondence that does not pertain to medical treatment of the patient may be kept in a separate section of the chart, as it does not have information that is included in the process of medical decisions. In addition, medical correspondence should be filed in the appropriate section of the chart depending on the type of document and the date.

Although correspondence does not always affect the care of the patient, it is just as important in maintaining accurate medical records for the patient. The medical record is considered a legal document and should be accurate and complete at all times. If the medical record was brought to court and a correspondence was missing from the file, the medical record would be considered incomplete and have a negative impact on the court proceedings. Any documents pertaining to the patient should be filed appropriately and immediately upon receipt to maintain an accurate medical record for the patient.

PROGRESS NOTES

Progress notes are the part of the medical record in which a physician, nurse, or other health care clinician records a patient's chief complaint, a brief description of the current illness, a history pertinent to the illness, and the findings from an examination. Progress notes serve as a summary of diagnostic tests, treatments, and outcomes. The progress notes will indicate a diagnosis, a prognosis, and treatment options. Each entry is dated and signed by the health care provider.

This progress note section of the medical record is especially important as it must comply with laws and regulations set forth by insurance carriers—private and government. **Current Procedural Terminology (CPT)** is a coding set for procedures and services performed by physicians and other health care providers in which codes have clear documentation guidelines on what the medical record must contain to justify the billing of a service or procedure. In addition, **International Classification of Diseases – Clinical Modification (ICD-diagnostic codes)** are also determined from the progress note as the provider documents the patient's diagnosis and signs and symptoms. Without proper documentation on the progress note, CPT and ICD- diagnostic codes cannot be determined and the revenue from the encounter will be lost. Billers and coders are not involved when the patient is present for his or her appointment; therefore, they rely on thorough documentation to get their codes accurate and complete for billing purposes.

Many types of progress notes exist, such as **Subjective, Objective, Assessment, and Plan (SOAP)** notes, consultation letters to other providers, dated paragraphs, and more. When documenting in the progress notes, be careful with abbreviations, document immediately, and do not wait or add anything at a later date. Add addendums when necessary, and date them accordingly so the document reflects when they were added. Although progress notes can come in different formats, the information they need to include regarding the patient is similar and should be a part of any progress note the health care facility utilizes.

Progress notes include:

Date

Chief complaint

History

Examination

Diagnostic tests ordered

Outcome of tests

Diagnosis

Treatment

Outcome of treatment

Signature

DOCUMENTATION RECORD FORMATS

When documenting in a patient's medical record, you should be sure that all information pertinent to the patient's treatment is thoroughly and accurately documented. By using predetermined formats to identify necessary information, the health care facility and the provider can identify the sections of the progress note to be included and not exceed the documentation requirements. There are required elements that must be included when a physician documents a patient's problems and diagnoses. Headings for these elements can be recorded on a physician progress sheet or preprinted templates for the history and examination portions to assist the provider in remembering to document. There are also different formats of documenting these elements, which allows providers to choose a method that is appropriate for them while still completing the requirements for the patient's medical record. Table 7-1 compares the elements of documentation when used with either SOAP or **Chief complaint, History, Exam, Details, Drugs, Assessment, and Return (CHEDDAR)** formats. When looking at this table, you can see that the same information is recorded—just in a different format.

Another way of documenting the elements is in a **problem-oriented medical record (POMR)**, in which each problem is listed with treatments and outcomes (see Figure 7-2).

TABLE 7-1: Documentation formats

Elements Included in Documentation Formats	SOAP Format	CHEDDAR Format
Chief complaint (CC): a statement in the patient's own words as to why he or she is in this health care facility. It can be a symptom, existing disease, or any other complaint.	S: Subjective	C: Chief complaint
History of the present illness (HPI): a chronological description of how this problem began and developed.		H: Histories

TABLE 7-1: continued

Elements Included in Documentation Formats	SOAP Format	CHEDDAR Format
Histories: **Past history (PH)** of the patient that includes disorders from birth, those that developed, allergies, and treatments directed at these disorders. A list of medications is taken. **Family history (FH)** looks for diseases that are known to run in families, such as cancer and heart disease. This section looks at parents, grandparents, and siblings. **Social history (SH)** includes a person's habits, such as smoking and alcohol. It may also include where you work and if you are married. For women, it includes how many pregnancies, live births, and/ or miscarriages. It would also include menstrual history and/or menopausal history.		
Review of (body) systems (ROS): This a series of questions aimed at eliciting information on the patient's signs, symptoms, and problems. The questions start at the top of the body and then go through the systems of the body.		
Physical examination (PE): The objective findings through direct examination or through diagnostic exams of the body's systems. A multisystem exam can be performed or limited to the affected area(s).	O: Objective	E: Examination
		D: Details
Diagnosis: An assessment by the physician based on the information gathered that gives an impression of the patient's problem. Additional diagnostic testing might have to be done to give a definitive diagnosis.	A: Assessment	D: List of medications and dosages
		A: Assessment and impression of what the diagnosis is
Treatment: A plan established that may include additional diagnostic tests, treatments to be provided, and medications to be given that are aimed at the problem.	P: Plan	R: Either a return visit or referral to another specialist
Prognosis: predicting the outcome after treatment.		

DATABASE

Medium-sized black-and-white spotted dog admitted ambulatory. Appears anxious. Vital signs include BP 120/80 left foreleg; pulse 100 per minute left front paw; respirations 36 per minute; nose is warm and dry.

CHIEF COMPLAINT: Can't eat.

HISTORY: No previous hospitalizations; born at home.

ALLERGIES: Cats, smoke.

VACCINATIONS: Rabies.

OCCUPATION: Mascot, Engine Co. #6 (delusions of grandeur).

EDUCATION: Obedience school drop-out.

HOBBIES: Baseball, collecting bones.

HOME: One room, unheated.

FAMILY: Whereabouts of siblings unknown; number of children unknown.

TYPICAL DAY: Very busy; spends day playing with firemen, sleeping, going for walks, and riding in fire truck.

PERSONAL HABITS: Sparky eats one meal per day, likes canned foods and cereals, dislikes vegetables.

FOOD ALLERGIES: Fish.

Sleeping habits include frequent naps; sleeps soundly. Hygiene: bathes once per month. Elimination: occasionally eats grass as a laxative (sometimes needs treatment for worms); voids frequently in small amounts, nocturia, housebroken.

PROBLEM LIST

DATE	PROBLEM #	PROBLEM DESCRIPTION	DATE RESOLVED
7/1/YYYY	1	Anorexia	
7/1/YYYY	2	Missing teeth	
7/1/YYYY	3	Unheated house	
7/1/YYYY	4	Delusions	
7/1/YYYY	5	Allergy (cats)	
7/1/YYYY	6	Allergy (smoke)	
7/1/YYYY	7	Pruritus (fleas)	

SOAP PROGRESS NOTE

7/1/YYYY

#2 Missing Teeth

S: Lost three teeth last week while playing baseball; doesn't remember where teeth went.

O: One incisor and one canine missing from upper jaw; one canine missing from lower jaw; sockets healing well.

A: Teeth could have been swallowed, accounting for opaque objects on X-ray film.

P: Diagnostic: discuss missing teeth with attending physician. Therapeutic: continue saline rinse. Educational: explain importance of dental hygiene and use of glove to catch baseball.

INITIAL PLAN

DATE	PROBLEM #	MEDICAL PLANS	NURSING PLANS
7/2/YYYY	7	DX: check for fleas	DX: observe for fleas; observe frequency of itching and areas of scratching
		RX: calamine lotion	RX: apply calamine lotion to affected areas of skin
		ED: pruritus	ED: communicate importance of *not* scratching

FIGURE 7-2 Problem Oriented Medical Record

MEDICATION RECORD

When referencing a patient's medical record, identifying medication history is extremely important for the treatment of a patient. In some medical records, the medication history is not always apparent. However, having a medication record can avoid mistakes for the health care facility and provider. The medication record is a form that lists the medication a patient is taking as well as the dose, frequency, and method of administration. It records the date the medication began as well as the date it was renewed and discontinued (see Figure 7-3).

The medication record will contain:

Medication

Date ordered

Date renewed

Date discontinued

Comments

MEDICATION RECORD

Patient Name _____

MR no. _____ Patient Phone no. _____

Pharmacy Name _____ Pharmacy Phone no. _____

Known Allergies or Drug Reaction to:

Medication Name	Allergic or Drug Reaction Manifestation with Date

Medication Name Dose, Amount and Method of Administration	Start Date	End Date	Dates of Refills				

© Cengage Learning 2013

FIGURE 7-3 Sample Medication Record

Creating a recognizable trail of medications for the patient can be beneficial for a patient's treatment. When the patient needs a refill, information regarding the medication can be obtained to compare to what the patient is requesting. If the provider considered adding a medication to the patient's treatment, having a separate list of currently prescribed medications can help the provider quickly identify any problems that may be associated with the new prescription. Although it may be time consuming to keep a separate log, in the end, this is beneficial for all involved.

DIAGNOSTIC TESTS

Many diagnostic tests are performed on patients to try and assess their signs and symptoms or the status of their conditions. Diagnostic testing is a routine part of a patient's visit when he or she has complaints that warrant further investigation. In many situations, the health care facility or

---

Addressograph

Betty A. Dent
92607
Aug 30 20XX

LABORATORY REPORT

SPECIMEN COLLECTED: **SPECIMEN RECEIVED:**

TEST	RESULT	FLAG	REFERENCE
Glucose			82-115 mg/dl
BUN			8-25 mg/dl
Creatinine			0.9-1.4 mg/dl
Sodium			135-145 mmol/L
Potassium			3.6-5.0 mmol/L
Chloride			99-110 mmol/L
CO2			21-31 mmol/L
Calcium			8.6-10.2 mg/dl
WBC			4.5-11.0 thous/UL
RBC			5.2-5.4 mill/UL
HGB			11.7-16.1 g/dl
HCT			35.0-47.0 %
Platelets			140-400 thous/UL
PT			11.0-13.0 seconds

End of Report

ALFRED STATE MEDICAL CENTER ■ 100 MAIN ST, ALFRED NY 14802 ■ (607) 555-1234

FIGURE 7-4A Laboratory Report

provider can determine a patient's treatment options when there is confirmation of the condition or illness through diagnostic testing. Because of the technological advances in medicine, many diagnostic tests have been able to further treatment for patients that was unexpected years ago. As with any medical correspondence, diagnostic testing results are returned to the health care facility for the patient's medical record and filed in the diagnostic testing section. This part of the medical record houses all the diagnostic tests a patient has had in connection with an illness or injury. These tests can be from a radiologist, a laboratory, a hospital, or a specialist. These records assist the physician in diagnosing and treating a patient as well as proving the medical necessity of a service or procedure. Diagnostic testing is an important section in the patient's medical record, and all documents must contain the patient's identifying information, including name, DOB, and physician. Figures 7-4A and 7-4B show two diagnostic test reports: a sample laboratory report and a sample radiology report.

Addressograph

Betty A. Dent
92607
Aug 30 20XX

RADIOLOGY REPORT

Clinical History/Indications:

Exam:

Date of Exam:

Reason for Exam:

Findings:

Impression:

Recommendation:

_____
Signature of Radiologist

ALFRED STATE MEDICAL CENTER ■ 100 MAIN ST, ALFRED NY 14802 ■ (607) 555-1234

© Cengage Learning 2013

FIGURE 7-4B Radiology Report

HOSPITAL RECORDS

Despite a patient being treated in a hospital, the hospital records need to be part of the patient's medical record at outpatient facilities, including the primary care physician and specialists. When a patient is admitted to a hospital, reports are included in the hospital's records as well as the physician's records in order for the provider to accurately follow up with, diagnose, and treat the patient. Maintaining a complete medical record for the patient means that hospital records should be included as part of a patient's medical record, especially if the provider was involved in the diagnosis and treatment of the hospital encounter. In some circumstances, the patient may have a hospital encounter that is not pertinent to that health care facility or provider, but that facility or provider may have access to the record in the event that the patient seeks treatment for the diagnosis at his or her health care facility at a later date. The hospital records section should be included in the patient's medical record, and all documents must contain the patient's identifying information, including name, DOB, and physician.

The reports in the hospital record that would also be in the physician office record are:

- History and physical for admission
- Admission and discharge record
- Face sheet
- Operative reports (if appropriate)
- Diagnostic services
- Procedures performed

History and Physical Report for Hospital Admission

Included in the hospital medical record for every patient who is admitted to the hospital is the history and physical (H&P), which explains the medical reason for the admission. The history part of this report documents the reason or chief complaint leading to the hospital admission. It also includes the patient's past, family, personal and social history as well as a review of the history of the patient's body systems. The physical portion of this report documents the physician's exam and findings of each pertinent body system. This report is a requirement from The Joint Commission for hospital admissions and is the property of the hospital despite being dictated by the provider. Figure 7-5 shows an example of a history and physical report.

Admission and Discharge Record or Face Sheet

As part of every hospital admission, there needs to be documentation of the admission and discharge record—also known as a face sheet. This is a summary of the patient's encounter from admission to discharge and includes the patient's medical status upon discharge. The discharge summary portion of the record includes the diagnosis before admission, the diagnoses upon discharge, the procedures performed, and diagnoses determined after the procedures were done. In addition, dates, codes for diagnosis, and procedures may also be on this form.

Also contained on this form is demographic information about the patient, such as address, birth date, social security number, marital status, name, address and telephone number of employer, and the admitting and discharge dates as well as the admitting physician. Financial information is also included, such as the insurance carrier, ID numbers, group numbers, and the subscriber. Finally, this form must include all diagnoses: the admitting diagnosis, the final diagnosis, and any secondary diagnoses. These diagnoses must have the appropriate ICD-diagnostic codes attached to them. The face sheet will include the condition of the patient at discharge and where the patient was discharged to (home, rehabilitative center, or another facility) (see Figure 7-6).

Betty A. Dent
92607
Aug 30, 20XX

HISTORY

CHIEF COMPLAINT:
Pain and restriction of motion of the right arm and a cut on the head.

PRESENT ILLNESS:
This 65-year-old Caucasian female was walking on the street when she slipped on some loose gravel and fell, landing on her right arm and striking her head against the curb. She sustained a laceration of her scalp and an injury to her right shoulder. She went home to change her clothes and started experiencing dizziness and blurred vision. She then went to the University Hospital Emergency Room by automobile where an x-ray of her right arm revealed a fracture involving the greater tuberosity of the humerus and a CAT-Scan of her head revealed a subdural hematoma.

PAST HISTORY:
The patient states that her general health has always been good except that in recent years she has suffered from spastic colitis. She had a flare-up of this condition about six months ago. Operations: T & A at age 13. A total abdominal hysterectomy in 1956. Social History: She smokes cigarettes occasionally and drinks alcohol socially only. Allergies: No known allergies.

FAMILY HISTORY:
Her father died at age 72 of a cerebrovascular accident. Her mother died at age 74 of a myocardial infarction. Three brothers, all deceased, two with cancer (age 67 and 71), and one with heart disease (age 60). Two sisters, alive and well, one has heart problems. No family history of tuberculosis or diabetes.

REVIEW OF SYSTEMS:
GENERAL: No fever, no chills, no night sweats, or weight loss.

HEENT: Blurred vision, headache, and head pain. No earaches, deafness, sore throats, hoarseness, or difficulty in swallowing.

CR: No chest pains, tachycardia, or ankle edema. No shortness of breath, chronic cough, or wheezing.

GI: Appetite good, slight nausea, no vomiting, diarrhea, constipation, or melena.

GU: No dysuria, hematuria or pyuria.

CNS: Dizziness reported. No fainting or seizures.

GYN: No spotting since her hysterectomy.

PHYSICAL EXAMINATION

GENERAL
This patient is a well-nourished, well-developed, 65-year-old Caucasian female who is awake, alert, and experiencing head pain, headache, dizziness, blurred vision, and slight nausea. She also is experiencing pain in her right shoulder when she attempts to move her right arm. Height 5'8". Weight: 155 lb. Blood pressure: 170/90. Temperature: 99°. Pulse: 100. Respirations: 20.

HEENT:
The pupils are dilated, equal, and react slowly. Extraocular movements are normal. Nasopharynx is clear. Upper and lower dentures. Ears are clear. There is a laceration measuring 2.3 cm on occipital region of scalp.

(continues)

FIGURE 7-5 Example of a History and Physical Report

Betty A. Dent
92607
Aug 30, 20XX

NECK:
Supple with a full range of painless motion. Thyroid is not enlarged. No lymphadenopathy and no venous engorgement.

CHEST:
Symmetrical with normal expansion. Breasts: No atrophy and no masses. Lungs: Clear to auscultation. Heart: Normal sinus rhythm, no murmurs, and no enlargement.

ABDOMEN:
Soft and nontender and somewhat obese. Liver, kidneys, and spleen are not palpable.

GENITALIA:
Normal external female.

RECTAL:
Deferred.

NEUROLOGICAL:
No motor deficits. Dizziness experienced without relation to head movement. Patient is oriented to person, place, and time. Slight drowsiness occurring.

MUSCULOSKELETAL:
There is a small bruise over the anterior aspect of the left knee. The hips, knees, and ankle joints are otherwise normal. Good peripheral pulses. The right upper arm is moderately swollen and discolored. There are no other gross deformities. The patient has considerable pain with any attempt at either active or passive movement of the right shoulder.

DIAGNOSIS:
1. Laceration—occipital region of scalp measuring 2.3 cm.

2. Subdural hematoma.

3. Relatively undisplaced fracture proximal right humerus (greater tuberosity).

4. Hypertension.

TREATMENT PLAN:
Suture scalp wound. Fracture treatment (without manipulation) with right arm placed in a long arm fiberglass cast. Admit patient to hospital observation unit directly from Emergency Department. Place patient under head trauma precaution and monitor blood pressure every hour.

Gerald Practon, MD

Gerald Practon, MD

mtf

D: 2-12-XX

T: 2-13-XX

FIGURE 7-5 continued

Alfred State Medical Center

100 Main St, Alfred NY 14802

(101) 555-1111

Inpatient Face Sheet

Patient Name and Address					Gender	Race	Birth Date	Patient No.
					Maiden Name	Employer		Occupation
Home Telephone Number: ( ) –								

Admission Date	Time	Room	Discharge Date	Time	Length of Stay	Employer Telephone Number		
					days	( ) –		

Guarantor Name and Address	Next of Kin Name and Address

Guarantor Telephone No.	Relationship to Patient	Next of Kin Telephone Number	Relationship to Patient
( ) –		( ) –	

Primary Payer	Primary Payer Policy No.	Secondary Payer	Secondary Payer Policy No.

Admitting Physician	Service	Admit Type	Room Number/Bed

Attending Physician	Admitting Diagnosis

Diagnoses and Procedures

ICD Codes

Principal Diagnosis	

Secondary Diagnoses	

Principal Procedure	

Secondary Procedures	

Signature of Attending Physician:

© Cengage Learning 2013

FIGURE 7-6 Face Sheet or Admission and Discharge Record

Operative Report

In the event that surgery was performed at the hospital during the patient's admission—whether inpatient or outpatient—the provider must generate a detailed operative report identifying all aspects of the operative procedure. The operative report has patient identification on the report; including name, DOB, and physician as well as a preoperative diagnosis, postoperative diagnosis, the approach, procedure done, findings, closure, homeostasis, and any complications. The physician's name, any assistant surgeon, and the anesthesiologist are also recorded on this report. Figure 7-7 shows an example of this report.

Addressograph	**OPERATIVE RECORD**	
Patient Number	Room/Bed	
Patient Name (Last, First, MI)	Date of Procedure	
Patient SSN	Time Started	Time Ended
Patient DOB Gender	Service	
Surgeon:	Assistant:	
Anesthetist:	Anesthetic:	
Preoperative Diagnosis:		
Postoperative Diagnosis:		
Procedure(s) Performed:		
Complications:		
Operative Findings:		

Dictation Date_____

Transcription Date_____

Signed _____

Form 4107, OCT 03

ALFRED STATE MEDICAL CENTER ■ 100 MAIN ST, ALFRED NY 14802 ■ (607) 555-1234

© Cengage Learning 2013

FIGURE 7-7 Operative Report

LAWS AND REGULATIONS

Within the medical field, there are always rules and regulations that need to be followed for the health care facility and the provider. There are a number of different entities that govern the content and release of medical records. There are documentation guides published by the **Centers for Medicare and Medicaid Services (CMS)** in the form of **national coverage determination (NCD)**, identifying which services or procedures Medicare will reimburse. Medicare publishes a Comprehensive Error Rate Testing report, and it can be accessed on Medicare's website at www.cms.gov/CERT

In addition to this website, there are many websites that can assist in learning the laws and regulations for your health care facility. While researching the websites, be sure to access only trustworthy websites that are provided by the government or known by your facility. Also, be sure the website source is current and not outdated.

The **American Medical Association (AMA)** publishes the CPT manual, a coding manual that lists codes for procedures and services performed in the outpatient setting. Each of the six sections is preceded by guidelines for using the codes. The **Healthcare Common Procedural Coding System (HCPCS)** coding book is another manual that can be utilized to identify rules and regulations to medical recordkeeping and documentation needs for billing and coding purposes. The HCPCS manual includes an **Internet-Only Manual (IOM)** of changes that have recently been made. Previous guidelines can be accessed online at www.cms.gov/Manuals/IOM. In addition, each insurance carrier has developed its own additional rules and regulations to documentation expectations, and each is obligated to provide the health care facility with information that identifies the requirements according to each one's policies.

Maintaining current information is pertinent to everyone involved. When the health care facility or provider identifies changes in the laws or regulations, it is their duty to ensure all administrative and clinical staff as well as management are trained accordingly.

SUMMARY

- The medical record is necessary to assure continuity of care between health care professionals as well as support compliance with coding and reimbursement policies.

- Medical records serve as a source of statistics, which are used to determine clusters of diseases as well as the need for additional health care services and facilities.

- The medical record has an administrative section that contains the patient registration, copies of the fronts and backs of insurance cards, and acknowledgment of the receipt of the notice of privacy. This section ensures compliance with confidentiality and HIPAA regulations.

- The medical and clinical portion of the medical record includes progress notes, a problem record, medication record, and all reports on diagnostic tests. The information in this section is important for the diagnosis, treatment, and evaluation of the outcome of illnesses.

- The medical record must be compliant with laws and regulations of the insurance carrier, the government, and the state in which the facility is located.

REVIEW EXERCISES

TRUE OR FALSE

1. _____ One purpose of the medical record is to provide continuity of care.

2. _____ The patient registration form contains the patient's history.

3. _____ The HIPAA permits the release of information for treatment.

4. _____ The notice of privacy states who will have access to patient information other than the health care provider.

5. _____ The patient's insurance card is only used to identify the patient.

6. _____ The medication record includes discontinued medications.

7. _____ A history and physical are required for all hospital admissions.

8. _____ A face sheet is another name for a history and physical.

9. _____ The medical record contains administrative and clinical portions.

10. _____ There are no laws governing medical records.

MATCHING

A   **Chief Complaint**

B   **History**

C   **Physical Examination**

D   **Diagnosis**

E   **SOAP**

F   **Problem-Oriented Medical Record**

G   **Notice of Privacy**

H   **AMA**

I   **Carrier**

J   **Prognosis**

1. _____ Statement of what is wrong in the patient's own words.

2. _____ American Medical Association.

3. _____ The insurance company.

4. _____ POMR.

5. _____ A patient's previous illnesses, injuries, or operations.

6. _____ Stands for subjective, objective, assessment, and plan.

7. _____ A requirement of the HIPAA.

8. _____ Predicting the outcome of a illness after treatment.

9. _____ The examination of a patient by a physician.

10. _____ Assessment of the patient.

CRITICAL THINKING ACTIVITIES

ACTIVITY 1

Underline 10 documenting errors or possibility of a document error in the following document. Identify the corrections on the lines.

Date: 7/1

Patient: Ken Smith   DOB: 2/2/11

The patient is here for an appointment for chest pain for three days. He denies any numbness in the arm. The patient went to MVP for an EKG, and the results were inconclusive.

Examination includes a repeat EKG, which shows some irregularities.

Patient has diagnosis from the irregular EKG and must be treated with medication.

Patient will go to TKS for a stress test and return for follow-up next week.

Signed: _ML_____   Date:

Corrections to errors:

1. _____

2. _____

3. _____

4. _____

5. _____

6. _____

7. _____

8. _____

9. _____

10. _____

ACTIVITY 2

Identify the following rules and regulations acronyms and write out what they mean.

1. AMA _____

2. CHEDDAR _____

3. NCD _____

4. DOB _____

5. CMS_____

6. IOM _____

7. POMR _____

8. HCPCS _____

9. SOAP _____

10. SOMR _____

ACTIVITY 3

Identify the three purposes of a medical record. Write a brief explanation of why they are important.

Purpose of a Medical Record

1. _____

_____

_____

_____

2. _____

_____

_____

_____

3. _____

_____

_____

_____

ACTIVITY 4

Explain the steps that are included in the creation of a medical record. Include the different sections and where they would be located in the medical record. Explain why the insurance card is considered part of the medical record in any type of health care facility.

_____

_____

_____

_____

_____

_____

_____

_____

_____

CRITICAL THINKING QUESTIONS

1. A patient does not want to receive or sign the acknowledgment of receiving the notice of privacy. Explain to the patient what information is in the notice of privacy and why it is important to him or her.

2. Compare the records that would appear in a physician's office record with a hospital medical record. Debate the pros and cons of working in each type of health care facility when working with medical records.

3. Debate the pros and cons of electronic medical records and paper medical records. Identify at least five reasons why one is better than the other.

4. Explain how the patient registration form is considered part of the medical record. Review reasons why the patient registration is considered confidential in conjunction with the medical record.

WEB ACTIVITIES

1. Research the medical record requirements for different health care settings for Medicare (http://www.cms.gov). List five requirements for Medicare.

2. Research the medical record requirements from The Joint Commission (http://www.jointcommission.org) for different health care settings. List five requirements from The Joint Commission.

3. Compare and contrast the differences in requirements between both organizations.

4. Research medical records documentation guidelines for your state. Identify the websites that provide appropriate information. Bookmark the websites for future use as a manager.

CHAPTER 8

MEDICAL RECORDS

MANAGING

Chapter 8 will Expand the fundamentals of medical records by looking at the manager's role in maintaining medical records, ensuring the content required is met for the patient's medical record. In addition, the manager will also be educated on legal and regulatory requirements for medical records to ensure they are also followed. Evaluating whether a medical record is complete will be emphasized and should be performed on a daily basis after patients are treated.

OBJECTIVES

Upon completion of this chapter, the student will be able to:

- Identify settings that have medical records.
- Identify reports within the medical record.
- Recognize deficiencies in medical records as defined by state, federal, or government agencies.
- Know how to manage medical records in each setting and ensure that the content meets regulatory standards.
- Create policies and procedures for medical record functions.

KEY TERMS

- Advanced beneficiary notice of noncoverage (ABN)
- Advanced directive
- Ambulatory surgical centers (ASC)
- Centers for Medicare and Medicaid Services (CMS)
- Electronic health record (E.H.R)
- Long-term care (LTC)

HEALTH CARE SETTINGS

There are many outpatient health care settings, and each health care setting is required to keep medical records on every patient. The need to have documentation has been identified, but the requirements at each facility are different based on the insurance carriers, the nature of the facility, and the state the facility is located in. The regulatory agencies that govern each setting require different content to be kept in a medical record. As a manager, looking for the required content and checking that entries and reports are signed, dated, and complete are important functions. Due to the changes in the medical field, you might endure challenges to stay current with the changes and to ensure all medical records guidelines are being met. Education is essential to staying up to date on the laws and regulations that are required by government and insurance carriers. The manager needs to become educated through workshops, seminars, online venues that are approved by government, and other local providers or facilities. Once the manager is up to date, the staff needs to be informed of the changes and trained accordingly. With medical records being required for every patient, developing the medical records guidelines is an ongoing process, and the manager should find ways to make it simpler if possible. Using a checklist, such as in Figure 8-1, ensures consistency and makes the process easier for training other employees.

PHYSICIAN OFFICE

As discussed in Chapter 7, physician offices have fewer regulatory agencies governing the content of the medical record. Despite these decreased rules, management is responsible for ensuring that the staff at the facility use thorough documentation and include all services, procedures, and diagnoses that pertain to the patient. Each practice will have a patient registration form as well as an acknowledgment of the receipt of the notice of privacy as required by HIPAA. Typically, this information is included in the administrative section of the medical record because it does not pertain directly to the patient's health status. However, in the clinical section, there will be progress notes that include the patient's subjective information about the patient's problems; an objective report of the physician's history and exam findings; and a copy of all diagnostic tests performed either in the office, at a freestanding radiology center or laboratory, or at the outpatient department of a hospital. A record of medications is kept that includes start and end dates, renewal dates, and any reactions from that medication. All entries must be signed and dated. The date must include the year. If multiple people make entries in the medical record, a "signature page" needs to be in the office documentation policies (see Figure 8-2). As a manager, you should sample medical documentation on a daily basis to notice the completeness and accuracy of the patient's medical records being submitted—whether paper or electronic.

Patient Name	☐
Date	☐
Medical Record No	☐
Documentation	☐
Form	☐
Signed	☐

FIGURE 8-1 Checklist for Medical Record

Printed Name of Personnel who document in the Medical Record	Signature of the person whose name is printed to the left
Dr. John Doe	*John Doe, MD*
Mary Smith RN	*Mary Smith, RN*
Jane Brown, RMA	*Jane Brown RMA*

© Cengage Learning 2013

FIGURE 8-2 Signature Sheet

Checklist for documentation for the physician office record

- ☐ Patient registration form complete
- ☐ Acknowledgment of the receipt of the notice of privacy
- ☐ Authorization for disclosure of health information (see Figure 8-3)
- ☐ Progress notes complete
- ☐ Diagnostic test reports
- ☐ Hospital records (if applicable)
- ☐ Medication record complete
- ☐ Other pertinent records

AMBULATORY SURGERY CENTER

Ambulatory surgery centers (ASC) perform surgical procedures in outpatient centers, which can be done on a same-day schedule. The facility is not an overnight facility and patients need to be discharged the same day. However, the documentation needed for the facility is similar to that of a hospital setting where surgeries are performed, especially if the facility is hospital owned. The documentation requirements will include an operative report with all requirements (refer back to Figure 7-7), including anesthesia reports as well as physician and nurses' progress notes. There will be a face sheet that includes the demographic information on the patient as well as billing and financial information. The agencies that provide regulatory guidance include **Centers for Medicare and Medicaid Services (CMS)**. Upon completion of medical record documentation in an ASC, the manager should be educated on the different rules and regulations that govern the facility and monitor patient documentation on a daily basis to ensure continuity.

Your Practice Name Here

Authorization for Disclosure of Health Information

Patient Name:_____

Date of Birth:_____ Phone:_____

Address:_____

City:_____ State:_____ Zip:_____

1. *I authorize the use or disclosure of the above named individual's health information as described below.*

2. *The following individual or organization is authorized to make the disclosure:*

Name:_____

Address:_____

City:_____ State:_____ Zip:_____

3. The type and amount of information to be used or disclosed is as follows: (include dates where appropriate)

    _____ Complete health records   _____ Lab results/X-ray reports

    _____ Physical exam   _____ Consultation reports

    _____ Immunization record

    _____ Other (please specify):_____

4. I understand that the information in my health record may include information relating to sexually transmitted disease, acquired immunodeficiency syndrome (AIDS) or human immunodeficiency virus (HIV). It may also include information about behavioral or mental health services and treatment for alcohol and drug abuse.

5. *This information may be disclosed to and used by the following individual or organization.*

Name:_____

Address:_____

City:_____ State:_____ Zip:_____

*For the purpose of*_____

6. I understand that I have a right to revoke this authorization at any time. I understand that if I revoke this authorization I must do so in writing and present my written revocation to the health information management department. I understand that the revocation will not apply to my insurance company when the law provides my insurer with the right to contest a claim under my policy. Unless otherwise revoked, this authorization will expire on the following date, event, or condition: _____ .

7. If I fail to specify an expiration date, event, or condition, this authorization will expire in <u>sixty days.</u> I understand that authorizing the disclosure of this health information is voluntary. I can refuse to sign this authorization. I need not sign this form in order to ensure treatment. I understand that I may inspect or copy the information to be used or disclosed, as provided in CFR 164.524. I understand that any disclosure of information carries with it the potential for an unauthorized redisclosure and the information may not be protected by federal confidentiality rules. If I have questions about disclosure of my health information, I can contact:

    _____ ,

    Privacy Officer for _____ .

_____   _____
Signature of patient or legal representative   Signature of witness

Date: _____   Date: _____

PLEASE NOTE: This information has been disclosed to you from confidential records protected from disclosure by state and federal law. No further disclosure of this information should be done without specific, written, and informed release of the individual to whom it pertains or as permitted by state law and federal law 42 CFR, part II.

FIGURE 8-3 Authorization for Disclosure of Health Information

> ### Checklist for a complete medical record at an ASC
>
> ☐ Face sheet
> ☐ Progress notes
> ☐ History and physical (H&P)
> ☐ Operative procedures and report
> ☐ Pre- and postanesthesia records
> ☐ Other pertinent reports to the procedures

FREESTANDING LABORATORY

A freestanding laboratory performs laboratory tests on patients as referred by their primary care physician. Management must be educated on the medical record policy of having a physician order and documenting the lab report according to guidelines. For lab reports to follow medical documentation guidelines, they must include the date, indication, specimen, test performed, results or findings, and signature. In addition to the administrative information found on the registration form, the medical record must contain the request from the physician, the test report, a signature (refer back to Figure 7-8A), and, whenever indicated for a noncovered service, a signed **advanced beneficiary notice (ABN)**. Figure 8-4 shows an ABN for an uncovered lab test. By monitoring the patient's medical record in the laboratory on a daily basis, management can ensure that the required information is included in the medical record for reimbursement and that the laboratory report is complete and accurate according to the guidelines.

> ### Checklist for a complete medical record at a laboratory
>
> ☐ Registration
> ☐ Request for test by primary care physician
> ☐ Signed test report
> ☐ ABN if indicated

FREESTANDING RADIOLOGY CENTER

A freestanding radiology center performs a variety of radiology procedures on patients as referred by their primary care physician or specialist. As part of management, you should realize the requirement for orders from a medical provider before the patient can have the test performed. The orders must state the type of radiology test, the views, and the potential findings or signs and

(A) Notifier(s):
(B) Patient Name: _____   *(C)* Identification Number: _____

ADVANCE BENEFICIARY NOTICE OF NONCOVERAGE (ABN)

<u>NOTE:</u> If Medicare doesn't pay for *(D)* _____ below, you may have to pay.

Medicare does not pay for everything, even some care that you or your health care provider have good reason to think you need. We expect Medicare may not pay for the *(D)* _____ below.

(D) _____	*(E)* Reason Medicare May Not Pay:	*(F)* Estimated Cost:
general health panel CPT 80050(2007)	*"This service and procedure is never a covered benefit under medicare"*	$ *xxx, xx*

WHAT YOU NEED TO DO NOW:
- Read this notice, so you can make an informed decision about your care.
- Ask us any questions that you may have after you finish reading.
- Choose an option below about whether to receive the *(D)* _____ listed above.
  Note: If you choose Option 1 or 2, we may help you to use any other insurance that you might have, but Medicare cannot require us to do this.

(G) OPTIONS: Check only one box. We cannot choose a box for you.
☐ OPTION 1. I want the *(D)* _____ listed above. You may ask to be paid now, but I also want Medicare billed for an official decision on payment, which is sent to me on a Medicare Summary Notice (MSN). I understand that if Medicare doesn't pay, I am responsible for payment, but **I can appeal to Medicare** by following the directions on the MSN. If Medicare does pay, you will refund any payments I made to you, less co-pays or deductibles.
☐ OPTION 2. I want the *(D)* _____ listed above, but do not bill Medicare. You may ask to be paid now as I am responsible for payment. **I cannot appeal if Medicare is not billed.**
☐ OPTION 3. I don't want the *(D)* _____ listed above. I understand with this choice I am **not** responsible for payment, and **I cannot appeal to see if Medicare would pay.**

(H) **Additional Information:**

This notice gives our opinion, not an official Medicare decision. If you have other questions on this notice or Medicare billing, call **1-800-MEDICARE** (1-800-633-4227/**TTY**: 1-877-486-2048).

Signing below means that you have received and understand this notice. You also receive a copy.

(I) **Signature:**	*(J)* **Date:**

Form CMS-R-131 (03/08)   Form Approved OMB No. 0938-0566

FIGURE 8-4 ABN for an Uncovered Laboratory Test

symptoms of the patient. The medical record would contain administrative information found on the patient's registration form, the request from the physician, and the test report, which includes the reason for the exam, the date the exam was done, the findings, impressions, and recommendations. It must be signed and dated by the radiologist. As management oversees the radiology center, it must monitor patient medical records on a daily basis to ensure that all criteria is met, including orders and reporting guidelines as per the medical record requirements (refer back to Figure 7-4B).

A checklist for a complete medical record in a radiology center includes:

☐ Registration

☐ Request from the physician

☐ Test results

OUTPATIENT HOSPITAL DEPARTMENT

There are many departments within a hospital that people come to for diagnostic exams but are not inpatient departments. Examples of some of these departments are the laboratory, the radiology department, and the cardiology department. Management within these departments must understand the difference between medical record requirements in each area. Within the radiology department documentation, guidelines will be slightly different from the cardiology department. Educating management within the hospital outpatient department is pertinent due to the hospital having more patient contact in some instances. Also, the rules for inpatient differ from outpatient, and staff may be more familiar with inpatient policies due to their training. These departments keep simpler records than the inpatient departments, which management should be aware of. The medical record includes a demographic record, such as the face sheet used in inpatient hospital records, billing information, the request for the diagnostic exam, and the test report.

The test reports must include the date, the name of the patient, the reason for the encounter, the referring physician, the record number, and a written report signed by a physician. Copies of these reports will also be kept in the patient's medical record at the primary care physician's office. The manager must ensure that the tests are completed and in the patient's medical record. In addition, a manager should monitor the patient's medical record on a daily basis to ensure the outpatient reports include the appropriate information on them depending on the type of service or procedure the patient encountered.

Checklist for a completed medical record for outpatient hospital departments

☐ Demographic record

☐ Billing information

☐ Request for exam

☐ Test report

LONG-TERM CARE AND REHABILITATION CENTER

Long-term care and rehabilitation facilities' medical records will have an initial assessment of the patient, monthly assessments by the nurse practitioner or physician, daily notes per shift, and a care plan.

Any rehabilitation therapy, such as physical therapy or occupational therapy, will have a report in the patient's record. Copies of blood tests, EKG tests, or other tests will also be a part of the long-term care facility's records.

Physicians who have patients in long-term care facilities will have copies of tests, reports, and entries on their visits, indicating their findings in the medical record. A manager must review the medical record to make sure the information is there. Therefore, management must be educated on what to request from the long-term care facility or rehabilitation center as a result of a patient seeking treatment. The appropriate medical documentation is part of the patient's medical record at the health care facility and will play an important role in future treatment for the patient. Management must educate staff on the need to obtain documentation from the facilities, with the patient's identifying information included, such as name, DOB, and physician.

> **The complete medical record in a LTC or rehabilitation facility includes:**
>
> ☐ The name of the facility the patient is in
>
> ☐ Initial assessment
>
> ☐ Admitting history
>
> ☐ Tests performed and their results
>
> ☐ Daily notes on progress reports as to visits to patients at a facility
>
> ☐ Monthly assessments

HOME CARE

A medical record for a patient in home care will include an initial assessment by a nurse, progress notes, medication record, documentation from the physician on the need for health care, the types of care received and treatments the patient will be on. Also included is the home health aide plan of care to meet the patient's needs, which includes short- and long-term goals. When requesting documentation about home care treatment, the manager must be aware of the medical record documentation requirements necessary for home care. The report for the patient's home care visits must be maintained at the health care facility in the patient's medical record. Understanding the requirements will allow management to monitor the medical records of patients on home care on a daily basis to ensure completion and accuracy for future treatment of the patient.

Checklist for contents of a home care patient's medical record:

☐ Initial assessment

☐ Progress notes

☐ Medication record

☐ Documentation from the physician on the need for home care

☐ Types of treatment provided, such as physical therapy

☐ Home health aide plan of care

HOSPITAL INPATIENT RECORD

Patients enter the hospital for many reasons. These reasons may include elective procedures, emergency procedures, medical conditions, and maternity. The basic medical record remains the same:

- An administrative section
- Medical and clinical section

For the hospital inpatient, the administrative section will contain a face sheet that has demographic information on the patient, financial information, and clinical information. It will also include a form called an **advanced directive** (see Figures 8-5 and 8-6). This gives the providers a written notice of the patient's wishes for end-of-life cases, including resuscitation.

In the medical and clinical sections of the medical record, the types of reports in the administrative, medical, or clinical sections change depending on the type of admission. For example, a patient in the hospital for surgery will have an operative note as well as pre- and postanesthesia reports. A patient admitted for a medical condition, such as asthma, would not have an operative or anesthesia report but will have medical reports and physician notes.

Parts of the medical record are used by risk managers, abstracted for coding and billing purposes, and examined by chart auditors, Medicare, and other third-party carriers.

Parts of the hospital inpatient record must also be sent to the patient's primary care physician or admitting physician. These parts include the admitting history and physical, any diagnostic tests performed, consultation reports, an operative report if the patient had surgery, and a discharge summary.

Because there are many departments for inpatient encounters, the manager must determine which medical documentation should appear in the medical record at the facility. Caring for patients after hospital admission is often done at the facility, as the primary care physician may be asked to follow up with the patient. Managers must educate their staff and themselves on the need for inpatient medical documentation in the patient's medical record as well as the requirements in order to provide future medical treatment for the patient.

Addressograph

ADVANCE DIRECTIVE ADMISSION
FORM & CHECKLIST

Your answers to the following questions will assist your Physician and the Medical Center to respect your wishes regarding your medical care. This information will become a part of your patient record.

	YES	NO	PATIENT'S INITIALS
1. Have you been provided with a copy of the information called "Patient Rights Regarding Health Care Decisions"?			
2. Have you prepared a "Living Will"? If yes, please provide a copy for your patient record.			
3. Have you prepared a "Health Care Proxy"? If yes, please provide a copy for your patient record.			
4. Have you prepared a Durable Power of Attorney for Health Care? If yes, please provide a copy for your patient record.			
5. Have you provided this facility with an Advance Directive on a prior admission and is it still in effect? If yes, Admitting Office will contact Health Information Department to obtain a copy for your current patient record.			
6. Do you wish to execute a Living Will, Health Care Proxy, and/or Durable Power of Attorney? If yes, Admitting Office will notify: a. Physician b. Social Service c. Volunteer Service			

ADMITTING OFFICE STAFF: Enter a checkmark when each step has been completed.

1. _____ Verify the above questions where answered and actions taken where required.

2. _____ If the "Patient Rights" information was provided to someone other than the patient, state reason:

_____

_____   _____
Name of Individual Receiving Information   Relationship to Patient

3. _____ If information was provided in a language other than English, specify language and method below.

_____

4. _____ Verify patient was advised on how to obtain additional information on Advance Directives.

5. Verify the Patient/Family Member/Legal Representative was asked to provide the Medical Center with a copy of the Advance Directive, which will be retained in the patient record.

6. _____ File this form in the patient record, and give a copy to the patient.

_____
Name of Patient or Name of Individual giving information, if different from Patient

_____   _____
Signature of Patient   Date

_____   _____
Signature of Medical Center Representative   Date

ALFRED STATE MEDICAL CENTER ■ 100 MAIN ST, ALFRED NY 14802 ■ (607) 555-1234

FIGURE 8-5 Advanced Directive

Checklist for documentation of an inpatient medical record:

☐ Face sheet

☐ Advanced directive

☐ Admitting history and physical

☐ Diagnostic tests

☐ Discharge summary

And as indicated:

☐ Operative report

☐ Anesthesia report

☐ Consultations

Do Not Resuscitate (DNR) Consent

I, _____ **do not authorize resuscitation in the event of cardiac or respiratory arrest**. I understand that this order remains in effect until revoked by me. I acknowledge that cardiopulmonary resuscitation (CPR) will not be performed if breathing or heartbeat stops. I understand this decision will **not** prevent me from obtaining other emergency care by emergency medical services personnel and/or care directed by a physician prior to my death. I understand I may revoke this DNR consent at any time by destroying this consent form.

_____   _____
Patient or Legal Representative Signature   Date

_____
Address of Patient

_____   _____
Attending Physician Signature   Date

_____
Address of Attending Physician

_____   _____
Witness Signature   Date

_____
Address of Witness

© Cengage Learning 2013

FIGURE 8-6 Advanced Directive Do Not Resuscitate (DNR)

RULES FOR DOCUMENTATION

There are many government agencies, regulatory agencies, laws, and standards that affect documentation in health care settings. The differences in the requirements result from the location of the facility as well as the type of health care provided. For example, a provider's office without radiology equipment would not need to follow the rules of a radiology center, hospital radiology department, or a physician's office that provides diagnostic radiologic services. Understanding the need for different guidelines helps assist managers in learning how to educate themselves as well as other staff members. In trying to understand the medical record requirements, managers can consult with local hospitals, management groups, and other similar facilities as well as network with insurance carriers and government agencies. These rules can be from the Centers for Medicare and Medicaid (CMS) under the conditions of participation in order to operate or The Joint Commission. To help you as a manager comply with all the various regulations, see the following template that gives a snapshot view of the medical record components and a checklist to use for compliance.

In addition to the required documentation in the medical record, there are components in the privacy portion of HIPAA that govern when and how to release information from the medical record. Management should also check with the state on how long to retain medical records as they are governed by each state.

THE FUTURE OF MEDICAL RECORDS

The medical field is growing rapidly, and like anything else, the time has come for changes. The medical record has evolved over the years, but facilities are still using paper medical records to track the progress of their patients. Although this has been accurate and comfortable for most, the requirements of medical record documentation are increasing in length, and mandatory guidelines for facilities can be difficult to follow with paper medical records. With governmental guidelines urging for quality patient care, the documenting in the medical record is becoming longer and requiring more time. In addition, the risk of missing vital information is higher. With the increase in expectations, the paper medical record is now taking longer to be thorough and accurate, which can result in a risk for medical malpractice for the health care facility and provider.

With the increase in requirements, the need to move to electronic becomes more appealing to the health care facility and the provider. When using electronic health records, there are positive and negative aspects. As the changes have evolved, many providers have moved to the electronic version and found the convenience of moving the patient history as helpful; however, in some cases, the history is copied to the new medical document but not reviewed for changes. This can be more damaging if the patient treatment depends on the history. On the other hand, having the ability to copy and paste the past history and use the same template each time saves time and ensures that each portion of the medical document is being completed. In addition, accessing the medical record is much easier than the paper chart that can only be accessed by one employee at a time.

Although the advantages exceed the disadvantages, the more prominent problem is the cost to transfer to electronic. With the government mandates for electronic health records (EHRs), there have been some incentives for health care facilities and providers to transfer now. Over the next couple of years, it is expected that more providers will see the advantages and make the change. With the intended changes to electronic versions of medical records, opportunities for IT employees also increase. If patient care is improved with electronic health records, then health care facilities and providers should make the move as soon as possible to maintain quality patient care.

Managers Checklist			Parts of the Medical Record	
Patient name	☑	☑	**Patient Registration**	**Insurance Cards**
Date	☑	☑	Name: *Jane Smith* MR #234	
Medical record number	☑	☑	Patient information: XXXXXX	Front: *Jane Smith*
			Insurance information: XXXX	
			Demographics: XXXXXXXXX	
				Back: XXXXXXXXXXXXX
Signed	☑	n/a	Signature: *Jane Smith* 3/4/XXXX	
Patient name	☐	☑	**Acknowledgment of the Notice of Privacy**	**Patient History**
Date	☐	☑	XXXXXXXXXXXXXXXXXXXXXX	Name: *Jane Smith*
Medical record number	☐	☑	XXXXXXXXXXXXXXXXXXXXXX	MR # 234
				Date: 3/4/XXXX
Signed	☑	☑	Signature: *Jane Smith* 3/4/XXXX	Signature: *Dr. John Doe*
Patient name	☑	☑	**Progress Notes**	**Laboratory Test**
Date	☑	☑	Name: *Jane Smith*	Name: *Jane Smith*
Medical record number	☑	☑	MR # 234	MR # 234
Tests ordered on file	☑	☑	Date: 3/4/XXXX	Date: 3/4/XXXX
			Lab test ordered:	Test name: XXXXXXX
			X-ray ordered:	Abnormal tests:
			RX prescribed:	
Signed	☑	☑	Signature: *Dr. John Doe*	Signature: *Dr. Jon Doe*
Patient name	☑	☑	**Radiology test**	**Medication Record**
Date	☑	☑	Name: *Jane Smith*	Name: *Jane Smith*
Medical record number	☑	☑	MR # 234	MR # 234
			Date: 3/4/XXXX	
			Test name: XXXXXXXXXX	
			Diagnosis: XXXXXXXXXX	
Signed	☑	☑	Signature: *Dr. John Doe*	Signature: *Dr. John Doe*

Medication Record table:

Date	RX	Initial	D/C	Notes
3/4/XXX	XXX	CC		

Template for a Snapshot of a Medical Record

ELECTRONIC HEALTH RECORDS

The **electronic health record (EHR)** will soon be the norm for most facilities. If we look at the changes in society as well as the advances in computer technology, the Internet, and the amount of knowledge on the World Wide Web, we can understand why. Transition to the electronic record will involve input from IT departments, physicians, other health care professionals, and financial personnel. All staff must have input for the implementation to be successful. The EHR must comply with all the privacy and security regulations of the HIPAA. The record will include all the administrative, medical, and clinical areas that the now-traditional paper medical record does. The ultimate goal is to not only house information on patients but provide such additional services as reminders on patients, alerts, and recall information as well as access patient information from multiple locations. Although there are cautionary measures to take, the move to an EHR is beneficial, and purchasing EHR software is something that should be pursued.

MEDICAL RECORDS

Medical records are vital to quality patient care, and the requirements for thorough and accurate documentation are increasing all the time. Patient medical records are accessed at each visit, providing a detailed history of exams, signs, symptoms, diagnostic testing, and outcomes in each document to ensure the patient treatment is appropriate. For this reason, the medical record must be kept current and accurate at all times.

Documentation made by administrative and clinical personnel and/or providers must be legible and identifiable. Staff must be cautious of abbreviations and use only the ones approved for use in the health care facility. Documentation must be made at the time of service or immediately following. If documentation is entered at a later time, the date and time must be entered and the reason why the documentation was late must be apparent, such as waiting for test results. Addendums can be done when accepted by the facility but must be dated and signed. Finally, be sure that staff members never document in a medical record for another staff member because you are putting themselves at risk for questions and concerns from management and the provider.

Signatures and dates need to be included as appropriate to identify who is making entries. Questions may arise or errors may occur, and without signatures, it is difficult to determine who is responsible for the documentation into the medical record. With paper medical records, signatures and dates should be included on each report; with electronic health records, employees should be logged into their own accounts when accessing or signing a patient's medical record, and they should not share their passwords with any staff members.

Whether it be a paper or electronic medical record, accuracy, timing, and completeness are pertinent. With the laws and regulations changing to improve patient care, management is responsible for overseeing the providers and administrative and clinical staff to ensure the guidelines are being met and that patients are receiving quality health care. In addition, they must also ensure there are no flags for malpractice within the facility.

SUMMARY

- Every health care facility keeps medical records, with each having various components.
- These components may be governed by various regulatory agencies, such as Medicare and The Joint Commission.
- To manage medical records, the medical manager must have a procedure in place to ensure consistency and compliance with each medical record.

- Using checklists helps the manager to ensure consistency in the review of medical records.

- Management must be up to date on new requirements on medical records to ensure they are up to date on governmental and agency requirements.

REVIEW EXERCISES

TRUE OR FALSE

1. _____ Only some health care settings have medical records.

2. _____ Only entries by a physician have to be signed.

3. _____ The medical record in a lab must contain a request slip from the physician.

4. _____ In an outpatient department, the only requirement in the medical record is the report.

5. _____ Long-term care records contain an initial assessment.

6. _____ Each facility decides what goes in the medical record.

7. _____ A checklist helps with consistency in the medical record.

8. _____ Retention laws are up to the states.

9. _____ The transition to electronic health records will be a team approach.

10. _____ Home care records require a referral from a physician.

MATCHING

A   ASC

B   HIPAA

C   Advanced Directive

D   LTC

E   Outpatient

F   EHR

G   CMS

H   Face Sheet

I   Home Care

J   Inpatient

K   Checklist

1. _____ Written directives on the patient's wishes for end-of-life care.

2. _____ Refers to long-term care facilities.

3. _____ Refers to centers for outpatient surgery.

4. _____ The move from paper medical records to electronic records.

5. _____ Departments within hospitals where people come to have diagnostic tests or treatments.

6. _____ A form that contains demographic, billing, and financial information.

7. _____ A medical record that contains a home health aide's plan of care.

8. _____ Requirements of the medical record for conditions of participation to operate.

9. _____ Governs when and how to release patient information.

10. _____ This medical record contains administrative, medical, clinical, advanced directive, and test information.

CRITICAL THINKING ACTIVITIES

ACTIVITY 1

Refer to the template of a snapshot view of the medical record components and a checklist to use for compliance, shown earlier in this chapter. Use the manager's checklist to look for consistency in the following medical record and then record any deficiencies.

Managers Checklist			Parts of the Medical Record	
Patient name	☐ ☐		**Patient Registration**	**Insurance Cards**
Date	☐ ☐		Name: Mary Smith MR #890	
Medical record number	☐ ☐		Patient information:	Front: XXXXXXXXXXXX
			Insurance information:	XXXXXXXXXXXX
			Demographics:	
				Back: XXXXXXXXXXXXX
Signed	☐ ☐		Signature: *Mary Smith*	
Patient name	☐ ☐		**Acknowledgment of the Notice of Privacy**	Patient History:
Date	☐ ☐			Name: Mary Smith MR #890
Medical record number	☐ ☐			Date: 9/9/XXXX
Signed	☐ ☐		Signature: *Mary Smith* Date:	Signature: *Dr. John Smith*
Patient name	☐ ☐		**Progress notes**	**Laboratory test**
Date	☐ ☐		Name: Mary Smith MR #890	Name: Mary Smith MR #890
Medical record number	☐ ☐		Date: 9/9/XXXX	Date: 9/9/XXXX
Tests ordered in chart	☐ ☐		Lab test ordered:	Test Name: XXXXXXXX
			X-ray ordered:	Abnormal tests:
Signed	☐ ☐		For Surgery:	
			Signature: *Dr. John Smith*	Signature: *Dr. Jon Jayson*
Patient name	☐ ☐		**Radiology test**	**Medication record**
Date	☐ ☐		Name: Mary Smith MR #890	Name: Mary Smith MR #890
Medical record number	☐ ☐		Test name: XXXXXXXXXXXXXXX	
			Diagnosis: XXXXXXXXXXXXXXX	
Signed	☐ ☐		Signature: *Dr. John Smith*	Signature: *Dr. John Smith*
Patient name	☐ ☐		**Admitting History and Physical**	**Operative Report**
Date	☐ ☐		Name: Mary Smith MR #890	Name: Mary Smith MR #890
Medical record number	☐ ☐		XXXXXXXXXX	Operation: XXXXXXXXXXXX
			XXXXXXXXXX	
			Diagnosis: XXXXXXXXXXX	Outcome: XXXXXXXXXXXX
Signed	☐ ☐			Diagnosis: XXXXXXXXXXX
			Signature: *Dr. John Smith*	Signature: *Dr. John Smith*

Medication record table:

date	RX	Inital	D/C	

Medical Record for Review

Patient name	☐ ☐	Discharge Summary	Pathology report
Date	☐ ☐	Name: Mary Smith MR #890	Name: Mary Smith MR #890
Medical record number	☐ ☐	Procedure: XXXXXXXXXXXXX	Test name: XXXXXXXXXX
Report in file	☐ ☐	Diagnosis: XXXXXXXXXXXXXX	Diagnosis: XXXXXXXXXXX
Signed	☐ ☐	Signature: *Dr. John Smith*	Signature: *Dr. John Smith*

© Cengage Learning 2013

Medical Record for Review (continued)

Discrepancies of Medical Record

_____

_____

_____

_____

_____

_____

ACTIVITY 2

Mark an X next to the following that demonstrate qualified signatures in a medical record.

1. _____ John Smith, M.D.   Date: 9/23/2011

2. _____ Mary Rouse, R.N.   Date: 7/15/2011

3. _____ Viv Courier, N.P.   Date: 12/2011

4. _____ R. Pew, P.A.

5. _____ Catherine Bernier, M.D.   Date: 5/22/2011

6. _____ George Wilder, N.P.   Date: June 6, 2011

7. _____ M.N., R.N.   Date 2/13

8. _____ Adam Pellerin   Date: March 5th

9. _____ Walter Tyler, M.D.   Date: August 1, 2011

10. _____ Peter Johnson, P.A.

ACTIVITY 3

There are times where your staff has to obtain additional medical documents from other facilities. List the steps involved in obtaining documentation that is at another location, including the types of facilities listed in the chapter.

Steps to Obtain Medical Documentation

_____
_____
_____
_____
_____
_____
_____
_____
_____
_____
_____
_____
_____

ACTIVITY 4

Explain the purpose of an advanced directive as it pertains to patient care. Identify which health care facility locations would use an advanced directive with a patient.

Advanced Directive

Purpose: _____

_____

_____

_____

_____

Locations: _____

_____

_____

_____

_____

CRITICAL THINKING QUESTIONS

1. Discuss how to handle an employee who is not documenting properly. A policy was created, and the employee has been trained not to use certain abbreviations due to the risk of confusion in the abbreviation.

2. Debate the pros and cons of creating and requiring the use of a checklist for employees to verify if the medical record is complete.

3. Explain how often medical record auditing should be done to determine if employees are following the documenting rules and regulations. Think about creative ways in which you can be alerted to correct errors immediately. Include ideas on how to remember to complete the auditing process.

4. Discuss the need for an in-service training when a policy is changed. Include small changes and large changes as well as staff involvement.

WEB ACTIVITIES

1. Research electronic medical records (EMR) and electronic health records (EHR) software online. Choose two options and then compare and contrast the differences. Choose two companies that offer the software and then compare and contrast the price and functions the software includes. As a manager, make a decision as to which option you may think is more appropriate. Write a brief description about why that was your choice.

2. Research governmental agencies online to find one government agency that lists its guidelines for medical records, documenting, or coding.

3. Research health care carriers online to find one carrier that lists its guidelines for medical records, documenting, or coding.

4. Identify the differences between governmental agencies and health insurance carriers. Include the pros and cons of each.

THINK LIKE A MANAGER

CREATE YOUR PRACTICE

Using the templates found in Appendix B and the information presented in this unit, complete the following interactive exercises:

1. Write a procedure on developing a consistent policy of review of the medical record.

2. Write a policy and procedure for ensuring consistency within the medical record. Include documenting, necessary requirements, and organization.

3. You have found when auditing a medical record that it is incomplete. Prepare a teaching session on what goes in the medical record and how to ensure its consistency. Create an outline, a sign-in sheet, and a handout.

4. Write a policy and procedure for maintaining consistency in a medical record with regards to an abbreviation policy, including approved abbreviations.

5. You have found when auditing a medical record that the use of abbreviations is inconsistent and impacting patient care negatively. Prepare a teaching session on how to ensure their consistency. Create an outline, a sign-in sheet, and a handout.

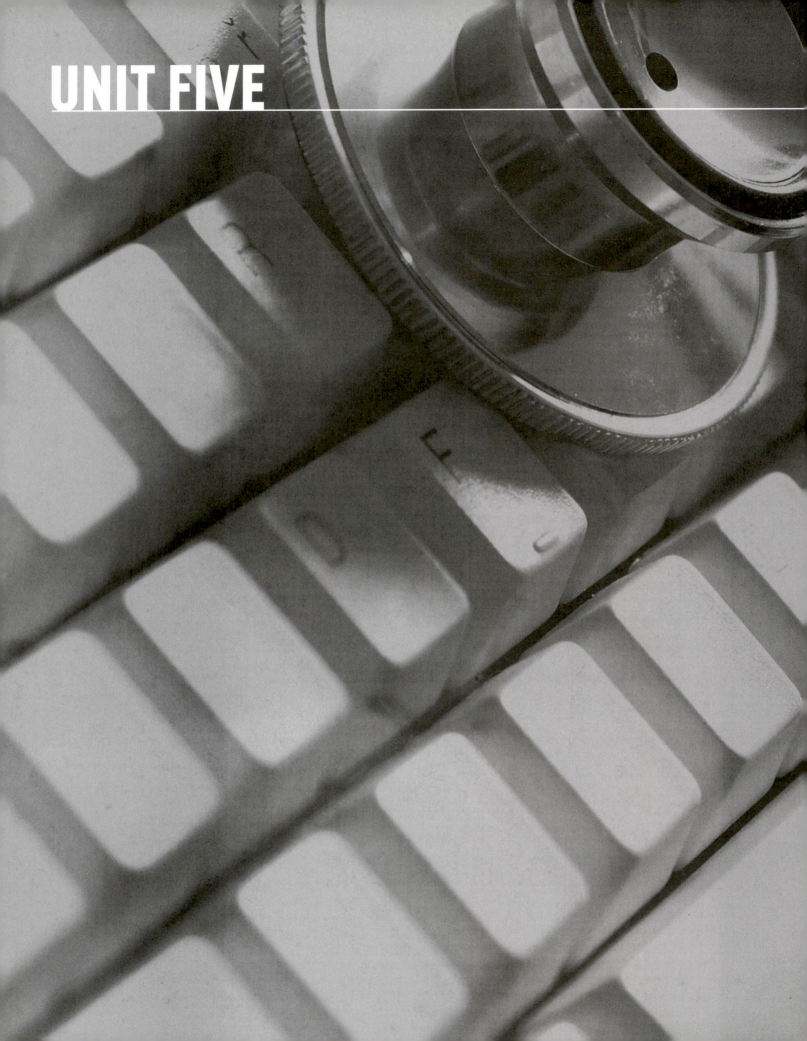

UNIT FIVE

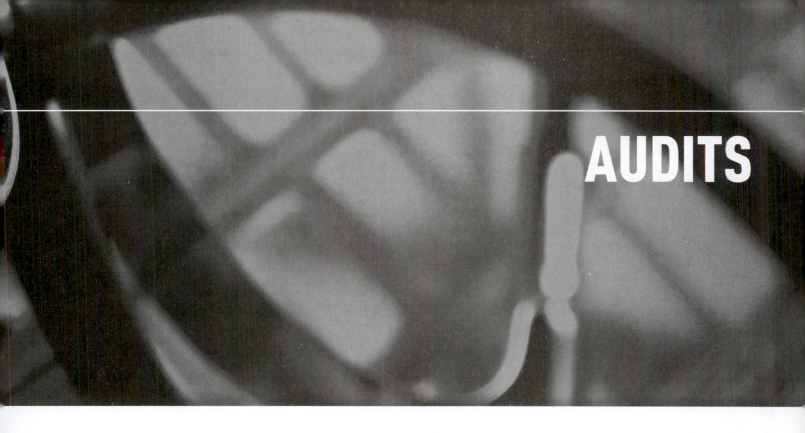

AUDITS

DUE TO THE compliance requirements in a health care facility, auditing is necessary to avoid inaccuracies with coding and billing, including linking codes correctly. Auditing is accomplished by examining specific activities for consultations, medical records documentation, appointment schedules, superbills, and financial information, including explanation of benefits. Internal and external audits are recommended, along with an audit schedule determined in advance.

AUDITS

- Conduct audits on a regular basis to maintain financial viability.
- Conduct audits of evaluation and management levels.
- Maintain policies and procedures on leveling evaluation and management services.
- Audit financial activities
- Audit the Explanation of Benefits for patterns of denial
- Maintain policies and procedures on medical necessity.
- Understand the need to audit often.
- Track inaccuracies.
- Evaluate employees and educate as needed.
- Educate employees about appropriate documentation guidelines.
- Educate employees on documentation requirements as they pertain to coding.
- Understand that the auditing process is involved but necessary.
- Determine an auditing schedule according to the health care facility.

CHAPTER 9

FUNDAMENTALS

Chapter 9 will discuss the fundamentals behind audits. The information will include the relationship between CPT, HCPCS, and ICD-9-CM or ICD-10-CM coding, the importance of linking procedures and diagnoses when billing an insurance company, and how to use EOBs or RAs as tools in auditing. Due to the increasing guidelines each year, auditing has increased in the health care facility. Outside auditors are requesting medical records for patients to determine if documentation is sufficient for the service and procedure codes chosen. Sample internal audits are an important aspect of the health care facility to avoid errors and prepare for external audit, which can result in penalties and jail time in some circumstances.

OBJECTIVES

Upon completion of this chapter, the student will be able to:

- Understand the fundamentals behind audits.
- Review CPT, HCPCS, and ICD-diagnostic coding guidelines.
- Discuss the parts of a claim form.

KEY TERMS

- Anesthesia
- Audit
- Certified registered nurse anesthetist (CRNA)
- Clean claim
- CMS-1500
- Comprehensive
- Coordination of care
- Counseling
- Detailed
- Evaluation and management (E&M)
- Examination
- Expanded problem focused (EPF)
- History
- Layered process
- Levels of E&M
- Linking
- Medical decision making (MDM)
- Modifier
- National provider identifier (NPI)
- Nature of presenting problem
- Place of service (POS)
- Problem focused (PF)
- Subscriber
- Time

INTRODUCTION

This chapter will review the elements included in an **audit**, which is the process of reviewing what was billed to the insurance carrier for reimbursement. Think of the patient who has had a procedure or service at a health care facility as the beginning of a **layered process** (see Figure 9-1). The first layer includes CPT codes for physician services, ICD-diagnostic codes (Note the 9th edition will be used until approximately October 1, 2013 and then the conversion to ICD-10) for diagnoses, and HCPCS codes for certain services and supplies. The CPT, ICD-diagnostic, and HCPCS codes are typically found on an encounter form and identified during the patient's encounter by the clinical staff. These codes are needed for the next layer: the **CMS-1500** claim form. In addition to the codes, the claim form has patient information, subscriber information, and insurance information, which are necessary to complete the next layer. This vital information can be obtained from the patient registration process, which includes demographics of the patient as well as the insurance information. Additional information needed for this layer are **place of service (POS)** codes, provider information, and fees, which are included in the health care facility computer system and automatically populated upon entry of the services, procedures, and diagnoses. Once the claim form is completed with the aforementioned elements, it is then submitted to an insurance carrier, which processes the claim and reviews the codes, the form, and the fees. Once the claim has been processed, payment is determined and sent to the provider with an explanation of benefits (EOB) or a remittance advice (RA). Whether a claim gets paid is determined by the following:

- The codes are correct and have been linked correctly.
- A Medicare national coverage determination (NCD) or local policy exists on that procedure.
- The claim form is completed correctly.
- The claim form is filed in a timely manner.

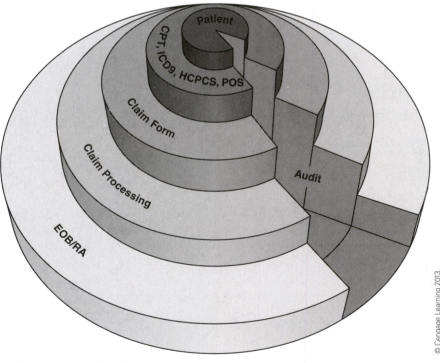

© Cengage Learning 2013

FIGURE 9-1 The Anatomy of an Audit

In this chapter, the fundamentals of each of the elements of an audit will be reviewed. Many functions of an office are included in the audit, such as the appointment book, the registration form, the encounter form, and medical documentation within the chart. During the patient's visit, all the steps need to be completed accurately to reflect the services and procedures provided to the patient and to avoid errors during an audit. Knowing your coding manuals will allow you to identify appropriate codes for a successful audit. How each of the elements becomes a part of an audit will be discussed in Chapter 10.

CPT CODES

CPT codes are a numerical system assigned to procedures and services provided in a health care facility. In order to report procedures and services to an insurance carrier or to bill a patient, the CPT coding system was developed to identify the procedures and services with a five-digit code rather than a lengthy description (see Figure 9-2). This allows the information to be put in numerical format but still inform the insurance carrier or patient about what was performed during the encounter. For example, 99201 is much shorter than writing "level I, new patient, outpatient office visit" on the claim form. The health care facility managers and providers are required to learn the CPT coding system and to understand each code in order to choose appropriate codes for the patient encounter as well as avoid errors during an audit.

Additionally, there are also two-digit **modifiers** that can be added to a CPT code to further modify the meaning, such as in the example of a surgical procedure. Generally a surgeon performs the preoperative, postoperative, and surgical procedures, which are represented by CPT codes. However, in the case where a different surgeon performs these functions, a modifier of –54 added to a surgical procedure CPT code indicates a surgeon performed only the surgical care. A modifier of –55 added to the same CPT code means a surgeon performed only the postoperative care, and a modifier of –56 added to the CPT code means a surgeon performed just the preoperative care. By adding appropriate modifiers to CPT codes, the health care facility and provider are indicating the code has been modified due to the patient's situation, and two digits can identify the change in treatment rather than using a sentence. In this case, knowing the modifiers is vital for the health care facility, management, and the providers due to the fact that an external audit can also determine the incorrect use of modifiers, resulting in penalties or jail time.

Section	Code Range
Evaluation and Management (E/M)	99201 to 99499
Anesthesia	00100 to 01999
	99100 to 99150
Surgery	10021 to 69990
Radiology	70010 to 79999
Pathology and Laboratory	80048 to 89356
Medicine	90281 to 99602
Category II	0001F to 6005F
Category III	0016T to 0170T

FIGURE 9-2 CPT Sections

The CPT manual is divided into six sections for which all codes will be audited during an internal or external audit:

- Evaluation and Management (E&M) Services
- Anesthesia
- Surgery
- Radiology
- Pathology and Laboratory
- Medicine

The nature of the facility determines which health care facilities can code from each section. All facilities use evaluation and management codes; however, anesthesiologists use the anesthesia section. In addition, for radiology, pathology, and laboratory, the facility must be approved prior to coding for these procedures. Although auditing involves all sections, evaluation and management are difficult to determine without proper documentation, and auditors spend a lot of time monitoring the CPT codes in the E&M section.

EVALUATION AND MANAGEMENT

The first section is Evaluation and Management (E&M), and this section provides CPT codes for services that range from office exams, hospital visits, consultation visits, case management, and observation. To determine the correct CPT code from this section, certain key facts must be known. First, is this patient a new patient or an established patient? E&M guidelines state that if a patient has not been seen in three or more years by any physician of the same specialty with in a group practice is considered a new patient. Second, at what health care setting did the physician see this patient? Settings include the physician offices, hospitals, long-term care facilities, assisted living, or home care. Third, is the status of the patient an inpatient or outpatient at the time of service? Even though the patient may be treated in a hospital setting, there are two statuses within the hospital, and inpatient E&M codes are different from outpatient E&M codes; therefore, this needs to be determined in order to choose the appropriate E&M code. New patient and inpatient codes have higher reimbursement, and choosing them inappropriately can flag an audit or result in a failed audit, including fines and jail time. Coders need to research medical documentation to achieve the appropriate codes for the patient encounter.

What you need to know for E&M coding:

New or established patient?

What health care setting?

Is the status of the patient inpatient or outpatient?

Within the E&M section are 20 types and different levels, and auditing involves a large amount of E&M codes due to the leveling requirements for some of the codes. The categories are all different and serve a purpose; however, reading the guidelines within the E&M section will assist the coder in his or her choices. In some code ranges, there are extensive guidelines, such as critical care, allowing the coder to make an educated decision based on the information provided as well as using an audit tool as a guide.

The E&M code categories in this section include:

- Office or Other Outpatient

- Hospital Observation

- Hospital Inpatient

- Consultations

- Emergency Department

- Critical Care

- Nursing Facility

- Domiciliary, Rest Home, or Custodial Care

- Domiciliary, Rest Home, or Home Care Plan

- Home

- Prolonged Service

- Case Management

- Care Plan Oversight

- Preventive Medicine

- Non-Face-to-Face Physician

- Special Evaluation and Management

- Newborn Care

- Inpatient Neonatal Intensive Care, Pediatric and Neonatal Critical Care

Once you determine the type of code to be used, the next step is to determine the level, which is usually accomplished with assistance from an audit tool. The tool should be similar to that of an auditor and provide a place to check off each item as you review your information. Determining the level is more complex because the process is accomplished through analyzing the patient's medical record, and documentation is sometimes not complete or accurate. Auditors must also review documentation when they perform an audit; therefore, coders have to ensure that code choices are generated from information in the patient's medical record to support them. Leveling for the codes that require it can be challenging, and this includes reviewing the patient's history and why he or she was seeking treatment, analyzing the exam and what happened during the visit, and determining the risk factor involved in the medical decision and diagnoses. When a patient visits the provider with an uncomplicated symptom that will resolve itself and not have much risk to his or her health, the level is low. However, when a patient seeks treatment for a more complex symptom that needs further workup and prescription treatment, the level is higher for the increased work and higher risk of death for the patient. With five **levels of E&M** in some of the code choices, determining the history, work involved, and risk category can be difficult and the coder will have to make an educated decision with an explanation of his or her code choice. E&M codes with five levels are based on history, exam, and medical decision making (MDM), such as 99211–99215. Other E&M codes have fewer levels, with specific verbiage helping with the choice of level, such as discharge having two levels based on time spent during the hospital discharge; for example, 99238 is 30 minutes and 99239 is more than 30 minutes (see Figure 9-3).

For accurate leveling of the E&M codes, seven components have to be viewed to determine which level of service was performed. The complete guidelines are accessible at the front of the E&M section of the CPT book and are very thorough in describing the leveling process; however, knowledge of the process must be known for an accurate understanding. It is important to use the current years CPT manual for accuracy. Auditors will use these guidelines when reviewing the provider's code choices.

E/M Code	History	Physical Exam	Medical Decision Making	Nature of Presenting Problem	Coordination of Care	Time Spent for Service
Office or Other Outpatient Services						
New Patient*						
99201	Problem-focused	Problem-focused	Straightforward	Minor or self-limited	Consistent with problem(s) and patient's needs	10 min. face to face
99203	Detailed	Detailed	Low complexity	Moderate	Consistent with problem(s) and patient's needs	30 min. face to face
99205	Comprehensive	Comprehensive	High complexity	Moderate to high	Consistent with problem(s) and patient's needs	60 min. face to face
Established Patient*						
99211	—	—	Physician supervision but presence not required	Minimal	Consistent with problem(s) and patient's needs	5 min. face to face
99213	Expanded Problem-focused	Expanded Problem-focused	Low complexity	Low to moderate	Consistent with problem(s) and patient's needs	15 min. face to face
99215	Comprehensive	Comprehensive	High complexity	Moderate to high	Consistent with problem(s) and patient's needs	40 min. face to face
Hospital Inpatient Services: Subsequent Care*						
99238	Hospital discharge day management	—	—	—	—	30 min. or/ less
99239	Hospital discharge day management	—	—	—	—	more than 30 min.

*Key component: For new patients with initial office and other outpatient services, all three components (history, exam, and medical decision making) are essential in selecting the correct code. For established patients, at least two of these three components are required.

FIGURE 9-3 Selection of E&M Codes

The seven components are:

- **History:** The chief complaint, a description of the present problem, a review of the patient's own history, and his or her social and family histories. The extent of the history in relationship to the presenting problem.

- **Examination:** A review of the affected body area or organ as well as other body systems that are affected by the current problem. The extent of the examination in relationship to the presenting problem.

- **Medical Decision Making (MDM):** The end result, which involves the number of diagnoses, the amount of tests and information to be reviewed, and the risk of morbidity or mortality.

- **Counseling:** A discussion with the patient and/or family about the diagnosis, treatments, options, and risk. The information must be specific to the presenting problem of the patient.

- **Coordination of Care:** The involvement of other agencies or health care professionals as they contribute to the patient's treatment plan at the request of the provider.
- **The Nature of the Presenting Problem:** The type of disease, illness, or condition the patient has presented to the facility with and the level of intensity required in treating the disease, illness, or condition.
- **Time:** Face-to-face contact during which the physician performs a history, an examination, and counsels the patient and/or family regarding the presenting problem and treatment.

The elements of an E&M code:

History

Examination

Medical decision making

Counseling

Coordination of care

Nature of presenting problem

Time

Many factors are involved in the coding process, and the choice will be determined based on the three key components of history, examination, and medical decision listed within the code choice in the CPT book. Although the coding is done by using seven components, when identifying the final decision, coders base it on the three key components; for example, 99212 lists a problem-focused history, problem-focused exam, and straightforward MDM. Included in the code description are instructions that state requirements that two of the three key components have to be met. Auditors will use this as a guide when reviewing their coding process; however, coders must realize that the current E&M guidelines need to be followed in addition to the information with the code.

The E&M three key components are:

- History
- Examination of the patient
- Medical decision making

Once information is gathered for the history and examination from the patient's medical record, the coder will then determine the level depending on the involvement of work and the presenting problem. Within the three key components, the history and examination have the same type of verbiage for identifying the four levels they represent. For example, 99213 includes expanded problem-focused history, expanded problem-focused exam, and low-complexity decision making. In this situation, the expanded problem focused means that there was more discussion than just the problem at hand, and other body systems may have been discussed, with the possibility that they have an effect on the problem. The deciding factor as to what to focus on has to do with the presenting problem and symptoms.

The four levels for the history and examination are:

- Problem focused
- Expanded problem focused
- Detailed
- Comprehensive

The information obtained in regards to diagnostic testing, further treatment, the risk of the patient, and the diagnosis is included in MDM. The levels of MDM also depend on the patient's presenting problem. The auditor will review all the information provided in the medical record to determine what was included in the MDM.

The four levels of Medical Decision Making are:

- Straightforward
- Low complexity
- Moderate complexity
- High complexity

The verbiage for these E&M codes is included in each code choice for the coder to use; for example, 99214 states detailed history, detailed exam, and moderate decision making. When choosing an appropriate E&M code, either two or three of the key components must meet or exceed the level you are choosing. Each E&M code choice will include how many factors are needed, allowing code choices to be made from the code description.

In addition to E&M coding and leveling, E&M modifiers are also used to identify information regarding the patient's encounter. Modifiers are key factors in coding for procedures and services. They are located in the CPT and HCPCS manuals and are added to codes to change the description, as discussed previously. In the CPT book, there are modifiers specific to the E&M chapter that modify the meaning of a code, such as modifier –25, which identifies a significant separate E&M service on the same day as a procedure by the same provider. This modifier is only added to E&M codes and only used when warranted. Modifiers are complicated to use, and understanding them is important to create appropriate coding practices with a positive outcome on audits.

E & M modifiers:

—24: Unrelated E&M service by the same physician during a postop period

—25 Significant, separately identifiable E&M service by the same physician on the same day as a procedure or service

—32 Mandated service

—57 Decision for surgery

Due to the nature of the E&M coding system and its everyday use by all medical providers, auditing has a strong focus on reviewing E&M codes. Most coders use an audit tool to level E&M codes in order to increase accuracy and avoid errors. There are audit tools specific to E&M that include areas for history, exam, and MDM. When the audit tool is used, the coder reads the E&M service documentation and puts a check mark next to the requirements that are met according to the guidelines. There are specific guidelines for choosing a level; however, auditors will often ask for clarification if they cannot understand how a level was chosen by the coder. Having a quality audit tool that represents what the auditor may utilize will be beneficial to your practice in avoiding any red flags or noncompliance.

The CPT manual includes guidelines at the beginning of the E&M and every section within explaining what factors determine the levels for the E&M codes. When referencing audit material, the guidelines are useful in determining the process of leveling E&M codes as well as the type of code to choose depending on the visit and the POS. Although an audit tool may be given to the staff, management should inform staff to also reference the guidelines in the CPT book when leveling E&M codes. There is an abundance of information that is necessary for the biller and coder in order to avoid fraud and abuse during an audit and maintain revenue for the facility.

ANESTHESIA

The second section of the CPT manual contains **anesthesia** service codes, which can only be used by an anesthesiology department, including the anesthesiologist and a **certified registered nurse anesthetist (CRNA)**. Anesthesia can be local, general, epidural, or regional. The anesthesia section is divided by body part or system and then the type of procedure (such as open, closed, or endoscopic procedure) further organizes this section. In instances where the anesthesia is performed by the surgeon, the surgeon is required to use the CPT surgical code with a modifier –47, indicating he or she administered anesthesia. Although this modifier does not occur frequently, the health care facility, management, and provider should be aware of this coding process to avoid any errors while coding or problems with audits.

Attached to anesthesia codes are two-digit modifiers called *physical status modifiers*. These modifiers indicate the patient's health status and help to determine the level of complexity of the service. When an anesthesiologist or CRNA performs an anesthesia procedure, he or she must append the appropriate modifier or identify what the status of the patient was while administering anesthesia. For auditing purposes, a physical status modifier on a patient that is not healthy must be clearly documented in the patient's medical record, including the anesthesia report.

Anesthesia P modifiers:

P1   Normal healthy patient

P2   Patient with mild systemic disease

P3   Patient with severe systemic disease

P4   Patient with severe systemic disease that is a constant threat to life

P5   Moribund patient who is not expected to survive without the operation

P6   A declared brain-dead patient who is having his or her organs removed for donor purposes

In addition to modifiers, anesthesia services can also have an add-on code of a qualifying circumstance for patients who have health complications. These are five-digit CPT codes that are used as secondary codes and can only be billed with the primary anesthesia codes. Understanding that qualifying circumstances add more reimbursement due to the patient's condition is important for the coder because he or she can be flagged for upcoding, which can generate a request for an audit.

Anesthesia qualifying circumstances:

+99100   Patient of extreme age: under 1 and over 70 years old

+99116   Complicated by use of total body hypothermia

+99135   Complicated by use of controlled hypotension

+99140   Complicated by emergency conditions

Coding for anesthesia involves a different process whether the anesthesia was administered by the anesthesiologist or the provider. Depending on the facility, the manager must be educated on the process to maintain appropriate procedures with staff and providers in the event that an audit is requested.

SURGERY

The third section of the CPT manual is considered the surgery codes; however, codes from this section do not indicate the patient had an operation. The procedures can be diagnostic or therapeutic and are performed on patients according to their signs, symptoms, and examination. Some procedures cannot be done in the office setting, and coders need to be careful not to code for unauthorized procedures in the office, such as major operations. Physicians from all specialties can use the surgery codes as appropriate; however, they must be careful with some of the more extensive codes, which require a license and certain qualifications for performing, such as cardiovascular surgery.

This is the largest section in the CPT book, and it is organized by body systems.

The surgery section includes:

- Integumentary
- Musculoskeletal
- Respiratory
- Cardiovascular
- Digestive
- Urinary
- Male/female
- Nervous
- Ocular/auditory

In most circumstances, the specialist will use the body system that relates to his or her specialty; for example, a dermatologist will use the integumentary section and the ophthalmologist will use the ocular section. When coding from the surgery section of the CPT book, coders will be responsible for particular codes that relate to their provider. They will also need to be aware of the different sections and guidelines in case there is a need to use codes from another section. For example, an orthopedic surgeon who does a major procedure may need to perform a layered closure, which is coded from the integumentary system, and the coder will also need to understand guidelines from that section. In each section of the surgery section, there is further division of the type of procedures performed within that body system. Understanding the meaning of the sections can help locate the appropriate codes for the type of procedure performed, determine which procedures are authorized in their location, and know what is included in the procedure description to avoid unbundling and alert an audit.

Within the body systems of the surgery section are subsections that include:

- Incision
- Excision
- Removal
- Repair
- Introduction
- Scope procedures

Most surgery codes are considered packaged and include a variety of services. A "package" can include the procedure, some local or regional anesthesia services, writing orders, postanesthesia evaluation, care on the day of the procedure, and routine follow-up services. Minor surgery has a 10-day global package, and major surgery has a 90-day global package for follow-up care; coding during the global period is limited to unrelated care. When a patient returns for normal checks of the wound, then the E&M is included and is coded with a 99024 for a postoperative visit with zero dollars. However, if the patient returns with something that is outside the normal care within the global package, then treatment is allowed and coding of the E&M with modifier –24 or procedures with modifier –79 is done to identify special circumstances. If something is coded outside the global package, the coder must be certain the documentation supports the additional coding for the auditor.

Multiple procedures at the same encounter or procedures during an E&M encounter are also coded differently due to the inclusion of one code to another. These are two other circumstances that require additional coding and modifiers. A CPT surgical code description is for that procedure to be done without additional services or procedures. In the situation where a patient has multiple services or procedures, the coder is able to code the multiple codes during the same encounter. With an E&M done during a procedure, the coder will add modifier –25 to the E&M service only and code the procedure by itself. When two procedures are performed together, the coder will add modifier –51 for related procedure or –59 for a distinct procedure to the lower priced procedure, as the reimbursement is lowered when these modifiers are applied. The coders must be certain not to add additional E&M and procedures that are not warranted and will be obvious during an audit.

The modifiers that were discussed for the CPT surgery section are two-digit codes that can be attached to a surgical procedure to indicate whether the surgery has been unpackaged and different physicians performed different components. In addition, procedures that are done separate from or unrelated to the initial procedure can be billed. When using modifiers, ensure they are specific to the type of code and special circumstances as auditors will watch for appropriate use and documentation.

Surgical CPT modifiers:

–54	Surgical care only
–55	Postoperative care only
–56	Preoperative care only
–62	Two surgeons
–66	Surgical team
–78	Return to the operating room for related procedure during postoperative period
–79	Unrelated procedure by the same physician during postop period
–80	Assistant surgeon
–81	Minimum assistant surgeon

When sample audits are conducted in the provider's office, be sure to also include the surgery CPT codes because their accuracy is just as important. Surgical CPT codes are only coded when appropriate for the encounter. In order to do well with an internal or external audit, coders will avoid coding anything included in another service or procedure, will code prior and during the global period for anything related and unrelated, and will use modifiers as necessary with additional coding. Working proactively and coding in a timely manner will allow for accuracy on the audits and increased revenue for the health care facility.

RADIOLOGY

The fourth section of the CPT manual contains radiology codes. The type of medical facility determines which type of radiology testing you will be coding; for example, an obstetric physician will typically perform ultrasounds in the office for patients. Although radiology CPT codes are used by many hospitals, they cannot be coded by every health care facility, as each must be licensed and certified to perform such services. There are unique requirements for radiology services that include equipment purchase, OSHA standards, equipment cleaning using approved chemicals, supplies, development of reporting measures, and more. The process is quite involved, and the health care facility that provides radiology services is educated on the coding process in advance. Coders must also be aware that each insurance carrier will require credentialing of radiology services for the procedures that are billed for patients.

The radiology sections include:

- Diagnostic radiology
- Diagnostic ultrasound
- Radiologic guidance
- Breast and mammography
- Bone/joint studies
- Radiation oncology
- Nuclear medicine

Radiology services have two components for reimbursement: a technical component and a professional component. The equipment, supplies, and personnel are considered the technical component, and the radiology CPT code will require a modifier of –TC added to the code. The radiologist, who reads, interprets, and reports the findings, will code for the professional component and add modifier –26 to the radiology CPT code. If one physician performs the technical and professional components, this is considered a global service and modifiers are not necessary for coding purposes. Auditing will be very precise with the components as they review who is entitled to reimbursement. In addition, internal auditing of the reporting process will be important to prepare for an external audit.

Modifiers for radiology CPT codes:

—26   Professional component

—TC   Technical component

Auditing for radiology is straightforward, as they are not leveled, such as with E&M codes. In addition, the code descriptions are easier and in some cases only pertain to certain providers who are licensed to offer radiology services in their facility. When auditing, they must ensure the health care facility is licensed and credentialed in the radiology services provided, as there are specific guidelines they are required to follow. Auditors must take into consideration the requirements to perform the radiology services before presenting to the health care facility for the audit of the coding process.

PATHOLOGY AND LABORATORY

The fifth section of the CPT manual is the pathology and laboratory section. Similar to the radiology section, the pathology and laboratory services and procedures need to be authorized in the health care facility. Pathology and laboratory CPT codes are specific, and staff should be educated on their allowance in the health care facility as well as the process involved in using the CPT codes. Many facilities do perform pathology and laboratory services and procedures in order to diagnose their patients. CPT codes included in this section are diagnostic and therapeutic tests that assist the medical provider in providing an appropriate treatment plan for their patient. This section has 18 subsections in which guidelines precede the section and provide additional information for correct coding and a successful audit.

The pathology and laboratory section includes:

- Organ or disease panels
- Drug testing
- Therapeutic drug assay
- Evocative/suppression testing
- Consultations (clinical pathology)
- Urinalysis
- Chemistry
- Hematology
- Immunology

- Transfusion medicine
- Microbiology
- Anatomic pathology
- Cytopathology
- Cytogenetic studies
- Surgical pathology
- In vivo laboratory procedures
- Reproductive medicine

There are three modifiers specific to the pathology and laboratory section. Similar to other modifiers, they are designed to add information to the CPT code that represents the pathology or laboratory services. In certain circumstances, modifiers are needed, and if they are not provided, the claim will be denied or paid at a lower rate. For example, with modifier –91, this states repeat lab, and if the lab was done more than one time, then the provider is entitled to reimbursement. In addition, modifier -92 is used with alternative laboratory testing platform such as with a kit. Without the modifier, the provider or health care facility would receive payment on the initial service only, and this would result in lost revenue.

Modifiers for pathology and laboratory CPT codes:

—90   Reference outside lab

—91   Repeat diagnostic laboratory test

—92   Alternative laboratory testing platform

Auditing is similar to radiology in that requirements are specific for the provider and health care facility. The approval process has to be conducted in order to use the CPT codes from this section. Usages of the codes in this section are pertinent to the health care facility according to what its diagnoses and treatment processes are for its patients. If the health care facility does not use pathology and laboratory results on a regular basis for determining patient treatment, then they will usually refer the patients to an outside laboratory. However, when the CPT codes are used in the health care facility and they are not used appropriately with modifiers when necessary, an audit could be flagged and the health care facility may receive penalties or even jail time.

MEDICINE

The sixth section of the CPT manual is called the medicine section. This section contains codes for services within specialties. Within this section are subsections and services for these specialties. There are also many diagnostic and therapeutic services and procedures. CPT codes are from all areas, and most providers or health care facilities use medicine codes. As stated with radiology as well as pathology and laboratory codes, there are certain approvals for some procedures that need to be done; for example, a stress test. Within this section, professional and technical components are billed accordingly and does not necessarily need a modifier. In the situation where the hospital owns the equipment and the physician dictates the report, there are two components in which each component has a CPT code. For example, with a stress test, there are two components: tracing or interpretation billed by the hospital (93016 and 93017) and report is billed by the physician (93018). During the auditing process, management must ensure the appropriate component is being billed for the service or procedure provided.

Some of these subsections and services include:

- Immune globulin
- Immunizations
- Psychiatry
- Biofeedback
- Dialysis
- Gastroenterology
- Ophthalmology
- Otorhinolaryngology
- Cardiovascular
- Pulmonary
- Allergy and clinical immunology

- Endocrinology
- Neurology and neuromuscular
- Genetics counseling
- Central nervous system assessments
- Hydration
- Infusion
- Chemotherapy
- Acupuncture
- Osteopathic/ chiropractic
- Moderate conscious sedation
- Medication therapy

Unlike the radiology and pathology and laboratory sections, the medicine section may require a modifier on the E&M code of 25 to report a procedure done at the same time. In addition, modifier −59 can also be used with multiple procedures if two procedures are done at the same time. Coders must be careful when coding multiple CPT codes in the same case in order to avoid red flags and an unnecessary audit.

Auditing CPT codes from medicine are important, and careful consideration needs to be given to the component your health care facility or provider is coding for. With multiple components, the global procedure or service may be billed without realizing and then the other facility will not be able to bill. An office policy or template with component codes may be helpful if they are used often.

ICD-9-CM CODING

Along with procedures and services, providers are responsible for determining the diagnoses of the patients. With some patients, a definitive diagnosis is made and coded by using the ICD-9-CM diagnostic codes. With some patients, they require further workups and are documented with suspected, ruled-out, or possible diagnoses, which cannot be coded in the outpatient setting. In this case, the patient would be given a diagnosis code that is consistent with the signs and symptoms, such as a fever and sore throat for someone with suspected strep throat. When coding from the ICD-9-CM manual, you need to follow many guidelines, and the coding process is more challenging than the CPT coding process. Guidelines are sometimes specific in identifying which order the ICD-9-CM codes must be presented in, and coders must be cautious when using these codes. Most codes do not require any particular order and are listed in order of presenting patient complaints. Identifying the appropriate ICD-9-CM code is crucial to an audit, as it justifies medical necessity for the procedure or service provided; therefore, billers and coders should check with providers or management if they are unsure.

The ICD-9-CM manual is divided into three volumes. Volume I is the alphabetic index for diagnoses, diseases, and disorders, and volume II is the tabular section that includes numeric codes and descriptions. Volume III is for hospital-based procedures only and does not involve diagnostic coding. Volume III also includes two sections that provide an alphabetic index and numeric tabular section for easier use in coding from this volume. For providers or health care facilities that do not use volume III, they may obtain an ICD-9-CM manual that only includes volumes I and II to simplify the coding process.

Within the alphabetic index, the ICD-9-CM manual includes specialized sections on neoplasms, adverse drug effects, and a hypertension table. The hypertension table and neoplasm table are located under their respective letters, allowing coders to view the codes at a glance to simplify the process. When using the alphabetic index, coders are not allowed to choose codes from this section and must reference the tabular list for their final selection. The alphabetic index is provided for searching ICD-9-CM codes when the number is not given; however, the tabular list has all the descriptions and guidelines needed to make an appropriate decision. At the end of the alphabetic index, the drug and chemical table is provided for coders to reference when patients have a reaction to a drug or chemical. The information included in the drug and chemical table can be found in the alphabetic index under poisoning; however, the table makes it easier for the coders to locate the necessary codes quickly. Although tables are provided in the alphabetic index, coders must not code from the tables, as this is still considered the index. Correct code choices must be obtained and verified in the tabular list in order to achieve a successful audit.

Many guidelines are included in the tabular list, which includes 17 chapters of numerical codes divided into three-digit categories. Upon finding the code number in the alphabetic index, coders will then find the number in the tabular list and read all guidelines that pertain to the code choice. Guidelines are located at the beginning of each chapter as well as the beginning of each three-digit category and reference inclusions, exclusions, alternative wording, additional fourth and fifth digits, and definitions. When auditing, if a coder used the alphabetic index, it will be obvious due to the lack of guidelines available.

The chapters of the tabular list are:

1. Infectious and parasitic diseases
2. Neoplasms
3. Endocrine, nutritional, and metabolic
4. Diseases of the blood
5. Mental disorders
6. Diseases of nervous and sense systems
7. Diseases of the circulatory system
8. Diseases of the respiratory system
9. Diseases of the digestive system
10. Diseases of the genitounrinary system

11. Complications from pregnancy, childbirth, and puerperium

12. Diseases of the skin

13. Diseases of the musculoskeletal system

14. Congenital anomalies

15. Conditions originating from the perinatal period

16. Symptoms, signs, and ill-defined conditions

17. Injury and poisoning

In addition to these chapters, there are two supplemental classifications, which include factors influencing health status and external causes. These are two additional sections located at the end of the tabular list and are referred to as the V and E codes in the ICD-9-CM manual. A V code is used when a patient is healthy and is seeking preventive care. The E codes are different from V codes in that they cannot be used alone and must include a primary code. They are used to help describe an injury or accident and are not necessarily used by everyone. The use of codes in these sections is very specific, and auditors will also require accuracy with the use of V and E codes.

Finding the correct codes can be challenging, and careful steps need to be taken to avoid red flags and a request for an audit. To locate a diagnosis code, you must identify the main term in the medical record. The main term is then located in the alphabetic index, where the coder will find a number next to the term. That number is looked up in the tabular section, and coders will read all the coding notes and conventions carefully so the correct code is chosen.

For example, the diagnosis for a patient with abdominal pain:

Pain is the condition, and the location of the pain is the abdomen.

1. Look up **pain** in the index.

2. Then, go through the listings until you get to **abdominal**.

3. The number next to abdominal is then used to go to the tabular section to find the correct code.

4. The code number is listed under the broad category of "other symptoms involving the abdomen and pelvis."

5. This particular code indicates the need for a fifth digit, which further identifies the section of the abdomen, if known.

Looking up abdominal pain in the index and tabular sections of ICD-9-CM manual:

Index

Pain(s)

    Abdominal 789.0

    Adnexa (Uteri) 625.9

    Arm   729.5

Tabular

    789 Other symptoms involving abdomen and pelvis

    Note the use of fifth digits:

        0 = unspecified site

        1 = right upper quadrant (of abdomen)

(Continues)

2 = left upper quadrant

3 = right lower quadrant

4 = left lower quadrant

5 = parabolic

6 = epigastric

7 = generalized

9 = other specified sites (or multiple sites)

During the patient's encounter, the provider will base the services and procedures on the signs, symptoms, and diagnoses. Performing services and procedures is a result of the patient's condition—whether healthy or sick—and they need to be justified with an ICD-9-CM code. All code choices need to be consistent with the official coding guidelines and must include the appropriate digits to identify the highest specificity. In addition, coders should not use ruled-out, suspected, or possible diagnoses, as this is not acceptable coding practice, and auditing for ICD-9-CM will result in finding occurrences where this has happened. Extensive training should be done with management, providers, coders, and billers to identify exact coding guidelines that should be identified in a successful audit. See figure 9-4 for the sections of the ICD-9-CM coding book.

Volume 1 Contains the Numeric Index	
Chapter	**Codes**
1. Infectious and Parasitic Diseases	001–139
2. Neoplasms	140–239
3. Endocrinologic, Nutritional, and Metabolic Diseases and Immunologic Disorders	240–279
4. Diseases of the Blood and Blood-Forming Organs	280–289
5. Mental Disorders	290–319
6. Disease of the Nervous System and Sense Organs	320–389
7. Diseases of the Circulatory System	390–459
8. Diseases of the Respiratory System	460–519
9. Diseases of the Digestive System	520–579
10. Diseases of the Genitourinary System	580–629
11. Complications of Pregnancy, Childbirth, and the Puerperium	630–677

FIGURE 9-4 ICD-9-CM Sections

12. Diseases of the Skin and Subcutaneous Tissue	680–709
13. Diseases of the Musculoskeletal System and Connective Tissue	710–739
14. Congenital Anomalies	740–759
15. Certain Conditions Originating in the Perinatal Period	760–779
16. Symptoms, Signs, and Ill-Defined Conditions	780–799
17. Injury and Poisoning	800–999
Supplementary Classification	
Classification of Factors Influencing Health Status and Contact with Health Service	V01–V86
Classification of External Causes of Injury and Poisoning	E800-E999
Appendices	
A. Morphology of Neoplasms	
B. Glossary of Mental Disorders	
C. Classification of Drugs by American Hospital Formulary Service List Number and Their *ICD-9-CM* Equivalents	
D. Classification of Industrial Accidents According to Agency	
E. List of Three-Digit Categories	
Volume 2 Contains the Alphabetic Index	
Section 1. Index to Diseases and Injuries	
Table of Hypertension	
Table of Neoplasms	
Section 2. Table of Drugs and Chemicals	
Section 3. Alphabetic Index to External Causes of Injury and Poisoning (E Codes)	

FIGURE 9-4 Continued

© Cengage Learning 2013

ICD-10-CM CODING

With so many advancements in the health care field, there is a new coding system for diagnoses, illnesses, and injuries, which will allow more detail when coding. The new ICD-10-CM coding system will transition completely in October 2014 for use by all providers and health care facilities. An increased amount of codes will allow for the coding of more descriptions, such as right, left, and bilateral, which will in turn allow the insurance companies and health care facilities to improve patient care overall. The auditing process will become more involved as additional documentation is needed in order to code for ICD-10-CM, and auditors will be looking for more detailed information within the patient's documentation.

Most of the features of the ICD-9-CM coding system will be maintained with the new ICD-10-CM coding. The conventions, symbols, and guidelines will remain the same for easier transition; however, the exclusions are set up differently, as there are two options now: an exclusion 1 and exclusion 2. The organization of the alphabetic index is set up the same, with the exception of the elimination of the hypertension table and the relocation of the neoplasm table at the end next to the table of drugs and chemicals. The tabular list has changes throughout, although the chapter titles are similar and the sections have remained the same for the most part. The designs of the ICD-10-CM codes will be alphanumeric instead of all numeric and include up to seven digits rather than five. The increased number of digits allows for more detail when coding. The ICD-10-CM coding system will have 21 chapters, which is 4 more than the ICD-9-CM due to the addition of the supplemental classification section and the external causes being assigned chapter numbers. The division of the chapters is similar to the ICD-9-CM; however, the additional chapters allow for breaking down the more detailed information that is going to be added.

The chapters of the tabular list are:

1. Infectious and parasitic diseases
2. Neoplasms
3. Diseases of the blood
4. Endocrine, nutritional, and metabolic
5. Mental and behavioral disorders
6. Diseases of the nervous system
7. Diseases of the eye and adnexa
8. Diseases of the ear and mastoid
9. Diseases of the circulatory system
10. Diseases of the respiratory system
11. Diseases of the digestive system
12. Diseases of the skin
13. Diseases of the musculoskeletal system
14. Diseases of the genitounrinary system
15. Pregnancy, childbirth, and puerperium
16. Conditions in the perinatal period
17. Congenital malformations and deformations
18. Symptoms, signs, and abnormal findings
19. Injury, poisoning, and external causes
20. External causes of morbidity
21. Factors influencing health status

When transition of the ICD-10-CM occurs, all health care personnel, including clinical and administrative, will be required to train on the new system. The new coding system will affect everyone involved in the care of patients, and the details involved in choosing the codes will have to be learned. Training will occur all over the country as everyone identifies his or her role in using the new ICD-10-CM codes, especially for the health care auditing personnel responsible for overseeing coding as an internal or external auditor. Auditors will continue to look at documentation, encounter forms, and appointment schedules; however, they will search for more detail included in the ICD-10-CM code choices to ensure they are appropriate. Internal auditing by management becomes more crucial now with the update of ICD-10-CM, and health care facilities, office managers, and providers must be proactive in researching the requirements ahead of time.

HCPCS

The Healthcare Common Procedure Coding System (HCPCS) includes codes for procedures, services, and supplies for physician and medical suppliers. The HCPCS manual is not used as often as the ICD-diagnostic and CPT code manuals, as there are fewer codes and some code choices are insurance-specific. In many situations, health care facilities use a handful of HCPCS codes and are able to obtain the codes from someone else rather than purchasing a HCPCS manual. The HCPCS codes are revenue based like CPT codes and need an ICD-diagnostic code to justify medical necessity.

Codes in the HCPCS coding manual are five digits and begin with a letter. Included in the HCPCS manual are 16 sections that begin with a letter and each letter represents a certain type of service or procedure in that section. For example, the section with the letter A represents ambulance transportation services and letter D represents dental procedures.

The sections of the HCPCS manual are:

- Transportation services
- Medical and surgical supplies
- Dental
- Durable medical equipment
- Drugs administered other than oral
- Orthotic procedures and devices
- Medical services
- Pathology and laboratory services
- Vision

Modifiers are also included in the HCPCS manual just like the CPT manual. They are two-digit alpha, numeric, and alphanumeric codes that are added to a five-digit CPT or HCPCS code to add additional information about the patients encounter. Modifiers are not coded for all services and procedures; however, they must be justified when used. During an audit, there must be sufficient patient documentation demonstrating the need for the modifier.

Some of the HCPCS modifiers include:

- AA
- CA
- E1–E4
- FA–F9
- GA
- GG
- GH
- LC
- LD
- LT
- RT
- QW
- TA–T9
- V5

Auditing HCPCS codes is important with respect to the insurance carriers, as each carrier has a preference as to which code set they require—either CPT or HCPCS. When an audit is conducted in a health care facility—whether internal or external—HCPCS codes are scrutinized as much as the other coding systems and documentation must be clear. During an audit, encounter forms, appointment schedules, and patient documentation will be compared to make sure appropriate codes are being used. Providers, management, billing, and coding staff should be trained on the use of HCPCS codes as they pertain to patient treatments.

THE CLAIM FORM

Once all the CPT, ICD-diagnostic, and HCPCS codes are chosen by health care providers, they are ready to submit a claim to the insurance carrier in order to receive reimbursement. The form used for physician services is called CMS-1500 and is developed by the Centers for Medicare and Medicaid Services (CMS). There are 33 blocks on the CMS-1500, and every carrier requires accuracy in completing the form. Although most of the guidelines are similar, insurance carriers have their own guidelines for completion, and they will deny the claim with any errors. A **clean claim** is a form that is submitted without errors and is usually paid within 1–3 weeks. After completion of the patient registration, the coding, and the billing, the CMS-1500 is created through various entries and ready for submission. Therefore, all staff members in the health care facility need to be accurate in whatever process they participate during and after a patient encounter. The first phone call to the office starts the process as the registration begins. All these components are part of the auditing process, including registration forms, appointment schedule, encounter form, and

CMS-1500 form. In order to maintain a successful audit, remember to complete all requirements timely and accurately.

This form was revised in 2005 to include fields for the new **national provider identifier (NPI)** number for providers next to each procedure code to identify the health care provider. The NPI numbers demonstrate one number that providers can use to identify themselves for all carriers rather than each carrier issuing a separate provider number, as previously done. The NPI number has made patient care much easier in relation to billing, reimbursement, approvals for services or procedures, referrals, and eligibility checks. As a result of using the NPI number, extra blocks were added to the claim form to accommodate for the number. For a look at the claim form, see Figure 9-5.

Although there are instructions in the blocks, not every insurance carrier requires the information. There are some carriers whose patients are self-insured, and they do not require the relationship blocks to be filled out. Use the claim form, along with insurance carrier guidelines, to get the most accurate claim when submitting for reimbursement. Remember: A clean claim is a paid claim!

LINKING

Code choice is one aspect of the reimbursement process, but in the end, it is necessary to link the codes to each other. **Linking** refers to showing the relationship and consistency of procedures, services, and POS on the claim form and justifying them as medically necessary with an appropriate diagnosis. All service and procedures need a reason to be performed to be approved for reimbursement from the insurance carrier. Each insurance carrier has specific rules, and the billing, coding, and office managers must be familiar with the rules of every insurance carrier. In addition, the location for services and procedures must also be consistent with every carrier. If services are performed at a hospital and then the hospital has an admission and discharge for the patient, the service or procedure codes must be an approved inpatient code for that date of service. In addition, the address for the facility must also be provided.

What insurance carriers look for on a claim include:

- Services listed in block 24D are linked to the diagnosis listed in block 21.
- Numbers from block 21 are related by an arrow to block 24E in each line with the service or procedure.
- The POS in box 24B is linked correctly to the place of service in which the CPT codes are approved.
- For the POS in block 24B, the facility name and address is in block 32.
- For any inpatient procedures, block 18 has an admission and discharge date.

Along with services, procedures, and diagnoses, you must ensure that patient and subscriber information is accurate. The first step to processing a claim is reviewing the patient information for eligibility. Any claim that has missing or inaccurate information will be denied. Every block on the claim form is important for the billing process, and whatever type of service or procedure is used, linking it to the appropriate information is necessary to avoid a red flag and have a successful audit.

Figure 9-6 demonstrates those areas that must be correctly linked.

CLAIMS PROCESSING

An insurance carrier is responsible for processing the claim and sending payment to the provider. The claim process is similar with each carrier, as payment depends on a number of approvals. After eligibility is determined by the insurance carrier, it begins to review the services and procedures for coverage options in the policy. When coverage has been approved, the linking of services, procedures, POS, and diagnoses are all reviewed. There are steps in the claim process that need to be taken in order to determine final payment to the provider or health care facility. Understanding the claim process is important to office staff and management, as this allows them to identify what

1500

HEALTH INSURANCE CLAIM FORM

APPROVED BY NATIONAL UNIFORM CLAIM COMMITTEE 08/05

| | PICA | | | | | | | PICA | |

1. MEDICARE   MEDICAID   TRICARE CHAMPUS   CHAMPVA   GROUP HEALTH PLAN   FECA BLK LUNG   OTHER
(Medicare #) (Medicaid #) (Sponsor's SSN) (Member ID#) (SSN or ID) (SSN) (ID)

1a. INSURED'S I.D. NUMBER   (For Program in Item 1)

2. PATIENT'S NAME (Last Name, First Name, Middle Initial)

3. PATIENT'S BIRTH DATE   SEX
MM   DD   YY   M   F

4. INSURED'S NAME (Last Name, First Name, Middle Initial)

5. PATIENT'S ADDRESS (No., Street)

6. PATIENT RELATIONSHIP TO INSURED
Self   Spouse   Child   Other

7. INSURED'S ADDRESS (No., Street)

CITY   STATE

8. PATIENT STATUS
Single   Married   Other

CITY   STATE

ZIP CODE   TELEPHONE (Include Area Code)
(   )

Employed   Full-Time Student   Part-Time Student

ZIP CODE   TELEPHONE (Include Area Code)
(   )

9. OTHER INSURED'S NAME (Last Name, First Name, Middle Initial)

10. IS PATIENT'S CONDITION RELATED TO:

11. INSURED'S POLICY GROUP OR FECA NUMBER

a. OTHER INSURED'S POLICY OR GROUP NUMBER

a. EMPLOYMENT? (Current or Previous)
YES   NO

a. INSURED'S DATE OF BIRTH   SEX
MM   DD   YY   M   F

b. OTHER INSURED'S DATE OF BIRTH   SEX
MM   DD   YY   M   F

b. AUTO ACCIDENT?   PLACE (State)
YES   NO

b. EMPLOYER'S NAME OR SCHOOL NAME

c. EMPLOYER'S NAME OR SCHOOL NAME

c. OTHER ACCIDENT?
YES   NO

c. INSURANCE PLAN NAME OR PROGRAM NAME

d. INSURANCE PLAN NAME OR PROGRAM NAME

10d. RESERVED FOR LOCAL USE

d. IS THERE ANOTHER HEALTH BENEFIT PLAN?
YES   NO   If yes, return to and complete item 9 a-d.

READ BACK OF FORM BEFORE COMPLETING & SIGNING THIS FORM.

12. PATIENT'S OR AUTHORIZED PERSON'S SIGNATURE I authorize the release of any medical or other information necessary to process this claim. I also request payment of government benefits either to myself or to the party who accepts assignment below.

SIGNED _____   DATE _____

13. INSURED'S OR AUTHORIZED PERSON'S SIGNATURE I authorize payment of medical benefits to the undersigned physician or supplier for services described below.

SIGNED _____

14. DATE OF CURRENT: ILLNESS (First symptom) OR
MM   DD   YY   INJURY (Accident) OR
PREGNANCY(LMP)

15. IF PATIENT HAS HAD SAME OR SIMILAR ILLNESS. GIVE FIRST DATE   MM   DD   YY

16. DATES PATIENT UNABLE TO WORK IN CURRENT OCCUPATION
MM   DD   YY   MM   DD   YY
FROM   TO

17. NAME OF REFERRING PROVIDER OR OTHER SOURCE

17a.
17b. NPI

18. HOSPITALIZATION DATES RELATED TO CURRENT SERVICES
MM   DD   YY   MM   DD   YY
FROM   TO

19. RESERVED FOR LOCAL USE

20. OUTSIDE LAB? $ CHARGES
YES   NO

21. DIAGNOSIS OR NATURE OF ILLNESS OR INJURY (Relate Items 1, 2, 3 or 4 to Item 24E by Line)

1. └____ . ____   3. └____ . ____

2. └____ . ____   4. └____ . ____

22. MEDICAID RESUBMISSION CODE   ORIGINAL REF. NO.

23. PRIOR AUTHORIZATION NUMBER

24. A. DATE(S) OF SERVICE						B. PLACE OF SERVICE	C. EMG	D. PROCEDURES, SERVICES, OR SUPPLIES (Explain Unusual Circumstances) CPT/HCPCS MODIFIER	E. DIAGNOSIS POINTER	F. $ CHARGES	G. DAYS OR UNITS	H. EPSDT Family Plan	I. ID. QUAL.	J. RENDERING PROVIDER ID. #
From To														
MM	DD	YY	MM	DD	YY									
1													NPI	
2													NPI	
3													NPI	
4													NPI	
5													NPI	
6													NPI	

25. FEDERAL TAX I.D. NUMBER   SSN EIN

26. PATIENT'S ACCOUNT NO.

27. ACCEPT ASSIGNMENT? (For govt. claims, see back)
YES   NO

28. TOTAL CHARGE
$

29. AMOUNT PAID
$

30. BALANCE DUE
$

31. SIGNATURE OF PHYSICIAN OR SUPPLIER INCLUDING DEGREES OR CREDENTIALS (I certify that the statements on the reverse apply to this bill and are made a part thereof.)

SIGNED _____   DATE _____

32. SERVICE FACILITY LOCATION INFORMATION

a. NPI   b.

33. BILLING PROVIDER INFO & PH # (   )

a. NPI   b.

NUCC Instruction Manual available at: www.nucc.org

APPROVED OMB-0938-0999 FORM CMS-1500 (08/05)

FIGURE 9-5 Claim Form

FIGURE 9-6 Linking Diagnosis, Service and Place of Service on the Claim Form

Date	Patient	Service	Charge	Allowed	Paid	Subscriber Responsibility	Comments
Oct. 31, 2011	John Doe	Exam	$75.00	$70.00	$60.00	$10.00	
Oct. 31, 2011	Mary Smith	Routine checkup	$75.00	00.00	00.00	$75.00	Uncovered service

FIGURE 9-7 Sample EOB/RA

is needed from the patient, documentation requirements, and expectations from the provider in order to receive appropriate payment for the encounter and have a good audit.

Once payment is decided, an explanation of benefits (EOB) is sent to the provider, along with payment, which details reimbursement made to the provider. The date of the service, procedures, or services performed, the charges, allowed charges, and payments are part of this explanation. This statement will also include amounts the patient owes the provider in copayments, deductibles, or coinsurance. In addition, the contractual adjustment is determined from the EOB as the charged amount minus the allowed amount. When a provider participates with the insurance carrier, most of the EOBs will have contractual adjustments included in the EOB as part of the claims process to avoid balances remaining on the account inappropriately.

If payment of a service or procedure has been denied, then the reason for the denial will also be indicated on the EOB. Refer back to Unit 3 for reasons that claims may be denied. Denials have to be scrutinized for accuracy and adjustments of denied services or procedures are not appropriate unless all possible scenarios for collecting payment have been ruled out. All aspects of the EOB must be understood by the manager as well as billing and coding staff. When the EOB is received, posting of the processed claim involves applying payments, making adjustments, and transferring balances to the patient. Understanding the EOB is another aspect of the audit process that will help staff to comprehend its importance. Figure 9-7 shows an example of what an EOB might look like. Patient John Doe had the service paid, while patient Mary Smith had the service denied.

SAMPLES OF GOOD AND BAD AUDITS

Although audits may seem overwhelming at first, internal audits are necessary for a health care facility to function smoothly. With routine audits, the facility will be able to identify any issues that may be occurring with the patient's accounts. Routine monitoring of the process will allow the office staff to make improvements as necessary.

Samples of a good audit include:

- E&M leveling above 90% accuracy
- POS appropriate on all claims
- Services and procedures performed were appropriate for facility
- All adjustments were necessary according to the EOB
- Medical necessity linked for all services and procedures
- ICD-diagnostic code specificity on all diagnoses

Samples of a bad audit include:

- E&M leveling below 80%
- POS inappropriate for services and procedures

- Unapproved services and procedures are performed
- Unnecessary adjustments were made, which results in lost revenue
- Services and procedures not medically necessary
- Additional digits missing on the ICD-diagnostic code

Audits can be performed internally within your own office or externally by an outside insurance carrier. Preparation for audits is time consuming; however, successful audits make it worth the effort. Having audit tools for E&M leveling, policies, and regulations in place can assist in the audit process. If medical billing and coding staff utilize tools approved by external auditors, then they are more likely to pass the audit. Periodic internal audits are a great way to experience auditing and be prepared. External auditors will let you know when they are preparing to come, and the health care facility will have time to prepare; however, the amount of time is not enough to decrease errors during the external audit. When an audit goes poorly, the health care facility may see penalties and even jail time for fraud or abuse. Auditing involves all aspects of patient care, including medical records, appointment scheduling, and claim submission, which means all aspects of patient care should be taken seriously by all staff, including providers and management.

SUMMARY

- CPT is a numerical coding system used by physicians for services and procedures performed. The CPT manual is divided into six chapters: evaluation and management, anesthesia, surgery, radiology, pathology and laboratory, and medicine. Guidelines precede each chapter and should be reviewed each year.

- ICD-diagnostic manual is a coding system divided into volumes I and II and are used for diseases, diagnoses, disorders, while volume III is for hospital-based procedures.

- HCPCS is a coding system for procedures, services, and supplies for physician and medical suppliers.

- The claim form, known as CMS-1500, is used to record CPT, ICD-diagnostic, and HCPCS codes for communication with the insurance carriers and for the determination of reimbursement.

- The EOB or the RA is used by the insurance carrier to communicate to providers what payments are made on the services and procedures submitted. It also provides the reason for why payment was denied.

- Audits are vital to the claims processing and should be performed by management on an ongoing basis according to the need of the practice—at least monthly.

REVIEW EXERCISES

TRUE OR FALSE

1. _____ There are six sections in the CPT manual.

2. _____ A new patient is one that was *never* seen in this physician's office.

3. _____ A chief complaint is part of the history component of the E&M section.

4. _____ There are 10 components that define a level of service in E&M.

5. _____ Modifiers are two-digit codes added to a five-digit CPT code.

6. _____ Two-digit codes used with anesthesia codes are called *P codes*.

7. _____ An X-ray exam of bones and organs is an ultrasound.

8. _____ Codes for services within specialties are found in the medicine section.

9. _____ There are six volumes for ICD-diagnostic codes.

10. _____ CMS-1500 is the name for Medicare.

MATCHING

A   E & M

B   EKG

C   Facility

D   Immunization

E   Linking

F   CMS-1500

G   POS

H   NPI

I   Modifier

J   P2

1. _____ Pt with mild systemic disease.

2. _____ Code for the place where the service took place.

3. _____ Claim form.

4. _____ ID number for a provider.

5. _____ Two-digit code that is added to a CPT code.

6. _____ First section of the CPT book.

7. _____ Polio vaccination.

8. _____ Diagnostic exam that looks at the electrical activity of the heart.

9. _____ When a diagnosis justifies a procedure to service.

10. _____ Place where the health care service took place.

CRITICAL THINKING ACTIVITIES

ACTIVITY 1

What part of the CPT manual will you find these services or procedures in? (Answers can be used more than once.)

A. Evaluation and management

B. Anesthesia

C. Surgery

D. Pathology and laboratory

E. Radiology

F. Medicine

_____ The patient had a chest X-ray.

_____ The physician performed a tonsillectomy on a child.

_____ The patient was referred to a specialist for consultation from the family physician.

_____ The anesthesiologist administered general anesthesia for a child who had a tonsillectomy.

_____ The blood was drawn and sent to the lab for a CBC (complete blood count).

_____ A urinalysis was performed.

_____ The physician saw a new patient in the office.

_____ Biofeedback was performed on a patient.

_____ The patient had a hysterectomy.

ACTIVITY 2

Link these services to the correct diagnosis:

1.	_____ Office exam	**A.**	_____ Pneumonia
2.	_____ EKG	**B.**	_____ Pharyngitis
3.	_____ Appendectomy	**C.**	_____ Appendicitis
4.	_____ Chest X-ray	**D.**	_____ Abdominal pain
5.	_____ Throat culture	**E.**	_____ Chest pain

ACTIVITY 3

Underline the main term used when looking up an ICD-diagnostic code in the index:

1. Abdominal pain

2. Tension headache

3. Gastric ulcer

4. Viral pneumonia

5. Fractured ankle

6. Urinary infection

7. Night blindness

8. Atypical chest pain

9. Nasal hemorrhage

10. Pilonidal cyst

ACTIVITY 4

Will the following need a CPT or ICD-diagnostic code?

1. _____ Office exam

2. _____ Diabetes

3. _____ Consultation

4. _____ Urinalysis

5. _____ Heart attack

6. _____ Asthma

7. _____ Radiation

8. _____ Strep throat

9. _____ EKG

10. _____ Tonsillectomy

CRITICAL THINKING QUESTIONS

1. Discuss the importance of choosing the additional digits for ICD-diagnostic coding system when necessary. Include the problems that will occur if the additional digits are not chosen for the codes.

2. Debate pros and cons of having one employee do all the billing and also perform his or her own audits. The jobs include coding, billing, payment posting, and auditing.

3. Explain the difference between diagnostic and procedure coding including information about monetary value.

4. Discuss the results of the undercoding and the overcoding of CPT & HCPCS codes. Include the possibility of fines, jail time, and shutdown of the health care facility.

WEB ACTIVITIES

1. Research the Medicare website for ICD-10-CM codes (http://www.cms.gov). Go to the home page, click on Medicare, scroll down to the Coding section, and then click on ICD-10. Periodically check on the implementation date and resources for ICD-10-CM.

2. Research a template online for a superbill or encounter form that will fit according to audit rules. Find two templates that you may use for your office and then compare these two options. Write down the pros and cons and then save one of the templates for future use.

3. Research online for the CMS-1500 claim form updates. Identify which years the CMS-1500 claim form has changed, particularly the year that the national provider identifier (NPI) number was added to the claim form.

CHAPTER 10

MANAGING

Chapter 10 will discuss specific audit activities revolving around CPT, ICD-diagnostic coding, HCPCS codes, billing, and reimbursement. The revenue cycle involves many processes that need to be precise to avoid penalties and fines with insurance carriers. Evaluation and management services, surgical records, general medical records documentation, and financial auditing will be examined. In addition, regulatory agencies pertaining to the auditing process will be identified.

OBJECTIVES

Upon completion of this chapter, the student will be able to:

- Manage audit activities for a medical practice.
- Use a checklist to audit E&M codes.
- Know what to look for when auditing consultations, surgeries, and preventative services.
- State how the OIG work plan impacts the audit process.
- Complete policies and procedures.

KEY TERMS

- Discharge summary
- Freedom of Information Act (FOIA)
- History and physical (H&P)
- Medically necessary
- Nonparticipating
- Office of Inspector General (OIG)
- Participating
- Postoperative
- Preoperative
- Recovery audit contractor (RAC)
- Skilled nursing facility (SNF)
- Social Security Act
- Timely filing

INTRODUCTION

The manager's role is extensive with respect to the audit process. Many insurance carriers, including Medicare, have increased their external auditing of health care facilities; in return, management must be proactive in its internal auditing process to be prepared. Management must take the initiative to recognize potential weaknesses in medical record documentation, train personnel, and perform ongoing self-audits of medical records and assigned codes.

EVALUATION AND MANAGEMENT ACTIVITIES

As described in Chapter 9, there are many factors to be considered when determining the code for an evaluation and management (E&M) service in the CPT code manual. While conducting an official audit is a complex and detailed activity, there are more routine self-audit activities that a manager can conduct on a regular basis that will help to ensure continuity and compliance. For services using an E&M code, a checklist can be created and used by the manager when reviewing medical record documentation.

Checklist for reviewing documentation when auditing E&M codes:

- ☐ Is the patient's legal name on all pages?
- ☐ Is the place of service consistent with the CPT code?
- ☐ If the place of service code is other than the office or the home, is the name and address of the other facility on the claim form?
- ☐ Does the documentation support the level and description of the E&M code?
- ☐ Are additional procedures and services bundled or coded separately?
- ☐ Does the additional service or procedure need a modifier?
- ☐ If diagnostic tests were performed and evaluated as part of the E&M service, are the reports in the patient's file and are they signed and dated?
- ☐ Did the provider communicate with other providers regarding the patient?
- ☐ What was included in the patient's treatment plan for prescriptions, diagnostic tests, therapeutic treatment, or additional health care?
- ☐ Does the date on the bill match the service date in the medical chart?

Modifiers are complicated, and management should be sure that billers and coders are aware of the appropriate usage of modifiers, as they can cause flags with the auditors if they are overused or incorrectly applied.

SELF-AUDIT TECHNIQUES

With all E&M services:

- ❑ Is the place of service (POS) consistent between the CPT code, the POS code on the claim form, and the location described on the claim form? For example, 11 is the place of service code for a physician office location, 21 is used for the inpatient hospital service, and 31 used for **skilled nursing facilities (SNF)** where patients are treated overnight but do not need hospital care. These correct POS must be linked correctly to the accurate E&M code. Figure 9-3 demonstrated the boxes that needed to be linked together.

- ❑ Does the diagnosis justify the procedure or service and is it linked correctly in column 24E?

- ❑ Is the appropriate provider assigned to the claim form as stated in the medical documentation—in blocks 24J and 31?

- ❑ Is the facility and provider authorized to perform those services or procedures, such as minor surgeries or radiology, in block 24B?

Consultation Self-Audit Techniques

If the E&M service is a consultation, does the audit of the service show:

- ❑ A request for the consultation from the patient's primary care physician?

- ❑ A written report for the consulting physician to the primary care physician?

- ❑ A recommendation for treatment based on the consultant's review of the patient's history, examination, and review of tests?

- ❑ Whether the service is in the physician's office or the hospital?

- ❑ A referral for services or procedures with an insurance that requires one?

The three Rs of a consultation:

- Request
- Report back to the patient's physician
- Recommendation for treatment

Hospitalization Self-Audit Techniques

If the E&M service is related to hospitalization, does the audit of the documentation include:

- The patient's name and medical record number on all pages of the medical hospital record?
- CPT codes from the inpatient hospital section?
- The POS code for hospital services in block 24B?
- The name of the hospital in block 32? (See Figure 10-1.)

Figure 10-1 demonstrates how to link the POS code, to name of facility and correct CPT code

- Dates of admission and discharge in block 18? (See Figure 10-2.)
- Hospital records on file in the patient's hospital and physician office chart signed by the provider?

FIGURE 10-1 Hospital Patient Linking POS code, Name of Facility Block 32 and a CPT Code for a Hospital Service

FIGURE 10-2 Date of Hospital Admission and Discharge in Box 18 and Box 32 Completed with Hospital Facility Name

Preventive Services Self-Audit Techniques

If the E&M service is for preventive service, does the audit of the documentation show:

- Consistency with the age of the patient and the code chosen?

- Whether the patient is new or established?

- If other services or procedures were performed with the preventive service? In this case, if they are separate billable procedures, a modifier must be used. For example, 99381 is the preventive code for a "new" patient receiving an initial comprehensive preventive medicine evaluation (age under one year), while CPT code 99382 is the code for a new patient between the ages of 1 and 4.

Common POS codes for professional service:

06: Indian health service freestanding facility

11: Office

12: Home

13: Assisted living facility

21: Inpatient hospital

24: Ambulatory surgical center

31: Skilled nursing facility

While conducting audits of E&M, the manager should consider the basics first before beginning a thorough review by using an audit tool. Thorough reviews are necessary and can be extensive; therefore, taking a sample for thorough review is appropriate if the basic questions are asked when coding and training. By using the aforementioned questions, if anything does not match, then that is an indication that further investigation is necessary. The more internal auditing you can do with the basic questions, the better results you will obtain with an external audit, and training of staff should include this information.

AUDITING THE SURGICAL FILE

If you are the manager in a surgical setting, auditing surgical activities revolve around three periods of time: **preoperative**, the operation, and **postoperative**. This is considered the global package, and all these services are included with one another for the same surgical procedure. When someone performs a major or minor surgical procedure, documentation on the preoperative and postoperative encounters are just as important as the operative report. The provider is obligated to report what occurred to create a need for the surgical procedure and what the health status of the patient was during the postoperative period. For coding guidelines in the health care facility, there are requirements in documentation and coding when performing minor and major surgical procedures that must be followed by the provider and audited by the manager.

PREOPERATIVE PERIOD

An audit in the preoperative (before surgery or surgical operation) period looks for documentation of:

☑ The reasons for surgery

☑ Diagnostic tests supporting the reason for surgery

☑ Preoperative history & physical (H&P)

☑ A signed consent form

☑ All diagnostic tests ordered prior to the surgery, clearing the patient

POSTOPERATIVE PERIOD

An audit of the postoperative period (after the surgical operation) looks for documentation of:

☑ A report of the operation following operative report guidelines

☑ An anesthesia report (if the setting is an ambulatory surgical setting or hospital)

☑ Any pathology reports done during the operation

☑ A discharge summary

Managers must ensure that providers in the health care facility are completing their documentation requirements in order to code the surgical procedure appropriately. Completed documents not only have requirements of information, but they must also all be signed by the provider. In some health care facilities, the coding staff is not permitted to code until documentation is received. In other health care facilities, the provider codes the procedures and submits the codes to billing. With both practices, this is acceptable; however, it is the responsible of everyone to have the documentation requirements met for all three surgical periods. Internal auditing of the documentation will allow for a positive external audit if one were to occur. Figure 10-3 demonstrates a sample operative report.

AUDITING FINANCIAL ACTIVITIES

When auditing financial activity, there are a number of duties that are performed in order to ensure money is collected appropriately. Financial activities involve work done with the income and expenses. Income is received via two types of payments to the office: patient payments and insurance payments. The success of the health care facility depends on the collection of money in a timely manner. The longer money is not collected, the more difficult it becomes to collect. Being proactive on the collection process with everyone is important for the health care facility. There are many ways in which a health care facility can operate with patient and insurance collections in order to maintain a positive income, and auditing their collection routines will allow for continued success. Creating an aging summary report of monies owed is one such way. Figure 10-4 shows an example of this summary report.

In dealing with patient collections, the office staff should collect balances at the time of service. It is easier to collect money with the patient there at the facility than at a later date. Trying to contact someone after the date of service can be challenging because everyone is usually busy. Staff should be proactive in collecting balances—whether previous or current—to maintain a positive revenue cycle. Rather than asking if they want to pay, ask how they will be paying, and that will reflect the idea that they have to pay. Also, offer the types of payments that you have available: cash, check, and credit card. For auditing purposes and to be sure money is being applied to the patient's account, require that all patients receive a receipt of payment at the time they paid. This

Addressograph	OPERATIVE RECORD

Patient Number	Room/Bed
Patient Name (Last, First, MI)	Date of Procedure
Patient SSN	Time Started	Time Ended
Patient DOB	Gender	Service

Surgeon:	Assistant:
Anesthetist:	Anesthetic:

Preoperative Diagnosis:

Postoperative Diagnosis:

Procedure(s) Performed:

Complications:

Operative Findings:

Dictation Date_____

Transcription Date_____

Signed _____

Form 4107, OCT 03

ALFRED STATE MEDICAL CENTER ■ 100 MAIN ST, ALFRED NY 14802 ■ (607) 555-1234

© Cengage Learning 2013

FIGURE 10-3 Sample Operative Report

will allow an auditor to ensure there is no mistake in the posting of the payment. Lastly, when calling to remind patients of their upcoming appointments, let them know they are obligated to make payment that day and then they will be prepared for the payment to occur. Taking these steps and being involved in the patient collection process can demonstrate appropriate records for a financial audit on patient collections.

Insurance payments are received in a different manner from patient payments. They take a little longer to receive and they have an explanation of benefits (EOB) included for details on the payment and denials. Tracking payments from insurance carriers can be more involved due to

Run Date: 12/31/20XX

AGING SUMMARY ONLY
FOR PATIENTS INCLUDED IN THIS REPORT (ONLY)

TOTALS FOR FRAN PRACTON MD

INSURANCE TYPE	PATIENTS	DEBITS	CREDITS	BALANCE DUE	CURRENT	AS OF 11/01/20XX	AS OF 10/02/20XX	AS OF 9/02/20XX
NO INS	7	23,850.00	0.00	23,850.00	23,850.00	0.00	0.00	0.00
MEDICARE	43	72,650.00	3,811.97	68,838.03	65,632.86	3,015.17	190.00	0.00
MEDICAID	22	35,880.00	1,000.00	34,880.00	33,140.00	1,740.00	0.00	0.00
MEDI-MEDI	45	86,785.00	3,567.13	83,217.87	80,080.00	2,715.02	260.00	162.85
PRIVATE	16	20,985.00	5,643.18	15,341.82	11,749.13	3,592.50	0.00	0.00
WORK COMP	1	5,950.00	4,810.00	1,140.00	1,140.00	0.00	0.00	0.00
PPO/HMO	34	45,140.00	17,102.45	28,037.55	25,803.86	2,233.69	0.00	0.00
TOTALS	168	291,240.00	35,934.73	255,305.27	241,396.04	13,296.38	450.00	162.85

TOTALS FOR GERALD PRACTON, MD

INSURANCE TYPE	PATIENTS	DEBITS	CREDITS	BALANCE DUE	CURRENT	AS OF 11/01/20XX	AS OF 10/02/20XX	AS OF 9/02/20XX
NO INS	2	4,750.00	0.00	4,750.00	4,750.00	0.00	0.00	0.00
MEDICARE	83	100,698.69	82,295.74	18,402.95	6,029.14	66.54	0.00	12,307.27
MEDICAID	34	79,555.00	63,755.00	15,800.00	4,880.00	3,750.00	0.00	7,170.00
MEDI-MEDI	72	131,520.01	108,973.55	22,546.46	2,453.34	0.00	0.00	20,093.12
PRIVATE	40	65,843.75	24,111.87	41,731.88	5,843.86	27,310.00	0.00	8,578.02
WORK COMP	3	5,240.00	3,640.00	1,780.00	790.00	0.00	0.00	950.00
PPO/HMO	30	40,505.07	31,227.59	9,277.48	1,880.00	702.13	0.00	6,695.35
TOTALS	264	428,292.52	314,003.75	114,288.77	26,626.34	31,828.67	0.00	55,833.76

Includes transactions with posting dates through 12/31/20XX.
Report compiled using all of the patients.
Includes patients with all insurance types.
There were no condition codes selected or de-selected for this report.
Includes the patients of both treating physicians.
Includes patients with all balances.
Aged by date of first billing with an aging date of 12/31/20XX.

FIGURE 10-4 Aging Summary Report

the nature of the claim form submission, the amount the patient may owe, the need for contractual adjustments, and the possibility of denials. When the payment is received, the amount of money is not the entire balance and the posting of the EOB has to be done with caution. The patient may owe some of the balance, such as a deductible, a copay, or coinsurance, and the insurance may have also denied some of the claim. For denials on the EOB, they are not automatically adjusted off because there could be recourse to get them paid. They could have an incorrect code or be missing a modifier. Making unnecessary adjustments can create a negative revenue cycle for the health care facility if they are not corrected and resubmitted appropriately and timely. The audit process for insurance payments and EOBs is much more involved and should be very precise as to what needs to be reviewed. The chance of error in adjustments is higher, and the auditing of the insurance payments will allow the health care facility to make appropriate changes to ensure that staff is educated on the process of posting payments.

EXPLANATION OF BENEFITS (EOB)

It is important for a manager to audit the EOB for patterns of denial by the insurance carrier. When working with denials on the EOB, the billing staff must immediately search for information that could get the claim paid rather than assuming the denial is an automatic adjustment. Claims may be denied for various reasons, including timely filing issues, not being a **participating** provider, missing information, and procedures and services that have not been linked with diagnoses proving medical necessity. Accepting these denials is not necessary, and research should begin immediately upon processing the EOB. Denials may have recourse as well as deadlines for resubmission and must be worked daily. If denials are left as uncollectable and adjusted off, this can result in unnecessary lost revenue for the health care facility.

> **Reasons for denial on the EOB:**
> - Timely filing
> - Not a participating provider
> - Not medically necessary
> - Missing information on the claim

As the manager, use the reasons for denial as the basis for training billing personnel and developing policies and procedures. Create a requirement of working on denials daily, and list techniques that can assist in finding appropriate information to recover the unpaid claims. Give specific examples, such as a claim denied for being over the filing limit on a patient who gave the wrong insurance card at the time of service. Then list the steps necessary in each situation to allow the staff insight on the best approach to collecting the denied claims on the EOB, such as submitting the claim form with a copy of the EOB from the original insurance carrier for proof of timely filing. Adjustments should be a last resort and in some cases require approval of management to be sure they are aware of all efforts taken to attempt the collection of revenue. With written policies and training, the staff will be ready to conquer all denials and approach them as collectable money in the beginning.

Timely Filing

Timely filing is a crucial factor when billing an insurance carrier because the result of missing a deadline is an adjustment and no reimbursement. No proof of previous submission to that insurance carrier or another insurance carrier can result in loss of payment because there is no recourse for timely filing because you forgot. However, management must train billing personnel to realize the exceptions and approaches to collecting reimbursement in certain circumstances.

If the issue was a timely filing one, then training would include:

Discussing the reasons for denial:

- ☒ Not knowing the insurance companies' timely filing limits
- ☒ Waiting until all services are done
- ☒ Waiting on the provider to submit the billing
- ☒ Not researching for additional information in a timely manner

Training will include what procedures to use to avoid timely filing issues and what exceptions can be submitted again with proof of timely filing from another carrier:

- ✓ Create a list of insurance carriers in the system.
- ✓ List the time frame for filing for each insurance carrier.
- ✓ List the telephone number for each carrier for additional questions.
- ✓ Prepare a list of reasons that could override the timely filing:
  - ○ Primary insurance carrier paid after filing limit of secondary
  - ○ Submission was timely but wrong patient information was entered
  - ○ Clearinghouse has report of timely filing and we can attach proof
  - ○ Liability carrier was listed as responsible but denied after the filing limit for the health carrier

Not a Participating Provider

When a provider is listed as **nonparticipating** on the explanation from the insurance carrier, this does not mean the claim will not be paid, and billing staff should investigate immediately. There are situations where the provider may be paid at a later date, and resubmission may be necessary. If the issue was that the provider is not listed as a participating provider, then training would include:

Discussing the reasons for this type of denial, and the reasons could include:

- ☒ The physician has not signed a contract with the insurance company.
- ☒ The agreement is pending credentialing or recredentialing of the physician.
- ☒ The service was outside the realm of the contract.
- ☒ It is a group practice and not all the physicians were participating.
- ☒ It is a group practice and the physician is not linked to the group appropriately.

Training will include understanding what insurance carriers are contracted with the health care facility and providers. In addition, the steps that may be taken if the provider is expected to be participating but the insurance carrier states otherwise:

- ✓ Create a list by physician of what insurance carriers they participate with.
- ✓ Include the effective date of agreement.
- ✓ Include specific services included or excluded from the agreement.
- ✓ Periodically review and update the contracts.
- ✓ Maintain group and individual contracts.
- ✓ If there is a discrepancy, contact the insurance carrier to correct it.
- ✓ Remember that contracts can be retroactive with some carriers.

Not Medically Necessary

Justifying the procedure or service provided to the patient during the encounter involves using the signs, symptoms, or diagnoses at the time of service. There are specific requirements for services and procedures as to what justifies the need. For example, the provider cannot perform a throat culture for a patient with an earache because this is not considered medically necessary. Identifying medical necessity is something that is determined by the provider and must also be done on the claim form to prevent denials on the EOB.

If the reason for denial is that the service is not medically necessary, the training needs to include the reasons a service may be called not medically necessary.

- ☒ Wrong CPT codes
- ☒ Incorrect ICD-diagnostic codes
- ☒ Incorrectly linking CPT and ICD diagnostic codes in block 24E
- ☒ A procedure or service performed without a medical condition warranting it
- ☒ The primary diagnosis not listed appropriately to identify the reason for the encounter

Corrected claims are possible when the medical necessity is not linked appropriately or the diagnosis is incorrectly coded, and training to identify and correct the issue will include:

- ✓ Review of CPT codes
- ✓ Review of ICD diagnostic codes
- ✓ Reading the medical documentation
- ✓ Understanding what linking is in block 24E of the claim form
- ✓ Reviewing the facilities services and procedures and understanding what each is
- ✓ Reviewing with the provider as to whether the information is accurate
- ✓ Contacting the insurance carrier for any rules on medical necessity
- ✓ Making necessary adjustments and sending a corrected claim to the insurance carrier

Missing Information on a Claim Form

If the reason for a denial is that the claim is missing information, then a review of the information needed on a claim form is necessary. Insurance carriers do allow for resubmissions and corrected claims, especially when the information provided is not enough. There is a timely filing limit for the resubmission, and the billing staff should be aware of the new filing limit in order to ensure they are meeting the requirements. They may require proof of the original submission depending on their system and how well it can identify both submissions. Billing should immediately resubmit a corrected claim with information stating what was corrected to allow for reprocessing.

Missing information that would cause a claim to be denied includes:

- ☒ Missing names and addresses of patient or subscriber
- ☒ Incorrect ID numbers
- ☒ Incorrect DOB
- ☒ Incorrect gender
- ☒ Other insurance information
- ☒ Forms not signed

Attempting to resubmit the claim should be initiated immediately and the training on recognizing and fixing the errors should include:

- ✓ Reviewing the claim and the medical record for errors
- ✓ Identifying the error and making appropriate corrections
- ✓ Regenerating the claim form and identifying the corrections
- ✓ Contacting the insurance carrier for appropriate corrected claim instructions

COPAYMENTS

Another important activity is to review the collection of copayments. Copayments must be collected at the time of service, as this is stated in the contract with the insurance carriers. For new patients, inform them of the facility policy of paying copayments upon arrival. It is not acceptable practice to routinely waive copayments. As a manager, training personnel and developing policies and procedures will be important for collecting these monies. This training must include an understanding as to the importance of collecting this payment to maintain a positive cash flow for the health care facility.

For example, if a practice sees an average of 200 patients a week and the average copayment is $20, $208,000 is collected in copayments each year.

In addition, the billing process is quite expensive because the staff has to review the account each time the statement is sent to the patient. The statements are all reviewed at 30-, 60-, and 90-day intervals. The staff will investigate for recent payment, and if the patient has neglected payment, they will include a notice for the patient with instructions. Mailing statements to patients is estimated to be about $7.00 per patient and can add up after a while. Collecting copayments at the time of service can prevent extensive work for the billing staff, lower the cost of sending statements, and increase overall income.

Training may include role-playing difficult collection situations or how to handle asking for money. Also, staff should identify which patients are allowed to be rescheduled, such as a patient with no life-threatening illnesses, and which patients need to be seen, such as a postoperative patient who is here for a wound check.

Some of these difficult situations can include:

- A patient who forgot his or her checkbook
- A patient who wants to pay next time
- An emergency patient
- An angry patient
- A patient who is a frequent offender

In all difficult situations, staff should remain calm, never raise their voices or argue with the patient, and try to encourage partial payments when it is not an emergency. Try to remind patients of copayments when doing appointment reminders. If policies are written, it is easier for staff to present the policies to the patient in writing to reiterate the seriousness. Figure 10-5 shows a Pay Now Policy letter. In addition, other staff members can also try to work with the patient using a different approach.

LAWS AND REGULATIONS

In every health care facility, laws and regulations are necessary to maintain patient integrity and quality health care. Knowing all the laws and regulations is the responsibility of managers, and they must educate themselves as well as all providers and staff. A manager must go through the abundance of information available and decide who needs to be educated on the material and how it pertains to them.

The largest resource of material on laws and regulations is the Internet, where managers can research for specific information. They must be certain to use an approved website that does not give false information. Another great resource is networking with local facilities that are similar to them. This approach can give the manager another connection to get questions answered and attend seminars and meetings together.

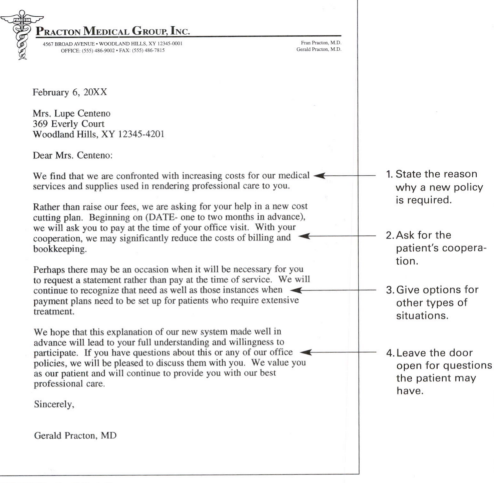

FIGURE 10-5 Pay Now Policy Letter

The letter content:

PRACTON MEDICAL GROUP, INC.
4567 BROAD AVENUE • WOODLAND HILLS, XY 12345-0001
OFFICE: (555) 486-9002 • FAX: (555) 486-7815

Fran Practon, M.D.
Gerald Practon, M.D.

February 6, 20XX

Mrs. Lupe Centeno
369 Everly Court
Woodland Hills, XY 12345-4201

Dear Mrs. Centeno:

We find that we are confronted with increasing costs for our medical services and supplies used in rendering professional care to you.

1. State the reason why a new policy is required.

Rather than raise our fees, we are asking for your help in a new cost cutting plan. Beginning on (DATE- one to two months in advance), we will ask you to pay at the time of your office visit. With your cooperation, we may significantly reduce the costs of billing and bookkeeping.

2. Ask for the patient's cooperation.

Perhaps there may be an occasion when it will be necessary for you to request a statement rather than pay at the time of service. We will continue to recognize that need as well as those instances when payment plans need to be set up for patients who require extensive treatment.

3. Give options for other types of situations.

We hope that this explanation of our new system made well in advance will lead to your full understanding and willingness to participate. If you have questions about this or any of our office policies, we will be pleased to discuss them with you. We value you as our patient and will continue to provide you with our best professional care.

4. Leave the door open for questions the patient may have.

Sincerely,

Gerald Practon, MD

© Cengage Learning 2013

Belonging to groups and subscribing to memberships is another way in which management can become educated on the many laws and regulations. Especially if they receive a monthly communication in which the manager can stay up to date on any changes that occurred in a 30-day time frame. The final suggestion for management to learn all the information is to attend seminars and workshops held on topics that are necessary to the health care facility and the manager. With many opportunities around us, managers can choose the workshops or seminars specific to their needs and be constructive in attending. Whichever method the manager chooses, he or she must ensure the laws and regulations that pertain to them are learned in detail in a timely manner. Being proactive with information will allow them to be successful in their audits from all insurance carriers.

OFFICE OF INSPECTOR GENERAL (OIG)

The **Office of Inspector General (OIG)** is responsible for performing audits and investigations. Every year, the OIG publishes a work plan that outlines areas that will be evaluated or inspected in the next year. The OIG work plan determines each year what areas of health care and other areas will be reviewed and audited. The plan varies from year to year and is determined by the need for making changes.

Areas that have been investigated include:

- [ ] In hospitals: unbundling of hospital outpatient services
- [ ] Physician practices: place of service (POS) errors
- [ ] Review of E&M services during global surgery periods
- [ ] Correct coding of consultation services

Managers should read the work plan prior to the start of the year and look for these areas in the place of practice. This plan can be found at http://oig.hhs.gov and then click on reports and then work plan.

Each year, the OIG identifies which areas will be reviewed more thoroughly for that year. With continued coding errors occurring, **the** OIG has an ongoing duty to monitor anything that has a red flag. The review of such coding discrepancies is a great way for providers and health care facilities to identify what they may be coding in error. Due to the ever-changing coding guidelines and rules, mistakes are made unconsciously, and the OIG is able to identify overuse or incorrect use and then assist the providers and health care facilities in correcting their mistakes. On-the-job training is important, and management must take the initiative to fully train billing and coding staff appropriately with every change that affects the practice. The OIG is behind management by identifying and auditing these techniques so they have the opportunity to make appropriate changes and follow protocol. There is a lot of work involved, and it is necessary to stay up to date.

CENTERS FOR MEDICARE & MEDICAID SERVICES (CMS)

CMS is responsible for regulating the coding rules for governmental plans and maintaining an honest system of reimbursement for the provider and health care facility. Due to the large volume of patients under governmental health plans, this has become a tremendous undertaking. CMS has grown as it increases regulations and works on changing health care. Detailed rules and regulations as well as information about CMS are located online for everyone to have access and be able to follow as appropriate. CMS also lists its fee schedule, which most providers and health carriers use as a guide to decide their own fee schedule. In order to regulate the governmental insurance industry, there are many acts that have been developed and approved, which include:

- [ ] Freedom of Information Act (FOIA)
- [ ] Health Insurance Portability and Accountability Act (HIPAA)
- [ ] Health Insurance Reform
- [ ] Social Security Act

In order to create a more cohesive union, CMS has hired **recovery audit contractors (RAC),** which are auditors that have been asked to audit health care facilities throughout the country. They began their auditing at the hospitals and have moved to physicians' offices, auditing all aspects of the Medicare patients and determining if fraud or abuse was involved, for which the provider or health care facility might receive penalties or jail time. The RAC is an outside contractor reimbursed by Medicare for auditing, and managers must be aware of the intentions and know when RAC is presenting to his or her facility.

Despite the insurance carrier, the manager is responsible for knowing all the laws and regulations that pertain to each carrier. This is an ongoing process for which they need to network and identify sources of information for each carrier. The Internet and the insurance contracts are great resources, but make certain to confirm the information with each insurance carrier. Education of the information is important within the health care facility because the provider and staff need to learn the laws and regulations that pertain to them. Management will receive a successful audit if it follows the laws and regulations appropriately.

SUMMARY

- E&M services, part of the CPT code manual, are one of the most audited areas, including office visits, preventive medicine, and consultations.

- Monitoring CPT codes to ensure there is an ICD-diagnostic code that correlates with the service and correctly links information on the claim form for medical necessity.

- Areas for which the manager should perform a self-audit include E&M, preventive, consultations, surgeries, and hospital services.

- The manager should review the OIG work plan each year to familiarize the areas targeted by the government for review.

- Managers should familiarize themselves with all rules and regulations that pertain to RAC audits and CMS, including audit tools that may be used by the auditors.

- Managers should perform audits on a monthly basis and use all documentation, including medical records, superbills, and EOBs, to audit for accuracy.

REVIEW EXERCISES

TRUE OR FALSE

1. _____ A correct POS code must be linked to a correct E&M code.

2. _____ The three Rs for a consultation are read, review, and recommend.

3. _____ Preventive service codes are age related.

4. _____ A report of an operation is part of the preoperative medical record.

5. _____ An audit of the preoperative medical record includes looking for a signed consent.

6. _____ Denials on an EOB include timely filing or missing information.

7. _____ A copay can be billed.

8. _____ If a claim form is missing information, the claim will be denied.

9. _____ Waived copayments is an acceptable practice.

10. _____ The OIG targets areas to be reviewed and investigated.

MATCHING

A   EOB

B   Preoperative

C   Postoperative

D   OIG Linking

E   Medically Necessary

F   Nonparticipating

G   H&P

H   SNF

I   Timely Filing

1. _____ A physician who has not signed an agreement with a insurance carrier to accept a set reimbursement fee.

2. _____ History and physical performed by a physician on a patient.

3. _____ Twenty-four-hour skilled nursing care in a nursing home.

4. _____ Not submitting a claim form in a predetermined time period.

5. _____ Before an operation.

6. _____ When a diagnosis corresponds to the need for a procedure or service.

7. _____ An explanation of benefits from an insurance carrier.

8. _____ After the operation.

9. _____ Work plan.

10. _____ Proving the medical necessity of a service.

CRITICAL THINKING ACTIVITIES

ACTIVITY 1

Identify five places of service codes that may be reviewed for an audit. Explain why the place of service and the procedure code need to correlate for appropriate coding and billing.

Place of Service Codes

1. _____

2. _____

3. _____

4. _____

5. _____

Explanation: _____

_____

_____

_____

ACTIVITY 2

Mark an M beside the Medicare-related rules and regulations that are affiliated with auditing.

1. _____ Freedom of Information Act (FOIA)

2. _____ Skilled nursing facilities (SNF)

3. _____ Health Insurance Portability and Accountability Act (HIPAA)

4. _____ History & physical (H&P)

5. _____ Health Insurance Reform

6. _____ Explanation of benefits (EOB)

7. _____ Current procedural terminology (CPT)

8. _____ Social Security Act (SSA)

9. _____ Recovery audit contractor (RAC)

10. _____ Medical necessity

ACTIVITY 3

Collecting copayments at the time of an encounter is important for the revenue cycle. Describe ways in which auditing can identify better methods in collecting timely copayments. Create scenarios by using the wrong technique and then the right technique for difficult situations in collecting copayments from patients.

Wrong Technique: _____

_____

_____

_____

_____

Correct Technique:

_____

_____

_____

_____

_____

_____

_____

ACTIVITY 4

As a manager, you will need a way to keep track of the auditing process. Create an audit checklist that would be used to ensure the auditing process is being followed.

Audit Checklist
☐ _____
☐ _____
☐ _____
☐ _____
☐ _____
☐ _____
☐ _____
☐ _____
☐ _____
☐ _____
☐ _____
☐ _____
☐ _____
☐ _____
☐ _____
☐ _____
☐ _____
☐ _____

CRITICAL THINKING QUESTIONS

1. Explain how the Office of Inspector General (OIG) work plans can assist in the auditing process. Use the current work plan referred to in this chapter to explain the relationship.

2. Discuss the documentation required for a surgical procedure. Include information about the preoperative and postoperative documenting requirements. Reimbursement for a surgery requires complete documentation.

3. Identify ways to be proactive with auditing techniques and with information that will allow them to be successful in their audits from all insurance carriers, including Medicare.

4. Debate pros and cons of recovery audit contractors (RAC) who have been hired by Medicare to audit providers of Medicare patients.

WEB ACTIVITIES

1. Research the Internet to find an appropriate audit tool that can be used for auditing E&M coding.

2. Locate the 1995 and 1997 E&M coding guidelines and then compare and contrast the differences.

3. Research medical auditor salaries to identify the salary range for the state you are in. Identify the experience and certification requirements. Use local facilities' job openings if necessary.

THINK LIKE A MANAGER

CREATE YOUR PRACTICE

Using the templates found in Appendix B and the information presented in this unit, complete the following interactive exercises:

1. Write a policy and procedure for auditing a hospital record.

2. Write a policy and procedure for auditing a surgical chart.

3. Write an in-service training session to teach your billing department how to recognize situations and prevent denials by an insurance company.

4. Write an employment advertisement to place in the classifieds of the local newspaper for an on-site medical auditor. Include the role, responsibilities, education, and salary.

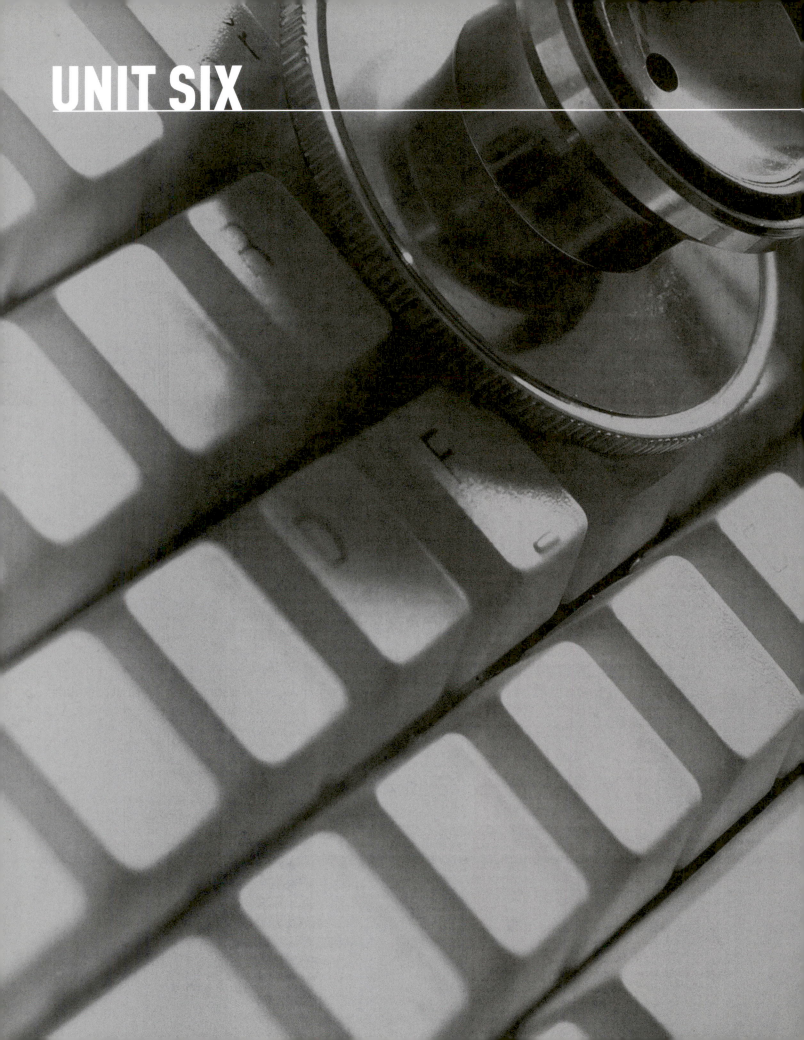

UNIT SIX

COMPLIANCE WITH REGULATORY AGENCIES

REGULATORY AGENCY RULES, laws, and regulations will impact the health care facility tremendously. Compliance is established by government agencies as well as insurance carriers and private organizations. Identifying compliance and understanding the expectations are part of the daily routine for management. Training and continuous monitoring is a management function, which also requires updates to be accessed.

COMPLIANCE WITH REGULATORY AGENCIES

- Manage the compliance of rules and regulations of all applicable agency.
- Conduct training continuously with employees.
- Maintain updates on compliance as the updates are released.
- Manage a compliance policy and procedure manual accessible to employees.
- Educate employees on all compliance regulations and the impact of those regulations.
- Educate employees on the audit process and how it affects compliance.
- Track noncompliance and address employees as necessary.
- Understand that noncompliance can result in fines, jail time, and/or closure.
- Determine the qualifications necessary to hire a compliance officer and trainer.
- Create a schedule of when compliance is recommended.

CHAPTER 11

COMPLIANCE WITH REGULATORY AGENCIES

FUNDAMENTALS

Chapter 11 will discuss the basics of compliance with regulatory agencies and governmental agencies. Following governmental rules and regulations is important to the function of a health care facility, and details will be identified. Patient and employee health safety will be reviewed as it pertains to the requirements. Voluntary standards will also be discussed as health care facilities choose to affiliate with outside organizations. In addition, billing, auditing, and laboratory expectations will be explained.

OBJECTIVES

Upon completion of this chapter, the student will be able to:

- Understand the impact of CLIA on physician office lab testing.
- State the role of the OIG to audit procedures.
- Identify the health care settings impacted by The Joint Commission.
- Know what OSHA is and how it protects employees.

KEY TERMS

- Ambulatory surgery centers (ASC)
- Centers for Disease Control and Prevention (CDC)
- Clinical Lab Improvement Act (CLIA)
- Centers for Medicare and Medicaid (CMS)
- Certificate of accreditation
- Certificate of compliance
- Certificate of waiver
- Engineering controls
- Exposure plan
- Federal register
- Hepatitis B vaccine
- Material safety data sheets (MSDS)
- Occupational Safety and Health Administration (OSHA)
- Office of Inspector General (OIG)
- Outpatient prospective payment system (OPPS)
- Personal protective equipment (PPE)
- Postexposure follow-up
- Provider-performed microscopy procedures (PPMP)
- Recordkeeping
- Recovery audit contractor (RAC)
- The Joint Commission
- Waived
- Work plan
- Work practice controls

INTRODUCTION

There are many agencies, organizations, and government bodies that create, implement, structure, review, and regulate the way health care operates. Management must understand what and who these entities are. Regulatory agencies are established to ensure that patient care and employee safety are respected. Explanations will be presented for each agency as well as the protocol to develop policies for staff.

Regulatory and compliance will include clinical and administrative duties that are performed in the health care facility. Clinical agencies include guidelines for performing laboratory tests, protection for clinical staff against patient body fluids, and patient health safety during treatment. Administrative agencies audit the billing procedure to ensure policy is followed, and all procedures and services are documented to protect patient health care and billing. The health care facility is a team and must work together to present quality care for patients; therefore, each department must be cautious and document everything timely and appropriately. Documenting accuracy should begin as soon as the patient telephones for an appointment (see Figure 11-1).

CLINICAL LAB IMPROVEMENT ACT (CLIA)

The **Clinical Laboratory Improvement Act (CLIA)** was passed by congress in 1988 to establish standards for all laboratory testing done, including testing in physician offices. The policy was developed to ensure accuracy, reliability, and timeliness of patient testing in every laboratory setting. Due to the nature of the testing in the laboratory, CLIA requires standards to be in place prior to implementing laboratory procedures in the health care facility. The qualifications are different depending on the extent of the laboratory procedures; for example, a specimen tested without a microscope has different expectations and does not require the qualifications of a licensed laboratory technician or physician pathologist. The complexity of testing the specimen affects the need for more requirements, thus the reason CLIA has initiated several types of approvals.

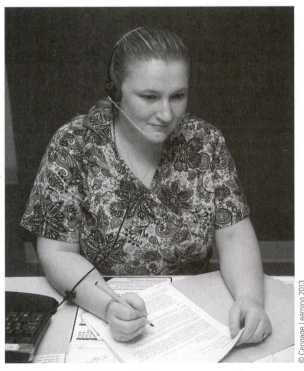

© Cengage Learning 2013

FIGURE 11-1 Operator Registering a Patient

The organization responsible for managing CLIA operations is the **Centers for Medicare & Medicaid Services (CMS)**, and its requirements are based on the laboratory testing and what is involved. CMS has developed many standards within the health care industry to protect patients and guide health care facilities in the functions necessary to display quality patient care during treatment. Some health care facilities consider the guidelines and standards a nuisance, and they are reluctant to research the necessary information; however, the intent of CLIA is to assist your health care facility in performing laboratory procedures accurately. When determining whether you want to perform laboratory procedures in your facility, using the CMS guidelines is a great way to begin your research. The CMS has an abundance of information at http://www.cms.gov/clia to assist in making your decisions and answer some of your questions. Take the time to research the information carefully before you begin the application process.

Once you determine that the facility is ready to proceed with laboratory testing on-site, the first approach to having laboratory tests performed in the health care facility is to apply for a CLIA number. Depending on the type of facility, the laboratory procedures on-site may not be worth the time and money. If the health care facility is small, the expense of having the laboratory and the time invested to obtain a CLIA number may not be worth the effort. For example, in an orthopedic office, a laboratory is not usually found; however, in a primary care or pediatrician office, the laboratory is used often and assists with diagnosing. Management would participate in the decision process of whether to have a laboratory and which laboratory procedures would be reimbursable. In addition, the need for the type of CLIA certification would also be decided. Does the laboratory tests you are requesting need a microscope for determining results? Are there chemicals involved in obtaining the laboratory results? These questions are important when deciding which category of laboratory tests the health care facility requires.

Figure 11-2 lists the categories of laboratory tests

After you have decided which lab category or tests to implement, the application process would begin. This process is very extensive and needs to be completed by management when any new

---

HEMATOLOGY

White blood cell (WBC) count	Hematocrit (Hct)
Red blood cell (RBC) count	Prothrombin time (PT)
Differential white blood cell count (Diff)	Erythrocyte sedimentation rate (ESR)
Hemoglobin (Hgb)	Platelet count

CLINICAL CHEMISTRY

Glucose	Potassium
Blood urea nitrogen (BUN)	Bilirubin
Creatinine	Cholesterol
Total protein	Triglycerides
Albumin	Uric acid
Globulin	Lactate dehydrogenase, LD (LDH)
Calcium	Aspartate aminotransferase, AST (SGOT)
Inorganic phosphorus	Alanine aminotransferase, ALT (SGPT)
Chloride	Alkaline phosphatase
Sodium	Phospholipids

SEROLOGY (IMMUNOLOGY/IMMUNOHEMATOLOGY) AND BLOOD BANKING

Syphilis detection tests (VDRL, RPR)	Rheumatoid factor (RA factor)
C-reactive protein test (CRP)	Mono test

FIGURE 11-2 Categories of Laboratory Tests

ABO blood typing

Rh typing

Rh antibody titer test

Cross-match

Direct Coombs' test

Cold agglutinins

URINALYSIS

Physical analysis of urine:

    Color

    Clarity

    Specific gravity

Chemical analysis of urine:

    pH

    Glucose

    Protein

    Ketones

    Blood

MICROBIOLOGY

Candidiasis

Chlamydia

Diphtheria

Gonorrhea

Meningitis

Pertussis

Pharyngitis

PARASITOLOGY

Amebiasis

Ascariasis

Hookworm disease

Malaria

Pinworm disease (enterobiasis)

CYTOLOGY

Chromosome studies

Pap test

HISTOLOGY

Tissue analysis

Biopsy studies

DNA

DNA testing compares individuals according to their individual genotype.

TOXICOLOGY

The toxicology department tests for chemicals, specifically for drugs and other toxins in blood.

Heterophil antibody titer test

Hepatitis tests

HIV tests: ELISA and Western blot

Antistreptolysin O (ASO) titer

Pregnancy tests

    Bilirubin

    Urobilinogen

    Nitrite

    Leukocyte esterase

Microscopic analysis of urine:

    Red blood cells

    White blood cells

    Epithelial cells

    Casts

    Crystals

Pneumonia

Streptococcal sore throat

Tetanus

Tonsillitis

Tuberculosis

Urinary tract infection

Scabies

Tapeworm disease (cestodiasis)

Toxoplasmosis

Trichinosis

Trichomoniasis

FIGURE 11-2 continued

testing is being requested. If the CLIA approval is one that requires a licensed technician, then the information regarding his or her qualifications would be attached when applying. The application process would be completed by management and include any necessary attachments and qualifications necessary. Management must ensure that laboratory tests are not performed until the entire application process is complete and an approval has been received.

A CLIA number is required by facilities that perform diagnostic or assessment tests on human specimens, such as blood and urine, and can be obtained through an application process. The types of tests performed will determine the type of certificate that must be attained. Upon acceptance by CMS, the physician is assigned a CLIA number, which is then placed on the CMS-1500 claim form in block 23. Figure 11-3 shows the form with the CLIA number. The CLIA number identifies the health care facility as a provider authorized to perform laboratory procedures and allows the provider to receive reimbursement. You must educate staff on the need for a CLIA number when billing and coding in order to maintain error-free claims; otherwise, reimbursement will be delayed. Working with CLIA approvals is a process that involves everyone in the health care facility, as laboratory procedures are performed and submitted for reimbursement.

The three different categories that a facility can apply for are:

1. Certificate of waiver

2. Certificate for provider-performed microscopy procedures (PPMP)

3. Certificate of compliance or certificate of accreditation

A **certificate of waiver** allows a medical facility to perform only those tests that are on the **waived** category list. The certificate consists of blood tests that have insignificant risk of error when being performed. When the approval is issued, it is only valid for two years and must be renewed to continue laboratory procedures. An updated list of tests can be found on the **Centers for Disease Control and Prevention (CDC)** website (http://www.cms.gov/clia).

In addition to a CLIA number, a modifier is associated with laboratory tests. Some of the laboratory tests on the certificate of waiver list require the use of modifier –QW, which is a HCPCS modifier stating that a CLIA-approved test has been performed. Waived tests do require modifier –QW attached to the CPT code to represent CLIA approval. The health care facility must be cautious in billing with modifier –QW when appropriate in order to receive reimbursement.

Waived tests include:

- **81002:** Dipstick or tablet reagent urinalysis
- **81025:** Urine pregnancy test
- **82270–82272:** Fecal occult blood test

Waived tests before 1996 include:

- **80101–QW:** Drug screen
- **81003–QW:** Bayer Clinitek50 urine chemistry analyzer
- **81007–QW:** Uriscreen
- **82055–QW:** Alcohol screen
- **82274–QW:** Fecal occult blood test
- **82962:** Blood glucose
- **83026:** Hemoglobin
- **84830:** Ovulation tests

1500

HEALTH INSURANCE CLAIM FORM

APPROVED BY NATIONAL UNIFORM CLAIM COMMITTEE 08/05

PICA ☐☐☐ — PICA ☐☐☐ — CARRIER

1. MEDICARE ☐ (Medicare #) MEDICAID ☐ (Medicaid #) TRICARE CHAMPUS ☐ (Sponsor's SSN) CHAMPVA ☐ (Member ID#) GROUP HEALTH PLAN ☐ (SSN or ID) FECA BLK LUNG ☐ (SSN) OTHER ☐ (ID)

1a. INSURED'S I.D. NUMBER (For Program in Item 1)

2. PATIENT'S NAME (Last Name, First Name, Middle Initial)

3. PATIENT'S BIRTH DATE MM | DD | YY SEX M ☐ F ☐

4. INSURED'S NAME (Last Name, First Name, Middle Initial)

5. PATIENT'S ADDRESS (No., Street)

6. PATIENT RELATIONSHIP TO INSURED Self ☐ Spouse ☐ Child ☐ Other ☐

7. INSURED'S ADDRESS (No., Street)

CITY STATE

8. PATIENT STATUS Single ☐ Married ☐ Other ☐

CITY STATE

ZIP CODE TELEPHONE (Include Area Code) ( )

Employed ☐ Full-Time Student ☐ Part-Time Student ☐

ZIP CODE TELEPHONE (Include Area Code) ( )

9. OTHER INSURED'S NAME (Last Name, First Name, Middle Initial)

10. IS PATIENT'S CONDITION RELATED TO:

11. INSURED'S POLICY GROUP OR FECA NUMBER

a. OTHER INSURED'S POLICY OR GROUP NUMBER

a. EMPLOYMENT? (Current or Previous) ☐ YES ☐ NO

a. INSURED'S DATE OF BIRTH MM | DD | YY SEX M ☐ F ☐

b. OTHER INSURED'S DATE OF BIRTH MM | DD | YY SEX M ☐ F ☐

b. AUTO ACCIDENT? ☐ YES ☐ NO PLACE (State)

b. EMPLOYER'S NAME OR SCHOOL NAME

c. EMPLOYER'S NAME OR SCHOOL NAME

c. OTHER ACCIDENT? ☐ YES ☐ NO

c. INSURANCE PLAN NAME OR PROGRAM NAME

d. INSURANCE PLAN NAME OR PROGRAM NAME

10d. RESERVED FOR LOCAL USE

d. IS THERE ANOTHER HEALTH BENEFIT PLAN? ☐ YES ☐ NO *If yes,* return to and complete item 9 a-d.

READ BACK OF FORM BEFORE COMPLETING & SIGNING THIS FORM.

12. PATIENT'S OR AUTHORIZED PERSON'S SIGNATURE I authorize the release of any medical or other information necessary to process this claim. I also request payment of government benefits either to myself or to the party who accepts assignment below.

SIGNED ____________ DATE ____________

13. INSURED'S OR AUTHORIZED PERSON'S SIGNATURE I authorize payment of medical benefits to the undersigned physician or supplier for services described below.

SIGNED ____________

PATIENT AND INSURED INFORMATION

14. DATE OF CURRENT: MM | DD | YY ◀ ILLNESS (First symptom) OR INJURY (Accident) OR PREGNANCY(LMP)

15. IF PATIENT HAS HAD SAME OR SIMILAR ILLNESS. GIVE FIRST DATE MM | DD | YY

16. DATES PATIENT UNABLE TO WORK IN CURRENT OCCUPATION FROM MM | DD | YY TO MM | DD | YY

17. NAME OF REFERRING PROVIDER OR OTHER SOURCE

17a. 17b. NPI

18. HOSPITALIZATION DATES RELATED TO CURRENT SERVICES FROM MM | DD | YY TO MM | DD | YY

19. RESERVED FOR LOCAL USE

20. OUTSIDE LAB? ☐ YES ☐ NO $ CHARGES

21. DIAGNOSIS OR NATURE OF ILLNESS OR INJURY (Relate Items 1, 2, 3 or 4 to Item 24E by Line)

1. ___ . ___ 3. ___ . ___

2. ___ . ___ 4. ___ . ___

22. MEDICAID RESUBMISSION CODE ORIGINAL REF. NO.

23. PRIOR AUTHORIZATION NUMBER

24. A. DATE(S) OF SERVICE From MM DD YY To MM DD YY	B. PLACE OF SERVICE	C. EMG	D. PROCEDURES, SERVICES, OR SUPPLIES (Explain Unusual Circumstances) CPT/HCPCS | MODIFIER	E. DIAGNOSIS POINTER	F. $ CHARGES	G. DAYS OR UNITS	H. EPSDT Family Plan	I. ID. QUAL.	J. RENDERING PROVIDER ID. #
1								NPI	
2								NPI	
3								NPI	
4								NPI	
5								NPI	
6								NPI	

25. FEDERAL TAX I.D. NUMBER SSN ☐ EIN ☐

26. PATIENT'S ACCOUNT NO.

27. ACCEPT ASSIGNMENT? (For govt. claims, see back) ☐ YES ☐ NO

28. TOTAL CHARGE $

29. AMOUNT PAID $

30. BALANCE DUE $

31. SIGNATURE OF PHYSICIAN OR SUPPLIER INCLUDING DEGREES OR CREDENTIALS (I certify that the statements on the reverse apply to this bill and are made a part thereof.)

SIGNED DATE

32. SERVICE FACILITY LOCATION INFORMATION

a. NPI b.

33. BILLING PROVIDER INFO & PH # ( )

a. NPI b.

PHYSICIAN OR SUPPLIER INFORMATION

NUCC Instruction Manual available at: www.nucc.org

APPROVED OMB-0938-0999 FORM CMS-1500 (08/05)

FIGURE 11-3 CLIA Number in Item 23 on the Claim Form

Providers with a certificate for **provider-performed microscopy procedures (PPMP)** can perform tests under the waived category as well as those classified as PPMP. When facilities are approved for PPMP testing, they are authorized to perform laboratory tests that are of medium difficulty and require the use of a microscope by an approved provider. During the application process, the provider is identified as the laboratory tester who will use the microscope to obtain results of specimens.

PPMP tests include:

- **81000–81001:** Urinalysis by dipstick or tablet reagent
- **81015:** Urinalysis; microscopic only
- **81020:** Urinalysis; two or three glass test
- **89055:** Fecal leukocyte examination
- **89190:** Nasal smears for eosinophils
- **G0027:** Semen analysis
- **Q0111:** Wet mounts, including preparations
- **Q0112:** All potassium hydroxide (KOH) preparations
- **Q0113:** Pinworm examinations
- **Q0114:** Fern test
- **Q0115:** Postcoital direct, qualitative examinations

The third category—**certificate of compliance** or **certificate of accreditation**—allows a facility to perform tests that are considered moderate or high complexity tests as well as tests from the waived and PPMP categories. The last category requires that laboratory tests are conducted by a fully accredited laboratory that includes a physician or pathologist on-site for obtaining results. The laboratory must go through an on-site investigation to determine whether the laboratory meets accreditation requirements to perform in this category.

Types of tests in category three include:

- Mohs surgery
- Examination and interpretation of tissue specimens

Along with accreditation under CLIA, appropriate disposal of materials is addressed in the application process, including fluid samples and bloody gauze. Management must realize biohazard materials cannot go into every day trash and must be disposed of differently. Containers identified

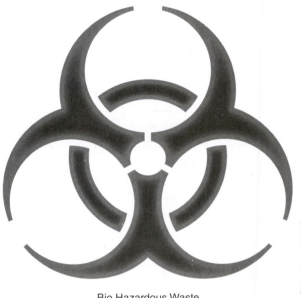

Bio Hazardous Waste

FIGURE 11-4 Biohazard Label

© Cengage Learning 2013

with a biohazard symbol for laboratory use and appropriate disposing of the material are required; see Figure 11-4 for examples of the label.

Monitoring laboratory procedures and ensuring that all approvals are in place and all standards are followed are ongoing processes that management needs to oversee in the laboratory. Performing laboratory procedures in your facility is a privilege and assists you in diagnosing and treating your patients promptly. With the extensive work involved and the risk to the laboratory personnel working with fluid samples, compliance with CLIA must be maintained at all times. Education about CLIA and approved laboratory specimens is ongoing, as updates come out yearly to improve the quality of patient care, and management must obtain the most up-to-date information in order to educate providers and staff.

CENTERS FOR MEDICARE AND MEDICAID SERVICES (CMS)

The **Centers for Medicare and Medicaid services (CMS),** as seen in other chapters, is a governmental health care program that has regulations that affect all aspects of medical care, including providers, facilities, services, medical records, billing, and reimbursement. Medicare regulations impact billing and proper use of codes for diagnoses, procedures, and services. Because of the high volume of patient care today, all providers are required to document the patient's history, the examination, findings, and the plan for treatment. The extensive documentation is the only access CMS has to verifying what was accomplished during the patient encounter. After the documentation identifies the procedures and services, medical necessity has to be determined through the linking of diagnoses. Following this step, the code bundles have to be reviewed to decide if the procedures or services are inclusive to each other. At the conclusion of this process, modifiers are added if necessary and only used with appropriate circumstances. In some situations, modifiers are used incorrectly to get services or procedures paid because Medicare will accept the modifier and not because it was a separate procedure or service performed. Careful consideration must be given to the documenting and coding process for Medicare providers as the RAC auditors make their way into the health care facilities nationwide.

As a result, fraud and abuse prevention and detection have become more complex and increasingly important to Medicare. Documentation is being monitored by Medicare through a group

BP✓	blood pressure check
C&C	called and canceled
C	canceled
Cons	consultation
CP	chest pain
CPE (CPX)	complete physical examination
ECG	electrocardiogram
FU	follow-up examination
Inj	injection
Lab	laboratory studies
NP	new patient
NS	no show
P&P	pap and pelvic
PT	physical therapy
Re✓	re-check
Ref	referral
RS	reschedule
Sig	sigmoidoscopy
S/R	suture removal
Surg	surgery

© Cengage Learning 2013

FIGURE 11-5 Sample Abbreviation List

of outside contractors called **recovery audit contractors (RAC)**. The auditors are responsible for verifying the medical document to ensure proper diagnoses and procedures are described. Included in this review is the accurate use of abbreviations, which can contribute to the possibility of a medical error and must be used carefully in a health care facility when treating patients; see Figure 11-5 for examples of common abbreviations.

From hospitals to offices to long-term care and **ambulatory surgery centers (ASC)**, Medicare has developed a policy, a statement, a directive, and a way of communicating how to comply with the rules. The policies are in place to protect the Medicare system and ensure that only the services and procedures performed are billed. With a high volume of Medicare and Medicaid providers, CMS guidelines are well known throughout the country. For management, there are many seminars online or local to attend for clarification and updates on the ever-changing CMS guidelines as well as how to locate the changes or updates pertaining to your health care facility. In addition, the rules and regulations can be found at http:\\www.cms.gov for further details of their expectations.

THE JOINT COMMISSION

The Joint Commission (formerly JCAHO) is an independent nonprofit organization that establishes standards in the practice and accreditation of health care facilities.

Affiliating with The Joint Commission is voluntary, and when a health care facility decides to take this step, it is considered to have higher standards for quality patient care.

The mission of The Joint Commission is: "To continuously improve the safety and quality of care provided to the public through the provision of health care accreditation and related services that support performance improvement in health care organizations."

The types of health care facilities affiliated with The Joint Commission include:

- Rehabilitation hospitals
- Critical access hospitals

- Medical equipment services
- Hospice services
- Home care organizations
- Nursing homes
- Long-term care facilities
- Behavioral health organizations
- Office-based surgery centers
- Independent or freestanding laboratories

The standards that The Joint Commission publishes deal with patient rights and patient safety as well as the control of infections. Included in the requirements is the sterilization of supplies and equipment, which can be done using an autoclave (see Figure 11-6). Specifics are identified by The Joint Commission as to what is expected of health care facilities with regards to the care of patients, and they are strictly monitored on a regular basis. Visits are made to the facility to ensure standards are being followed in every department, and changes are made when appropriate to avoid safety issues in the future. When The Joint Commission visits the health care facility, it will give you advanced notice of the visit and explain its intentions for visiting. When it arrives, the inspection process will include the review of documentation, policies and procedures, and any errors that may have occurred during patient care. All documentation and logs are required to be up to date, with dates and signatures for any type of entry. All requirements are reviewed for compliance, and the health care facility is given a report and an opportunity to amend the issues. The Joint Commission will follow up for a final report and results.

At the end of each year, the Joint Commission standards are updated for the next year based on the issues presented in health care, including a review of all types of health care facilities. When patient accidents or exposures to infections occur (see Figure 11-7 for examples), The Joint Commission

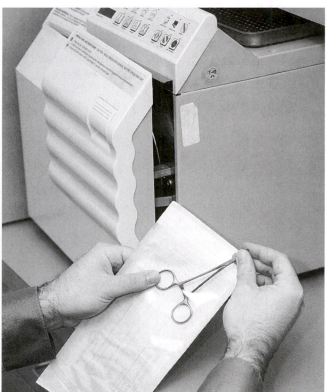

© Cengage Learning 2013

FIGURE 11-6 Autoclave for Sterilization

Disease	Infectious Agent	Mode of Transmission
Anthrax	Bacillus anthracis	Inhalation
Botulism (food poisoning)	Clostridium botulinum	Ingestion
Chlamydia (sexually transmitted disease)	Chlamydia trachomatis	Sexual contact
Clostridial myonecrosis (Gas gangrene)	Species of gram-positive Clostridia	Wound entry
Escherichia coli	Gram-negative bacilli	Ingestion, wound entry
Gonorrhea (sexually transmitted disease)	Neisseria gonorrhoeae	Sexual contact
Legionnaires disease (pneumonia)	Legionella pneumophila	Inhalation
Meningococcal meningitis	Neisseria meningitidis, Streptococcus pneumoniae, or Haemophilus influenzae	Direct contact, inhalation
Nosocomial (hospital-acquired) infection	Gram-negative bacteria	Normal flora transmitted during illness/procedures; opportunistic pathogens transmit during debilitated condition
Pneumococci	Streptococcus pneumoniae	Respiratory (inhalation)
Pulmonary tuberculosis	Mycobacterium tuberculosis	Inhalation
Samonellosis (food poisoning)	Salmonella	Ingestion
Shigellosis (bacillary dysentery, diarrhea)	Shigellae	Fecal-oral
Staphylococcal infection (abscesses, food poisoning, urinary tract infections)	Staphylococci	Direct contact, ingestion, inhalation, bloodborne, vectors (animals)
Streptococcal infection (strep throat, otitis media, pneumonia)	Hemolytic streptococci (usually beta-hemolytic group A)	Inhalation
Syphilis (sexually transmitted disease)	Treponema pallidum	Sexual contact
Tetanus (lockjaw)	Clostridium tetani	Wound entry
Tuberculosis	Mycobacterium tuberculosis	Inhalation
Typhoid fever (enteric fever)	Salmonella typhi	Fecal-oral

FIGURE 11-7 Examples of Infectious Bacterial Diseases

will review the problems and make suggestions accordingly, requiring changes in the rules and regulations. Any problems at your health care facility should be reported to The Joint Commission and documented to educate staff and make them aware of the problem to avoid it occurring in the future. The Joint Commission approaches these changes to protect patients and promote high standards of quality patient care for affiliated organizations. Complete details of the changes can be accessed at http://www.jointcommission.org, and management must be aware of the health care facility's affiliation with The Joint Commission and remain up to date with the requirements and changes.

OFFICE OF INSPECTOR GENERAL (OIG)

The **Office of Inspector General (OIG)** develops projects each year with regards to program audits, program inspections, investigating potential areas of fraud or misconduct, and resolving fraud and abuse cases. Each year, the OIG publishes the proposed plan in the **federal register**, which is an online publication of governmental rules and regulations. When determining which area to work on for the year, the OIG reviews previous years for prior audits and concerns and can continue previous work tasks as indicated. Fraud and abuse can be a result of uneducated employees, and the OIG's initiative is to create a working audit system, allowing attention to be brought to areas susceptible to fraud and abuse—whether intentional or unintentional.

One such publication of the OIG is the yearly **work plan**, which identifies particular areas that need to be audited for fraud and abuse by health care facilities. Every fall, the OIG publishes a new work plan, which states what areas are going to be reviewed, audited, and reported on. Areas reviewed for fraud and abuse included billing companies, physical and occupational therapy, and payments to providers who perform initial preventive physical examinations. The identification of fraud and abuse was consistent with the inappropriate billing of services and procedures in which health care facilities may not be aware. By creating the work plan, the OIG has promoted the improvement of billing services and procedures for every type of health care facility to remain compliant.

For the 2012 work plan, some of the areas the OIG will be for looking include:

- Hospitals
- Home health care
- Nursing homes
- Physicians
- Part D prescriptions
- Medical equipment and supplies

HOSPITALS

With regards to hospital regulations, areas that have been reviewed by the OIG work plan are hospital-owned physician practices and their accreditation process. They want to ensure that the provider-based practice is not trying to get out of the **outpatient prospective payment system (OPPS),** which is a bundled payment made to the hospital for services under CMS reimbursement. When the OPPS is determined for a patient encounter, many services and procedures are bundled in the payment and are not allowed to be coded separately. A hospital-based physician practice can bill the CMS fee for service and they are not paid under the OPPS. If a hospital runs a physician-based practice, it needs to follow appropriate regulations that demonstrate it is an authorized physician office and not a hospital-based facility paid under an OPPS system.

In order to function as a hospital-owned practice, the health care facility needs to obtain licensing as a physician-based facility. The process is involved, and all required applications must be submitted with documentation. Information must be given on the providers that will practice as well as the type of facility they are attempting to establish. The OIG work plan will review the federal requirements for becoming a hospital-owned physician practice, along with the information for accreditation and licensing. This work plan was created to ensure that the health care facility has completed the application process and been approved. The primary goal is to be certain the health care facility is not required to bill under the OPPS as per the regulations. The 2012 work plan shows a plan that is concentrating on compliance issues as well as safety, quality and billing practices.

HOME HEALTH CARE

With respect to the home health care services, the OIG has reviewed Medicare Part B payments for home therapy services to patients. When services and procedures are provided in the home, billing, coding, and documentation are crucial for CMS patients. OIG has developed a work plan to audit the medical records and identify whether the billing they are doing is appropriate for the services and procedures provided. Because therapies are paid under the Medicare Part B policy for CMS providers, the OIG set up a work plan to detect any inappropriate billing. Some of the issues that may be looked at could include deciding if the therapy was administered, if the therapy was adequate for the clinician and patient needs, if it was performed by a licensed clinician, and if the modalities were appropriate for the diagnosis. The development of this work plan is initiated to assist home health providers with completing documentation and developing an appropriate tool for controlling the services and procedures as appropriate for Medicare Part B payments. New to the 2012 work plan for home care agencies is the documentation of patient outcome and assessment data.

NURSING HOMES

In the nursing home setting, skilled nursing facility, or rehabilitation center, the payments for consolidated billing were reviewed by the OIG work plan. With the development of consolidated billing to reduce the patient stay and provide a less expensive hospital stay, the system was implemented to reimburse the health care facility with one lump sum. The fees were based on certain types of treatment specific to the needs of the patient. When the billing and coding are completed, all services and procedures need to be reviewed for the possibility of a service or procedure being outside the package. Careful attention needs to be given to the consolidated package and the alternative billing to be sure they are not inclusive of one another. The OIG has set up a work plan to identify the need for monitoring services and procedures billed outside the package that are not allowed to be billed separately. This approach will allow nursing homes and skilled nursing facilities to be certain they remain in compliance with their consolidated billing rules. The 2012 work plan reviews the compliance safety and quality plan that should be in place.

PHYSICIANS

For physicians, the continuous place of service errors, E&M services during the global surgery period, and Medicare payments for colonoscopy are some of the areas that have been scrutinized. For example, if place of service problems have been noted on denials of payment on an explanation of benefits, then this area needs to be reviewed and fixed. By identifying potential errors in coding and billing in the physician's office, the OIG is able to prepare the work plan for the manager to follow ahead of time. They are also able to assist the physician's office with proper techniques so it can avoid noncompliance. The plan is published in the fall and gives the health care facility time to correct any problems and deficiencies.

Management must be proactive in determining the OIG work plan ahead of time so it is prepared for the changes and ready to make adjustments. The yearly work plan can be accessed at http://www.oig.hhs.gov under Reports & Publications; scroll down to find the "Work Plan" link. Areas that pertain to your setting should be reviewed and discussed. What is your policy or procedures? Have there previously been errors in these areas? With so many health care facilities billing for patient care, the OIG has helped identify potential red flags and made it apparent as to what may be inappropriate. Their intent is to assist health care facilities in improving the practices to remain within the rules and regulations. By following the OIG work plan schedule, management can initiate proper techniques and be prepared for audits.

OCCUPATIONAL SAFETY AND HEALTH ADMINISTRATION (OSHA)

The **Occupational Safety and Health Administration (OSHA)** details the types of protections that employers need to provide their employees to protect them from exposure, including those who are exposed to patients' fluids, such as blood and urine. When you work with patients, situations arise where patient fluid is exposed, and the rules and regulations are in place to ensure employers are maintaining a safe environment for their employees, especially clinical staff. Although the rules mostly apply to clinical situations, administrative employees need to be supervised under OSHA; thus, they also require training during orientation. The training of OSHA requirements is an ongoing process for managers, and they must be knowledgeable about the OSHA expectations for each employee hired. Notification should be given to the employees when training is necessary, as management will track accordingly.

Knowing all safety requirements is overwhelming for health care facilities, as each one operates differently, and OSHA has varying rules and regulations depending on the function. OSHA has established qualifications based on the type of facility and the treatment of the patient. Management should be aware that each type of facility, employee, and department may require different training, and OSHA will identify the requirements for each. The risk of exposure determines what type of training and requirements are necessary. Some of the diseases health care employees can be exposed to are noted in Figure 11-8, including some suggested methods to follow for extra precaution.

The regulations required by OSHA include:

- **Exposure Plan:** An exposure plan is a written plan that outlines the ways a health care facility protects its employees from exposure to blood-borne pathogens. The plan should be created ahead of time and followed regularly. Health care employees should be informed of the importance and potential for injury or illness if the exposure plan is not followed appropriately. The plan details what types of equipment is used for particular patient treatment or diagnosing and is updated yearly to reflect new and safer methods.

- **Engineering Controls:** Engineering controls are the devices that are used to comply with the exposure plan. They can include sharp containers, needleless systems, and self-sheathing needles. They must be identified by the health care facility, and the employee must be trained in their use. Contact information must be accessible for health care employees in the event they have issues with the engineering controls and they need assistance in any way. Compliance by all employees is necessary to remain safe and follow OSHA standards.

- **Work Practice Controls:** Work practice controls are the procedures used to reduce exposure. These controls include washing hands, disposing of sharps, packaging for lab specimens, handling laundry, and cleaning surfaces and materials. As with the engineering controls, health care employees must be trained thoroughly despite their knowledge from previous employers. Training at each health care facility is mandatory, and documentation of participation is required by OSHA.

- **Personal Protective Equipment (PPE):** Personal protective equipment covers the employee when treating patients and includes gloves, gowns, masks, and goggles. When bodily fluids are involved in patient care, the more a health care employee is covered, the less chance for exposure. The PPE provides the employee coverage so he or she does not contract bodily fluids, including saliva or blood. OSHA requires extra protection to reduce exposure and keep employees safe.

- **Hepatitis B Vaccine:** Due to the risk of exposure and the possibility of spreading, hepatitis B needs to be contained. OSHA has created a regulation that requires the hepatitis B vaccine be made available to all health care employees within a given time period—usually about 10 days. This allows the employee protection to reduce the risk of contracting hepatitis B from patients.

- **Postexposure Follow-Up:** Postexposure follow-up is to be given to any employee who has been exposed to hazardous materials, such as blood-borne pathogens or any other fluids. After such exposure, the health care employee is urged to seek medical attention—depending on the type of exposure—to be monitored. Follow-up is at no charge to the exposed employee and includes medical evaluation, testing, prophylactic treatment, counseling, and further follow-up. Information must be reported back to the health care facility to document for OSHA; however, the information in the postexposure plan regarding the employee is always confidential.

- **Labels, Signs, and Material Safety Data Sheets (MSDS) Information:** Labels and signs are a way of visually indicating a hazardous material, such as blood, chemicals, or infectious materials. MSDS forms are from companies and suppliers on items that could be hazardous if not used correctly, such as testing materials and

Disease	Agent	Transmission	Symptoms	Diagnosis	Treatment	Comments	Patient Education
Acquired immunodeficiency syndrome (AIDS)	Human immunodeficiency virus (HIV)	• Bloodborne • Sexual contact • Intrauterine • Lactation	Opportunistic infections, **lymphadenopathy**, fatigue, malaise, fever	CD4 percentage level less than 14%	Palliative care and treatment for **opportunistic infections**, antiviral drugs	World Health Organization (WHO) estimates 36 million people infected with HIV	1. Careful infection control and **asepsis** to reduce contact with pathogens that cause opportunistic infections 2. Use of latex condoms in conjunction with effective spermicide 3. Support groups/education
Hepatitis B	Hepatitis B virus (HBV)	• Bloodborne • Sexual contact • Intrauterine • Human bites	Fatigue, malaise, **anorexia**, headache, liver tenderness and enlargement, fever, jaundice	Serum antibody tests; liver function studies elevated	Immunization of all those at risk for exposure; palliative therapy, monitor bilirubin levels, bed rest, frequent low-fat, high-carbohydrate diet for those infected	May lead to liver cancer or cirrhosis; 100 times more infectious than AIDS; report to public health authorities	1. Follow-up required to monitor liver function studies 2. Close personal contacts of patient should receive HB vaccine or HBIG (HB immunoglobulin) 3. Teach infection control to patient to prevent spread to close contacts 4. Avoid alcohol, sedatives, or aspirin during acute phase
Hepatitis C	Hepatitis C virus (HCV)	• Tattooing • Body piercing • Sexual contact • Blood and body fluids • Needle exchange	Few or none for years or decades; progresses to chronic liver disease	Blood test for HCV; liver enzymes; liver biopsy	Medication combination of peginterferon with ribavirin; liver transplant	Most serious type of hepatitis; 5 million cases in the United States; may surpass mortality rate of AIDS if not contained; unknown to general public; progresses to cirrhosis or cancer; no vaccine	1. Ultimate defense is knowledge and awareness 2. Use protection during sexual contact 3. Be aware that ink used for tattooing can be contaminated with the virus 4. Do not use other people's toothbrush or razor 5. Do not donate blood 6. Zero alcohol consumption because of liver stress 7. Get hepatitis A and B vaccines 8. Testing is important

FIGURE 11-8 Examples of Common Infectious Diseases

Disease	Agent	Transmission	Symptoms	Diagnosis	Treatment	Comments	Patient Education
Tuberculosis (TB)	Mycobacterium tuberculosis bacillus	• Inhalation of contaminated airborne mucous droplets • Possibly ingestion	Productive cough, fatigue, fever, weight loss (older adults: behavior changes, anorexia, weight loss), night sweats	Sputum culture for M. tuberculosis, Mantoux skin test (PPD), chest X-ray, pleural needle biopsy	Antituberculosis agents, airborne transmission-based precautions, until drug agents started	Increase in incidence of TB, especially among persons with AIDS and the homeless; may be drug resistant; health care professionals should have annual skin testing; report outbreaks	1. Encourage hand washing and proper sputum tissue disposal 2. Promote compliance with medications 3. Encourage close contacts to have skin tests 4. Well-balanced diet
Gastroenteritis	Bacteria or viruses (i.e., staphylococci, Clostridium, botulinum, E. coli, shigella)	• Ingestion of contaminated food or water	Nausea, intestinal cramps, vomiting, diarrhea, dehydration, respiratory failure, death	Culture of feces, vomitus, or suspected food or water	Fluid balance restoration, medications, emergency treatment as required	Report outbreaks to local authorities; especially dangerous in children and older adults	1. Teach proper food handling 2. Carefully washing hands before handling all food 3. Report to physician all signs of dehydration 4. Gastroenteritis usually communicable via feces for up to seven weeks after exposure
Influenza	Influenze viruses A, B, or C, haemophilus (bacteria)	• Inhalation • Aerosolized • Mucous droplets	Acute upper/lower respiratory infection, severe cough, fever, malaise, sore throat, **coryza**	Tissue culture of nasal or pharyngeal secretions	Palliative therapy, active immunization (annual vaccine recommended for persons at risk [older adults, heart patients] for complications from infection)	Report cases to local health authority; may be fatal in older adults and children; may cause meningitis; may easily become epidemic	1. Bed rest for two to three days after fever decline 2. Force fluids 3. Report signs of secondary infections (pneumonia, otitis media) 4. Vaccine available
Chickenpox	Varicella-zoster virus	• Direct and indirect contact with respiratory droplets	Sudden-onset fever, malaise, **maculopapular-vesicular** skin rash	Vesicular fluid tissue culture during first three days after eruption; serology: increased anti-bodies two weeks after rash; **lesion** appearance characteristic of varicella	**Acyclovir** helpful to reduce severity of disease; zoster immunoglobulin (ZIG) for high-risk persons only within 96 hours of exposure; palliative therapy	Vaccine (varicella virus vaccine live) available in United States for children older than 12 months	1. Communicable one to two days before rash until lesions crust 2. Avoid scratching lesions to prevent secondary infection and scarring 3. Benadryl and calamine lotion for itch 4. Acetaminophen for fever

FIGURE 11-8 continued

Disease	Agent	Transmission	Symptoms	Diagnosis	Treatment	Comments	Patient Education
West Nile Virus	Virus	• Infected mosquito	Central nervous system; fever, headache, coma, convulsions, paralysis; 80% of people infected show no signs or symptoms	West Nile Virus IgM Capture ELIZA	None; supportive only	Potentially serious illness	1. Use insect repellent with DEET 2. Wear long sleeves and pants when outside, especially at dawn and dusk 3. Get rid of mosquito breeding sites by emptying standing water in flowerpots, buckets, and barrels 4. Keep children's pools empty and on their sides when not in use
Severe acute respiratory syndrome (SARS)	Virus	• Close person-to-person contact • Kissing • Sharing eating or drinking utensils • Perhaps respiratory droplets	High fever, headache, cough, shortness of breath, diarrhea	SARS serum antibodies validated by Centers for Disease Control and Prevention	None; supportive only; may treat pneumonia with anti-biotics but will not cure patient	Potentially serious illness; currently no known SARS transmissions; last transmission was in China, April 2004,;because no one knows if SARS will recur, early recognition of cases and appropriate infection control are essential to control outbreaks; Transmission-Based Precautions (Isolation): airborne and direct contact	1. Travel to a previously SARS-affected area (China, Hong Kong, or Taiwan) or close contact with an ill person who has such a travel history 2. A diagnosis of pneumonia raises the suspicion of exposure to SARS 3. Avoid close contact such as kissing, hugging, sharing of eating or drinking utensils

FIGURE 11-8 continued

even alcohol. MSDS forms should be accessible to health care employees if there is hazardous material on-site in the event there is an emergency and they need treatment for coming in contact with the material. The MSDS allows the treating providers to identify the type of treatment needed if necessary and then educate employees on the expectations of possible side effects.

- **Training:** Employers must provide extensive training to health care employees upon initial hiring, when new products or procedures are implemented, and then annually. The training will include the dangers of blood-borne pathogens, preventive practices, and postexposure procedures. The information must reference OSHA requirements and the results of noncompliance for the health care facility and employee. Training should be documented when the employee attends, and employees need to fully understand or communicate with a compliance officer for anything they are unfamiliar with. The manager is responsible for ensuring that the employees understand OSHA requirements as well as having everyone attend future training as required.

- **Recordkeeping:** Detailed records are kept on employees, including training and reporting injuries, such as a sharps injury log. Recordkeeping is the method in which OSHA justifies compliance, and the health care facility can demonstrate compliance during an investigation. OSHA is not able to be present at the health care facilities; therefore, they rely on documentation. The training requirements, engineering, and work practice controls as well as postexposure follow-up are all monitored by OSHA. In addition, reporting exposure or injury is also required and should be documented appropriately. Recordkeeping is vital to the health care facility, and the manager is responsible for ensuring that recordkeeping practices are in place and easily understood by all employees.

The manager will be responsible for training and understanding the guidelines for OSHA during his or her hiring process. Maintaining the current updates will also be part of the job. The complete details and information can be found on OSHA's website at http://www.osha.gov. When managers get the updates, they are required to update providers and other staff members immediately to remain compliant with OSHA. If they are noncompliant, there is a chance they could face penalties, jail time, or even closure of the health care facility; therefore, ongoing training and education are necessary.

SUMMARY

- CLIA has established standards for the performance of laboratory testing. The physician's office and outpatient settings must apply for one of the levels of CLIA-impacted testing. In order to obtain a CLIA number, the staff and health care facility must be qualified. The CLIA number, given after approval of the application, must be placed on the insurance claim form.

- CMS publishes rules, regulations, and guidance for all health care facilities that treat Medicare and Medicaid patients. All regulations are mandatory, and Medicare will perform audits to ensure they are being followed. The standards are implemented to avoid fraud and the abuse of Medicare and Medicaid patients.

- The Joint Commission establishes standards that hospitals, long-term care facilities, and other health care settings should follow. Enrollment is voluntary, and health care facilities that enter into a relationship with The Joint Commission show a higher standard for quality patient care and respect.

- The OIG develops projects each year in the areas of audit, inspections, and potential areas of fraud or misconduct. According to the previous year's billing practices, a decision is made to monitor the area of weakness. A work plan is established, and the health care facility is obligated to monitor the functions under review.

- OSHA establishes practice controls to protect workers from hazards during employment. Standards are mandatory, and staff must be trained on all policies and procedures. If the health care facility is found noncompliant with the OSHA expectations, there is potential for fines, jail time, and even closure of the health care facility.

REVIEW EXERCISES

TRUE OR FALSE

1. _____ CLIA established standards for performing lab tests in a physician's office

2. _____ Any physician can perform any test with a certificate of waiver.

3. _____ Medicare is just an insurance company for people over 65.

4. _____ The Joint Commission has regulations that impact many health care facilities.

5. _____ The work plan is published by The Joint Commission.

6. _____ The hepatitis B immunization must be offered to all employees.

7. _____ Personal protective equipment includes gloves, masks, and gowns.

8. _____ The Joint Commission standards do not apply to nursing homes.

9. _____ All health care settings have the option of complaining about regulations.

10. _____ Only managers need to know about regulations.

MATCHING

A CLIA

B PPE

C Waiver

D OSHA

E QW

F PPMP

G Work Plan

H Exposure Plan

I MSDS

J The Joint Commission

1. _____ Performing a urinalysis is considered this type of testing.

2. _____ Designed to protect the employee against hazards or injury.

3. _____ A-two digit modifier attached to a CPT code to indicate its waived category status.

4. _____ Gloves, masks, gowns, and goggles.

5. _____ Tests with a microscopic component.

6. _____ Established standards for laboratory testing.

7. _____ A yearly outline of areas to be scrutinized for fraudulent activities.

8. _____ A written plan to protect employees from exposure to hazardous materials.

9. _____ A form that lists the hazardous substances in materials.

10. _____ Publishes standards for many health care settings.

CRITICAL THINKING ACTIVITIES

ACTIVITY 1

When it comes to OSHA regulations, there are requirements for different types of controls that must be introduced to the health care facility. Explain the difference between engineering controls and work practice controls. List five of each to identify what is involved.

Difference: _____

_____

Engineer Controls	Work Practice Controls
1. _____	1. _____
2. _____	2. _____
3. _____	3. _____
4. _____	4. _____
5. _____	5. _____

ACTIVITY 2

As a manager, there is an approval process that must be understood when performing laboratory tests at the health care facility. Identify the order of the steps 1-8 when obtaining CLIA approval and a CLIA number. Use 1 for the first step and 8 for the final step.

_____ Code the CLIA approved tests and bill the insurance carrier.

_____ Receive a CLIA approval number.

_____ Provide appropriate signatures if you are not the signer of the application.

_____ Add the CLIA number to CMS-1500 claim form block 23.

_____ Mail the application and all attachments to CMS.

_____ Download the application from online or obtain it from CLIA.

_____ Perform CLIA-approved tests.

_____ Attach appropriate documents to the application for proof of credentials.

ACTIVITY 3

Identify the following rules or regulations with its affiliation. Use an O for OSHA or a C for CMS. There may be some that do not require an answer.

1. _____ CLIA

2. _____ MSDS

3. _____ Recordkeeping

4. _____ The Joint Commission

5. _____ PPMP

6. _____ Federal register

7. _____ Mohs surgery

8. _____ PPE

9. _____ Exposure plan

10. _____ Certificate of waiver

CRITICAL THINKING QUESTIONS

1. Discuss the importance of obtaining a Clinical Lab Improvement Act (CLIA) number prior to performing labs in the health care facility. Include the risk of fines, jail time, or closure.

2. Debate pros and cons of performing laboratory or radiology tests in a small physician's office. Explain how the decision can affect the revenue cycle if the tests do not get covered or generate enough income.

3. Discuss the Centers for Medicare & Medicaid Services (CMS) regulations and why requirements are different for the ambulatory surgical centers (ASC) than for the physician's office.

4. Identify the benefits of a hospital being accredited by The Joint Commission. Review the standards they require and how they pertain to patient care.

WEB ACTIVITIES

1. Research the Office of Inspector General (OIG) website (http://www.oig.hhs.gov) to list the areas of concern for Medicare physicians and other health professionals as described in the current work plan.

2. On The Joint Commission website (http://www.jointcommission.org) access the current year's patient safety goals and then discuss two of them.

3. Search for an updated list of tests that can be found on the Centers for Disease Control and Prevention (CDC) website (http://www.cdc.gov). In the search box, type CLIA. Search for PPMP tests and then list five that need this type of certification.

CHAPTER 12

COMPLIANCE WITH REGULATORY AGENCIES

MANAGING

Chapter 12 will discuss managing compliance with regulatory agencies by identifying what the manager should know as it applies to the specific health care setting in which he or she is employed. The review of all regulations will be included, keeping in mind different healthcare settings have different regulations. This chapter will also highlight activities that a manager will need to know relating to the regulatory agencies, including the risk of a fine or jail time if not in compliance.

OBJECTIVES

Upon completion of this chapter, the student will be able to:

- Review a CLIA application for laboratory testing.
- Review the OIG work plan.
- Ensure the safety of staff in the workplace by complying with OSHA standards.
- State the patient safety goals, which are part of The Joint Commission standards each year.

KEY TERMS

- Action plan
- Biohazards containers
- Clinical Lab Improvement Act (CLIA)
- Exposure plan
- Eyewash station
- The Joint Commission
- National coverage determination (NCD)
- National patient safety goals (NPSG)
- Office of Inspector General (OIG)
- Occupational Safety and Health Administration (OSHA)
- Personal protective equipment (PPE)
- Provider
- Sentinel event
- Sharps container
- Work plan

INTRODUCTION

As a manager, knowing the regulations and regulatory agencies that impact your health care setting is of the utmost importance. During training, the responsibility to comply with regulations will be reviewed. Establishing a plan or inquiring about a current plan is in your best interest and should be done immediately. Compliance with the regulatory agencies, especially government agencies, is mandatory and should be addressed immediately.

Developing a compliance plan is the best approach. After you review the requirements from each agency, the current compliance plan should be referenced. In a health care facility where there is no compliance plan, seeking professional advice about developing a plan would prove beneficial. In addition, you should realize that health care facilities that are noncompliant may face penalties or jail time if necessary. As we review the information necessary to comply with regulations, keep in mind that not all the regulations apply to your facility and you may have to adjust the compliance plan accordingly.

CLINICAL LAB IMPROVEMENT ACT (CLIA)

In certain health care facilities is a desire to perform laboratory tests for patients. With primary care physicians or pediatricians, having a laboratory perform services and procedures will allow the providers to diagnose and treat patients during their encounters. Doing the laboratory tests on-site allows for immediate treatment of a problem that may be diagnosed. For example, a pediatrician can perform a strep test and order antibiotics prior to the patient's discharge. In this case, the treatment of the patient is during the encounter, and calling the patient afterward is not necessary. When circumstances arise that may benefit from laboratory testing on-site, management and providers must decide if this is the right plan of action for the health care facility. After you investigate the costs of equipment as well as reimbursement, if a determination is made to pursue an on-site laboratory, the next step needs to be taken.

For health care facilities to perform clinical laboratory tests, an application for certification form must be completed. Management must complete the application and include all necessary information required. The types of laboratory procedures physicians want to perform on-site determine how much information is needed. For example, if the health care facility wants to perform small surgeries with pathology, as discussed in Chapter 11, there needs to be an approved laboratory employee qualified to perform such tests. For this to occur, appropriate paperwork will have to be forwarded as proof of the qualifications. Understanding the entire process and necessary steps is important for the manager as he or she decides to pursue laboratory testing in the health care facility. In addition, you should know what type of laboratory testing your facility wants to perform so the application is completed accurately the first time. Figure 12-1 shows a sample of the application. The form can be downloaded from http://www.cms.gov/clia; scroll down to **Clinical Lab Improvement Act (CLIA)** and then click "CLIA."

Upon acceptance, the health care facility and provider will be assigned a CLIA number by CMS. The manager must keep track of the CLIA number, as this needs to be used on claims that go to the insurance carrier. By identifying your CLIA number, the claims will be processed timely for reimbursement. In addition, if there is ever an audit or a need for additional laboratory approvals, maintaining the CLIA number will allow any further activity to be conducted easily. Applying for a CLIA number for basic laboratory testing may be what you want at first, but then there may be a need to expand the CLIA approval. Maintain all records in order to set up a compliance plan for the laboratory, training all staff as appropriate to perform laboratory tests. Always remain in compliance with documentation, safety regulations, and a detailed compliance plan available at all times.

DEPARTMENT OF HEALTH AND HUMAN SERVICES
CENTERS FOR MEDICARE & MEDICAID SERVICES

Form Approved
OMB No. 0938-0581

CLINICAL LABORATORY IMPROVEMENT AMENDMENTS (CLIA)
APPLICATION FOR CERTIFICATION

I. GENERAL INFORMATION

☒ Initial Application ☐ Survey

☐ Change in Certification Type ☐ Other Changes

CLIA Identification Number

_____ D_____
(If an initial application leave blank, a number will be assigned)

Facility Name

Your Practice

Federal Tax Identification Number
000 X 42000

Telephone No. *(Include area code)* Fax No. *(Include area code)*
999.88XX

Facility Address — *Physical Location of Laboratory* *(Building, Floor, Suite if applicable.)* Fee Coupon/Certificate will be mailed to this Address unless mailing address is specified

123 main st

Mailing/Billing Address *(If different from street address, include attention line and/or Building, Floor, Suite)*

Number, Street *(No P.O. Boxes)*
Your Town, USA 00000

Number, Street

City	State	ZIP Code

City	State	ZIP Code

Name of Director *(Last, First, Middle Initial)*

For Office Use Only
Date Received _____

II. TYPE OF CERTIFICATE REQUESTED *(Check one)*

☒ Certificate of Waiver *(Complete Sections I–VI and IX–X)*

☐ Certificate for Provider Performed Microscopy Procedures *(PPM) (Complete Sections I–X)*

☐ Certificate of Compliance *(Complete Sections I–X)*

☐ Certificate of Accreditation (Complete Sections I through X) and indicate which of the following organization(s) your laboratory is accredited by for CLIA purposes, or for which you have applied for accreditation for CLIA purposes

☐ The Joint Commission ☐ AOA ☐ AABB
☐ CAP ☐ COLA ☐ ASHI

If you are applying for a Certificate of Accreditation, you must provide evidence of accreditation for your laboratory by an approved accreditation organization for CLIA purposes or evidence of application for such accreditation within 11 months after receipt of your Certificate of Registration.

According to the Paperwork Reduction Act of 1995, no persons are required to respond to a collection of information unless it displays a valid OMB control number. The valid OMB control number for this information collection is 0938-0581. The time required to complete this information collection is estimated to average 30 minutes to 2 hours per response, including the time to review instructions, search existing data resources, gather the data needed, and complete and review the information collection. If you have any comments concerning the accuracy of the time estimate(s) or suggestions for improving this form, please write to: CMS, Attn: PRA Reports Clearance Officer, 7500 Security Boulevard, Baltimore, Maryland 21244-1850.

Form CMS-116 (10/07)

Page 1 of 4

FIGURE 12-1 Application for Certification, pages 1-4

III. TYPE OF LABORATORY *(Check the one most descriptive of facility type)*

- ☐ 01 Ambulance
- ☐ 02 Ambulatory Surgery Center
- ☐ 03 Ancillary Testing Site in Health Care Facility
- ☐ 04 Assisted Living Facility
- ☐ 05 Blood Bank
- ☐ 06 Community Clinic
- ☐ 07 Comp. Outpatient Rehab Facility
- ☐ 08 End Stage Renal Disease Dialysis Facility
- ☐ 09 Federally Qualified Health Center

- ☐ 10 Health Fair
- ☐ 11 Health Main. Organization
- ☐ 12 Home Health Agency
- ☐ 13 Hospice
- ☐ 14 Hospital
- ☐ 15 Independent
- ☐ 16 Industrial
- ☐ 17 Insurance
- ☐ 18 Intermediate Care Facility for Mentally Retarded
- ☐ 19 Mobile Laboratory
- ☐ 20.Pharmacy
- ☒ 21 Physician Office

- ☐ 22 Practitioner Other *(Specify)*
  _____
- ☐ 23 Prison
- ☐ 24 Public Health Laboratories
- ☐ 25 Rural Health Clinic
- ☐ 26 School/Student Health Service
- ☐ 27 Skilled Nursing Facility/ Nursing Facility
- ☐ 28 Tissue Bank/Repositories
- ☐ 29 Other *(Specify)*
  _____

IV. HOURS OF LABORATORY TESTING *(List times during which **laboratory testing** is performed in HH:MM format)*

	SUNDAY	MONDAY	TUESDAY	WEDNESDAY	THURSDAY	FRIDAY	SATURDAY
FROM:		4	8	10	9	8	8
TO:		5	7	8	6	2	1

(For multiple Sites, attach the additional information using the same format.)

V. MULTIPLE SITES *(must meet one of the regulatory exceptions to apply for this provision)*

Are you applying for the multiple site exception?

☒ No. If no, go to section VI.   ☐ Yes. If yes, complete remainder of this section.

Indicate which of the following regulatory exceptions applies to your facility's operation.

1. Is this a laboratory that has temporary testing sites?

   ☐ Yes ☒ No

2. Is this a not-for-profit or Federal, State or local government laboratory engaged in limited (not more than a combination of 15 moderate complexity or waived tests per certificate) public health testing and filing for a single certificate for multiple sites?

   ☐ Yes ☒ No

   If yes, provide the number of sites under the certificate _____ and list name, address and test performed for each site below.

3. Is this a hospital with several laboratories located at contiguous buildings on the same campus within the same physical location or street address and under common direction that is filing for a single certificate for these locations?

   ☐ Yes ☒ No

   If yes, provide the number of sites under this certificate _____ and list name or department, location within hospital and specialty/subspecialty areas performed at each site below.

If additional space is needed, check here ☐ and attach the additional information using the same format.

NAME AND ADDRESS/LOCATION		TESTS PERFORMED/SPECIALTY/SUBSPECIALTY
Name of laboratory or Hospital Department		
Address/Location *(Number, Street, Location if applicable)*		
City, State, ZIP Code	Telephone Number ( )	
Name of laboratory or Hospital Department		
Address/Location *(Number, Street, Location if applicable)*		
City, State, ZIP Code	Telephone Number ( )	

FIGURE 12-1 continued

In the next three sections, indicate testing performed and annual test volume.

VI. WAIVED TESTING

Indicate the estimated TOTAL ANNUAL TEST volume for all waived tests performed _1000_
☐ Check if no waived tests are performed.

VII. PPM TESTING

Indicate the estimated TOTAL ANNUAL TEST volume for all PPM tests performed _____

For laboratories applying for certificate of compliance or certificate of accreditation, also include PPM test volume in the "total estimated test volume" in section VIII.
☒ Check if no PPM tests are performed

VIII. NONWAIVED TESTING (*Including PPM testing*)

If you perform testing other than or in addition to waived tests, complete the information below. If applying for one certificate for multiple sites, the total volume should include testing for ALL sites.

Place a check(✓)in the box preceding each specialty/subspecialty in which the laboratory performs testing. Enter the estimated annual test volume for each specialty. Do not include testing not subject to CLIA, waived tests, or tests run for quality control, calculations, quality assurance or proficiency testing when calculating test volume. (For additional guidance on counting test volume, see the information included with the application package.)

If applying for a Certificate of Accreditation, indicate the name of the Accreditation Organization beside the applicable specialty/subspecialty for which you are accredited for CLIA compliance. (The Joint Commission, AOA, AABB, CAP, COLA or ASHI)

SPECIALTY/ SUBSPECIALTY	ACCREDITING ORGANIZATION	ANNUAL TEST VOLUME	SPECIALTY/ SUBSPECIALTY	ACCREDITING ORGANIZATION	ANNUAL TEST VOLUME
HISTOCOMPATIBILITY		_____	**HEMATOLOGY**		_____
☐ Transplant	_____		☐ Hematology	_____	
☐ Nontransplant	_____				
			IMMUNOHEMATOLOGY		_____
MICROBIOLOGY		_____	☐ ABO Group & Rh Group	_____	
☐ Bacteriology	_____		☐ Antibody Detection (transfusion)	_____	
☐ Mycobacteriology	_____				
☐ Mycology	_____		☐ Antibody Detection (nontransfusion)	_____	
☐ Parasitology	_____				
☐ Virology	_____		☐ Antibody Identification	_____	
			☐ Compatibility Testing		
DIAGNOSTIC IMMUNOLOGY		_____			
☐ Syphilis Serology	_____		**PATHOLOGY**		_____
☐ General Immunology	_____		☐ Histopathology	_____	
			☐ Oral Pathology	_____	
CHEMISTRY		_____	☐ Cytology	_____	
☐ Routine	_____				
☒ Urinalysis	_____		**RADIOBIOASSAY**		_____
☐ Endocrinology	_____		☐ Radiobioassay	_____	
☐ Toxicology	_____				
			CLINICAL CYTOGENETICS		_____
			☐ Clinical Cytogenetics	_____	

TOTAL ESTIMATED ANNUAL TEST VOLUME _____

Form CMS-116 (10/07)

FIGURE 12-1 continued

IX. TYPE OF CONTROL

VOLUNTARY NONPROFIT
01 Religious Affiliation
02 Private
03 Other _____
(Specify)

FOR PROFIT
04 Proprietary

GOVERNMENT
05 City
06 County
07 State

08 Federal
09 Other Government
_____
(Specify)

X. DIRECTOR AFFILIATION WITH OTHER LABORATORIES

If the director of this laboratory serves as director for additional laboratories that are separately certified, please complete the following:

CLIA NUMBER	NAME OF LABORATORY

ATTENTION: READ THE FOLLOWING CAREFULLY BEFORE SIGNING APPLICATION

Any person who intentionally violates any requirement of section 353 of the Public Health Service Act as amended or any regulation promulgated thereunder shall be imprisoned for not more than 1 year or fined under title 18, United States Code or both, except that if the conviction is for a second or subsequent violation of such a requirement such person shall be imprisoned for not more than 3 years or fined in accordance with title 18, United States Code or both.

Consent: The applicant hereby agrees that such laboratory identified herein will be operated in accordance with applicable standards found necessary by the Secretary of Health and Human Services to carry out the purposes of section 353 of the Public Health Service Act as amended. The applicant further agrees to permit the Secretary, or any Federal officer or employee duly designated by the Secretary, to inspect the laboratory and its operations and its pertinent records at any reasonable time and to furnish any requested information or materials necessary to determine the laboratory's eligibility or continued eligibility for its certificate or continued compliance with CLIA requirements.

SIGNATURE OF OWNER/DIRECTOR OF LABORATORY *(Sign in ink)*	DATE

Form CMS-116 (10/07)

© Cengage Learning 2013

FIGURE 12-1 continued

CENTERS FOR MEDICARE & MEDICAID SERVICES (CMS)

There are many programs and regulations within CMS. Although CMS is a governmental program, contracting with CMS to become a **provider** is when you have to follow its regulations. However, CMS does set the stage for other insurance carriers and knowing the expectations of CMS are important for a health care facility manager. When you work in a health care facility, CMS regulations will be discussed in detail on an ongoing basis and especially when updates are made.

For those facilities that provide services to Medicare patients, you should know about the programs and their purposes. When treating patients with a governmental insurance policy that is under CMS jurisdiction, the health care facility must identify the coverage allowances and give the most appropriate treatment options. For example, if diagnostic testing is being considered but the patient does not have coverage, he or she can be informed of the potential balance. Management and the health care providers will work with patients to educate them regarding CMS programs and regulations.

Some of these many programs include:

- Programs about Medicare, such as enrollment and prescription drugs
- Programs about Medicaid, such as coverage and enrollment
- Programs related to the Children's Health Insurance Program (CHIP), such as low-cost health insurance for children
- Regulations and guidance manuals, including national coverage determination policies
- Training programs
- Education programs through the Medicare learning network
- Additional information about HIPAA, CLIA diseases, and current news

National coverage determination (NCD) policies are a unified policy from Medicare on whether a service or procedure will be covered under CMS. Management will need to review NDCs on a regular basis for information on services and procedures pertinent to the health care facility. The Medicare website (http://www.cms.hhs.gov) provides links to coverages, policies, and HIPAA and CLIA information. Accessing the website is the best approach to obtaining current information due to the amount of information available on CMS policies and regulations. In addition, forms can also be downloaded as needed. Education and training are vital to understanding CMS; therefore, management, staff, and providers should be trained on a regular basis.

THE JOINT COMMISSION

The Joint Commission is involved with creating standards for health care facilities to follow in order to create a safe environment for patients. Participating with The Joint Commission is an accreditation that health care facilities must earn. Hospitals and long-term care facilities are two facilities that fall under regulations. Understanding The Joint Commission requirements is important to management in order to maintain the accreditation by creating policies and following standards on a daily basis. Management training should include the necessary information for any health care facility desiring to maintain accreditation under The Joint Commission. Training should include access to the standards and information on policy creation as it pertains to The Joint Commission.

You should realize that goals are revised every year and serve as a basis for measuring performance. Within the standards, you will find **national patient safety goals (NPSG)**, which is designed to help create a new method of changing something that can promote better patient care. Based on the goals for the current year, management will be responsible for developing policies that promote procedures to meet these goals.

The 2012 patient safety goals are designated for:

- Ambulatory care
- Behavioral health care

- Critical access hospitals
- Disease-specific care
- Home care
- Hospitals
- Laboratory
- Long-term care
- Office-based surgery

Some of these goals are aimed at correct patient identification, communication, medication safety, health care–associated infection, reducing patient falls, and the involvement of patients in their care. In 2012, one of the goals is to improve the effectiveness of communication. This goal especially refers to the taking of telephone orders for the reporting of critical test results. The rationale behind this goal is that ineffective communication is the most common cause of a **sentinel event** which occurs when the actions of an employee causes serious harm or death to a patient. Let us look at an example:

> A physician is waiting for important test results that will help to diagnose a patient's cause of severe chest pain. If the patient was having a heart attack but the test results were inadvertently recorded as negative, the patient will not get the care needed to treat the heart attack and avoid serious illness or death.

To ensure that information is correctly sent and received, the following actions should always take place. Management is responsible for developing policies to be followed by all staff.

Creating policies and procedures:

1. The staff person who is receiving the results of tests must document the following:

   Patient's name

   Date

   Test

   Test report

   Complete results

   Who reported those results

2. The results should be read back and confirmed as accurate.

3. Results are immediately reported to the physician, with the patient's record attached, to avoid a delay in diagnosis and treatment.

In-service training should be given initially and as needed. The importance of communication to be accurate, understood, confirmed, and relayed in a timely fashion cannot be emphasized enough.

The Joint Commission is also responsible for monitoring sentinel events as they occur. A sentinel event is considered to be an adverse outcome of a patient's illness or condition and is directly related to this condition. The Joint Commission has high standards, and with the risk of a sentinel event or the occurrence of one, it will initiate an investigation.

A sentinel event includes a wide range of situations, such as:

- Suicide while receiving care
- Surgery on the wrong person or wrong body part
- Leaving a foreign object in a patient after surgery
- Death of a full-term infant

- Infant discharged to the wrong family
- Falls resulting in death or permanent loss of function

When a sentinel event happens in the health care facility, an analysis report and plan must be created by management and submitted to The Joint Commission. The Joint Commission reviews the plan and follows up until it is satisfied that the **action plan** will prevent further events. Management will be responsible for implementing the plan and following protocol to meet the standards.

Let us look at this example:

A patient is admitted to a hospital for surgery. The patient falls, resulting in partial paralysis.

The steps the facility will have to take include:

1. What happened: Report the event.
2. Prepare an analysis that includes:
   a. Why
   b. What changes occurred
   c. Associated factors
   d. Risk factors
   e. Findings
   f. Resources used or needed
3. An action plan is created that includes;
   a. The changes to be implemented
   b. Who is responsible for implementing these changes
   c. A timeline for implementation
   d. Measure effectiveness: examples of testing this plan

The Joint Commission's framework for reviewing sentinel events:

What happened

Questions concerning what happened and details

Findings

Root cause

Action taken to reduce further incidents

Measure of effectiveness

To help prevent sentinel events, you should implement policies and procedures as well as offer in-service training. A template with the policy requirements could be developed if there is an option to do so. In addition, ongoing monitoring should be conducted to identify anyone who is not following directions and policies. Identifying any problems and being proactive will prevent future incidences and investigations from The Joint Commission.

OFFICE OF INSPECTOR GENERAL (OIG)

As discussed in Chapter 11, the **Office of Inspector General (OIG)** publishes a **work plan** every year that outlines the areas to be targeted in the next calendar year. By reviewing the current work plan for each year, the manager can review the policies and procedures of the facility, especially those areas to be targeted. Health care facilities have many regulations to follow, and management must be familiar with all requirements and create policies and procedures as necessary.

Previously, one of the areas targeted was the correct use of place of service (POS) codes.

As the manager, you should:

1. Review applicable place of service codes for your facility.
2. Review the explanation of benefits from the insurance companies.
3. Note any denials due to place of service codes being incorrect.
4. Cross-reference place of service codes with procedure codes and the name and address of the facility.
5. Plan an in-service training on how to code the place of service accurately.

Understanding the need for the OIG to create a work plan is important for managers, as they are attempting to create uniformity and accuracy with patient treatment. Identifying the areas of expected review allows management to be proactive in making changes on a regular basis. When the OIG sets up a work plan, it is creating its review from potential red flags and inappropriate billing. Immediate attention should be given to the OIG work plan in order to maintain compliance.

OCCUPATIONAL SAFETY AND HEALTH ADMINISTRATION (OSHA)

The purpose behind the **Occupational Safety and Health Administration (OSHA)** in the health care facility is to create an environment that allows for everyone to remain safe. Policies and procedures also need to be created for compliance with OSHA. OSHA expectations are different for every environment, and your expectations will be specific for the type of health care facility you are employed at. When researching OSHA requirements, you should understand that OSHA has set standards for every type of business. Careful consideration should be given to identifying the requirements necessary for your health care facility in order to ensure you have chosen the appropriate OSHA standards.

In 1984, OSHA first created safety standards for sterilization of the facility to reduce the exposure to hazards and create a cleaner environment. In 1991, OSHA issued guidelines for health care workers requiring employers to reduce exposure by providing personal protective equipment, free vaccinations, and protection against diseases that are blood borne, such as AIDS and hepatitis. To assist you and the health care facility in complying with OSHA standards, policies and procedures should be in place, along with checklists for compliance. In addition, an option should be given for employees to report to management if a violation has occurred. For those policies that have been updated, changed, or recently created, management is responsible for obtaining

The Work Practice or Standard	Completed	Not Completed	Comments	Other
Is PPE required for the employee's job provided?				
Employee trained in procedures for safety?				
Employee is trained in safety items, such as eyewash station or sharps containers?				
Employee trained in use of the fire extinguisher?				
Employee has had a hepatitis vaccination?				

© Cengage Learning 2013

FIGURE 12-2 An OSHA Checklist

new information and making appropriate adjustments as necessary. One approach to maintaining mandatory OSHA requirements and ensuring every employee is trained is to keep a separate OSHA binder with policies and checklists accessible to everyone.

An OSHA checklist could look something like Figure 12-2.

Training employees about OSHA is a requirement for a health care facility manager and should be ongoing, including directions on reporting violations to management. Whether the management does training or assigns qualified personnel to train staff, management is responsible and must do follow-up to ensure compliance. Health care facilities that are found in violation will be given penalties and possible shut down. There may be an opportunity to make corrections and request a revisit by OSHA to verify compliance and recover. However, keep in mind that violations can be reported by employees to OSHA and that possibility must be considered. OSHA standards should be monitored on a daily basis due to the high expectations. OSHA is very powerful, and OSHA safety standards must be met in every health care facility with continued education and training.

PERSONAL PROTECTIVE EQUIPMENT

Purchasing **personal protective equipment (PPE)** for the health care facility for staff is a requirement of OSHA. Because of the possibility of staff being exposed to bodily fluids while working with patients, PPE will allow staff to reduce any risk of transfer. PPE includes gloves, gowns, goggles, and other protective coverings that protect staff when treating patients. When you are drawing blood or giving vaccinations, gloves protect from blood transfer, and using goggles while checking a patient's mouth will reduce the spread of saliva. The type of equipment needed depends on the procedures or setting. Figures 12-3A and 12-3B shows different examples of using personal protective equipment.

SAFETY

Safety procedures developed by OSHA are in place to reduce risk of injury, protect staff from being injured, and provide assistance in the event of an accident. Safety procedures include the use of sharps containers, biohazard bags, and eyewash stations. A sharp is a needle, butterfly, or another "sharp" item. After a sharp is used on a patient, it is discarded in a puncture-proof

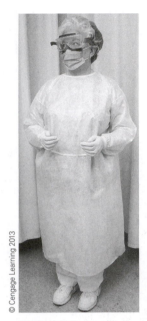

FIGURE 12-3A Employee Wearing Personal Protective Equipment: goggles, mask, gown, gloves

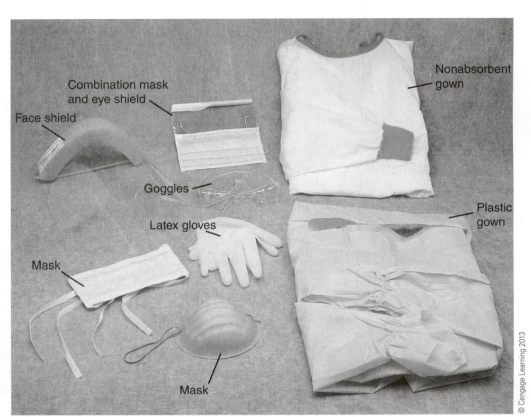

FIGURE 12-3B Personal Protective Equipment (PPE)

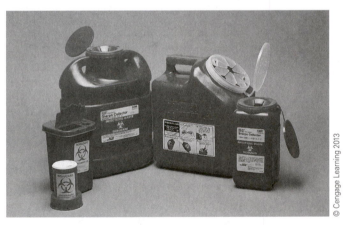

FIGURE 12-4 Examples of Sharps Container

sharps container. Figure 12-4 shows an example of a sharps container. These containers come in different sizes and shapes. They are usually bright red, but they could be other colors, such as yellow. They will have a biohazard label on them. Once a sharps container is full, a registered waste management company is contracted to remove it. A careful log and an invoice are kept of this activity, and management should follow up on this procedure daily.

BIOHAZARD BAG AND BOX

Another safety precaution required by OSHA is the use of **biohazard containers**, including safety bags or boxes for discarding hazardous material. A biohazards box is used for other hazardous

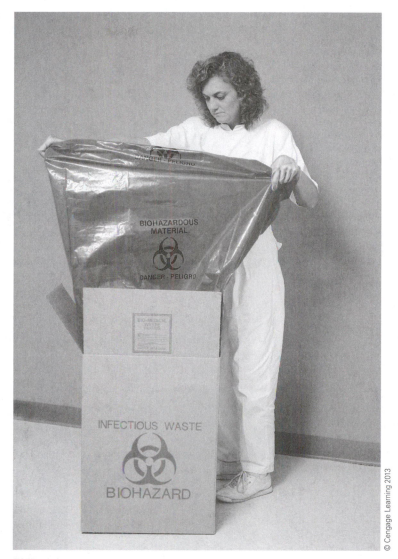

FIGURE 12-5 Biohazards Bag and Box

materials, such as blood-soaked gauze pads or any bandages off a patient's body. The box is lined with a red bag and also has a biohazard label on it.

When this box is full, it is weighed and labeled and is picked up by your contracted medical waste company, which is also carefully logged. Management must have a plan of action in place for someone to monitor the appropriate disposal of biohazard material. Figure 12-5 shows a biohazard box and bag.

EYEWASH STATION

According to OSHA, every health care facility—whether working with hazardous substances daily or not—should have an **eyewash station** in the event that a staff member has an accident. It is hooked directly to an existing faucet and should be visible and easily accessible. It is designed to aim water at both eyes in the event a hazardous substance gets in the eyes. The eyes should be flushed for 15–20 minutes and/or until the employee can get further help. In the event there is an accident and the eyewash is used, management must be notified immediately to address the situation. Figure 12-6 shows an eyewash station.

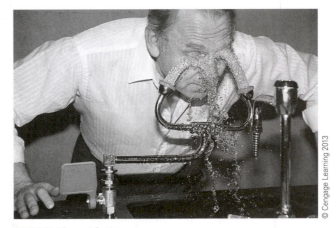

FIGURE 12-6 Eyewash Station

FIRE EXTINGUISHERS

Every health care facility must have fire extinguishers throughout the facility, as dictated by OSHA standards. Each employee—whether clinical or administrative—should be trained in identifying where they are and how to use them. A yearly in-service training session should be done on the use of these fire extinguishers. Management must expect all employees to use a fire extinguisher as necessary. Figure 12-7 shows a fire extinguisher.

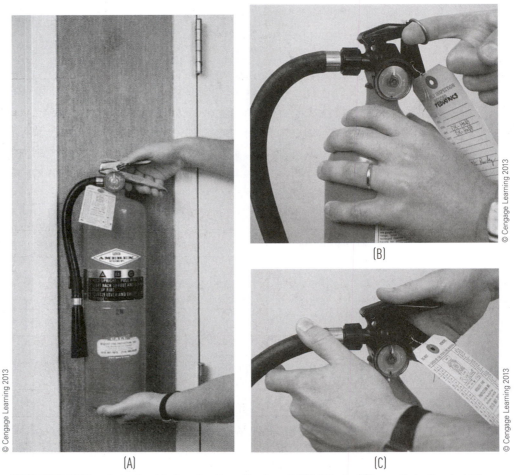

(A)

(B)

(C)

FIGURE 12-7 A-C (A) Know the location of the fire extinguisher and how to use it. (B) Pull the ring. (C) Squeeze the handle and point the hose at the base of the fire.

Category of Personnel	Do the Tasks This Personnel Perform Put Them at Risk of Coming in Contact With Blood, Urine, or Other Body Fluids?	Is There a Risk of Exposure for This Task?	What Measures Are in Place to Protect This Person?
• Medical • Clinical • Administrative • Clerk • Receptionist • Maintenance • Volunteer	• Yes • No • N/A	• Yes • No • N/A	• PPE • Masks, gloves • Sharps container • Immunization • Other

FIGURE 12-8 Sample Exposure Control Plan

© Cengage Learning 2013

EXPOSURE PLAN

An exposure control is also required by OSHA. This **exposure plan** includes identifying classifications of personnel and their risk of exposure to infectious materials. In this process, identifying tasks that personnel perform enables a plan to be put in place for the health care facility to protect employees when performing these tasks. Additionally, having a follow-up plan if employees are exposed to an infectious material is needed. A follow-up plan must include the steps to take as well as the requirement to get management involved in the event of an exposure. Figure 12-8 outlines the parts of an exposure plan.

Policies and procedures must be in place to train new personnel as well as update current employees in safety each year. These policies should include the purpose of protecting employees, copies of vaccination records, and the use of PPE and safety training. Policies and procedures will also be modified based on job descriptions. For example, a medical assistant will need training on the use of PPE and the use of sharps and sharps containers as well as biohazard bags and boxes. Nursing personnel will not only need to know what medical assistants do but also how to use the eyewash station and helping with hepatitis immunizations.

Administrative and billing personnel who do not have contact with patients and hazardous waste may only need to know how to use the fire extinguisher. Management will be responsible for organizing policies and procedures and developing a training curriculum to meet everyone's needs. The use of checklists will allow for easier monitoring and review within each department of the health care facility.

SUMMARY

- The manager is responsible for knowing what regulatory agencies and policies impact the health care setting in which he or she manages.

- CLIA regulations affect health care facilities performing laboratory testing. A facility must complete an application for certification and upon acceptance will be issued a CLIA number. This number is to be used on claim forms.

- CMS impacts all health care providers who treat Medicare and Medicaid patients. The many regulations and policies are posted on its website and are updated regularly. The manager must keep up with the changes for compliance.

- The Joint Commission rules and standards are updated yearly. The manager must be well versed on sentinel events, patient safety goals, and other areas applicable to the health care setting.

- The OIG publishes programs, activities, and a work plan each year. The OIG utilizes audit activities, inspections, and studies to evaluate potential areas of noncompliance in each health care setting.

- OSHA has mandatory standards and measures to protect health care employees against exposure to infectious materials. The manager must ensure training, safety measures, consistency, and safety precautions in the practices of the health care setting.

REVIEW EXERCISES

TRUE OR FALSE

1. _____ The 2012 patient safety goals included effective communication.

2. _____ A sentinel event can result in death.

3. _____ Effective information should be emphasized starting at orientation.

4. _____ An action plan for The Joint Commission must include a timeline and a testing of the plan.

5. _____ Birth of a live full-term infant is a sentinel event.

6. _____ A fire extinguisher should be in all health care facilities.

7. _____ An eyewash station is not required in health care facilities.

8. _____ A physician's office will be assigned a CLIA number for performing waived tests.

9. _____ When an adverse event happens, it must be reported to The Joint Commission.

10. _____ Billers need to know OSHA standards to work.

MATCHING

A **Ineffective Communication**

B **Sentinel Event**

C **Action Plan**

D **POS**

E **Work Plan**

F **Safety Procedures**

G **Exposure Plan**

H **OSHA**

I **NCD**

J **CMS**

1. _____ Includes changes, a timeline, and testing.

2. _____ Place of service codes.

3. _____ Sharps containers, biohazard bags and boxes, and an eyewash station.

4. _____ Classifies the risk of exposure to employees.

5. _____ Medicare.

6. _____ Hepatitis immunization.

7. _____ A 2012 patient safety goal.

8. _____ Adverse outcome.

9. _____ A unified policy from Medicare on billing a service.

10. _____ One of the most common causes of a sentinel event.

CRITICAL THINKING ACTIVITIES

ACTIVITY 1

Create a list of 10 safety standards that are monitored under OSHA and then explain the protection provided by each. This does not have to be in the medical field.

1. _____
2. _____
3. _____
4. _____
5. _____
6. _____
7. _____
8. _____
9. _____
10. _____

ACTIVITY 2

Put an "S" next to the situations that are considered sentinel events. If it is not a sentinel event, leave it blank.

1. _____ Diabetes in a child

2. _____ Suicide while in the psychiatric ward as inpatient

3. _____ Infection of wound

4. _____ Surgery on the wrong person

5. _____ Leaving sponge in patient after gallbladder removal

6. _____ Death of a full-term infant

7. _____ Rash due to antibiotics

8. _____ Surgery performed on right knee instead of left knee

9. _____ Patient fall in physician's office, resulting in a laceration

10. _____ Pneumonia due to bronchitis

ACTIVITY 3

Compare and contrast the three different plans that were discussed about compliance, the action plan, exposure plan, and work plan. Then, list five items under each that pertain to each plan.

Comparison: _____

_____

_____

_____

_____

Action Plan	Exposure Plan	Work Plan
1. _____	_____	_____
2. _____	_____	_____
3. _____	_____	_____
4. _____	_____	_____
5. _____	_____	_____

ACTIVITY 4

Identify three different CMS insurance programs that patients may have as an insurance policy. Discuss the ways in which the administrative and clinical staff may have to educate patients under the CMS program about their policy. Include resources that the staff can reference to assist in this process.

1. _____

2. _____

3. _____

Education by staff _____

_____

_____

_____

_____

_____

_____

_____

CRITICAL THINKING QUESTIONS

1. Explain the importance of creating policies, putting them in writing, and having a policy book available to staff at all times.

2. Discuss the potential for issues if compliance in-service training sessions are not provided immediately when changes are discovered. As a manager, define a timeline you feel is appropriate for in-service training to be held.

3. Discuss the purpose of national patient safety goals (NPSG) and who handles the implementation. Identify ways you know to create a better environment for patient safety.

4. Debate pros and cons of administrative personnel not having the same requirements as clinical personnel in OSHA standards. Use at least three situations where there could be a need for additional protection.

WEB ACTIVITIES

1. As a manager, the health care facility may benefit from being affiliated with The Joint Commission. Research The Joint Commission's website (http://www.jointcommission.org) to find out the enrollment qualifications and process.

2. Search online stores that sell safety equipment required by OSHA. Find pricing for at least 10 items required by OSHA for a health care facility and then compare those items with equipment on another online site. Choose the least expensive for the entire order or decide if it is worth it to order from two places.

3. Research the Centers for Medicare & Medicaid Services (CMS) website (http://www.cms.gov) for information on national coverage determination (NCD) policies. Check how the website works and then bookmark it to access it later.

THINK LIKE A MANAGER
CREATE YOUR PRACTICE

Using the templates found in Appendix B and the information presented in this unit, complete the following interactive exercises:

1. Write a policy and procedure for employee exposure control for compliance with OSHA standards.

2. Perform in-service training for a medical assistant to cover the OSHA exposure control requirements. Include clinical and administrative standards for your state.

3. Write a policy and procedure for effective communication when recording critical test results.

4. Perform in-service training for all employees on effective communication when recording critical test results.

5. Write a policy and procedure for developing an action plan after a sentinel event (such as a patient falling).

6. Write an exposure plan for protecting clinical employees from blood-borne pathogens. Include information necessary to keep employees safe from patient's blood or body fluids.

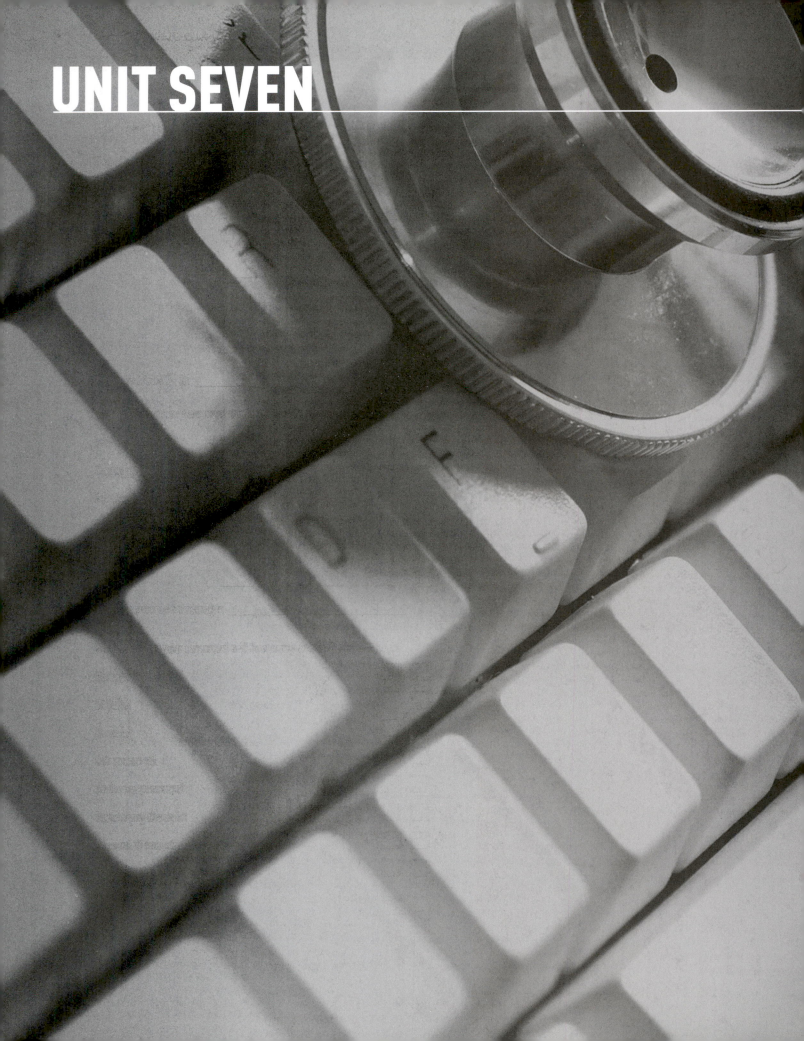

UNIT SEVEN

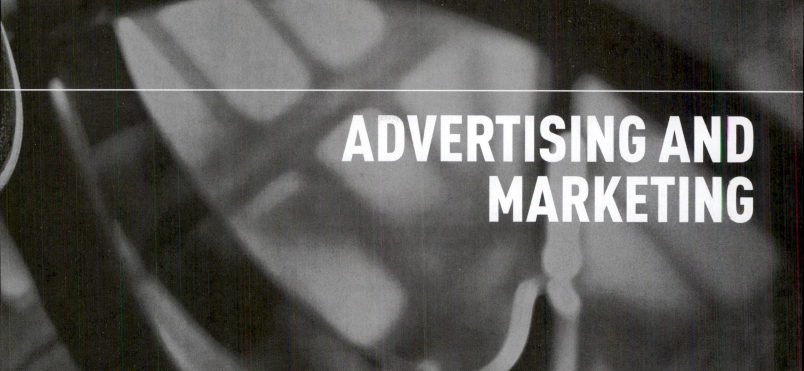

ADVERTISING AND MARKETING

THE SUCCESS OF a health care facility depends on advertising and marketing, and these techniques will be analyzed, along with the costs. Identifying the target audience and conducting a market analysis are important prior to pursuing an advertising technique to ensure the advertisement is appropriate. Expenses, options, and free advertising are all considered, but remember to include labor hours in your budget. Essentially, the bottom line is to get a return on your investment, and the health care facility manager will be responsible for maintaining advertising and marketing within the budget.

CHAPTER 13 Fundamentals: Advertising and Marketing

CHAPTER 14 Managing: Advertising and Marketing

ADVERTISING AND MARKETING

- Manage overall marketing and advertising as necessary for the health care facility.
- Conduct a market analysis when determining advertising needs.
- Determine a target audience when deciding to advertise or market.
- Manage choices about advertising techniques based on expenses.
- Educate employees about the advertising techniques and free advertising options.
- Manage advertising campaigns, designs, and costs.
- Manage an advertising budget as necessary.
- Develop a market plan
- Develop a patient survey form

CHAPTER 13

ADVERTISING AND MARKETING

FUNDAMENTALS

Chapter 13 will discuss the fundamentals of advertising and marketing in a medical practice, with the intent to increase revenue. Several advertising techniques will be identified, along with what is involved for each process. Identifying a plan that is appropriate to the health care facility will be discussed. In addition, the relationship between advertising and marketing will be reviewed with regards to how advertising can affect revenue.

OBJECTIVES

Upon completion of this chapter, the student will be able to:

- Understand the different forms of advertising.
- Discuss how advertising will market your practice.
- Understand how advertising will affect your revenue.
- Evaluate advertising and determine the success rate.

KEY TERMS

- Advertising
- Bottom line
- Brochure
- Design elements
- E-mail lists
- Labor hours
- Marketing
- Media advertising
- Networking
- Online social networks
- Professional organizations
- Target audience

INTRODUCTION

While you determine a location for the practice or provider, market research is important to be sure the business will be successful. Prior to establishing an office or clinic, you should determine the need for the type of provider in that area. The provider should have a marketing strategy to identify the market need and develop ideas of how to approach the area with success. **Marketing** is determining if the health care facility will be successful in that area and how it can advertise to promote its services. A market plan is a vital step to increasing revenue for the practice and should also include advertising techniques that can promote the health care facility.

ADVERTISING TECHNIQUES

Advertising is a way to generate information regarding the health care facility in order to promote future business. Many types of advertising techniques exist, and determining the appropriate techniques can be challenging. When you first approach advertising, be sure to have complete understanding of the options available. Research on advertising techniques and success rates in the area should be done beforehand. Discussing advertising opportunities with surrounding health care facilities will allow you to get an idea of which techniques may bring a positive outcome.

The type of facility should be considered prior to initiating advertising. As discussed in previous chapters, health care facilities can be very different in the way they operate their businesses, and their expectations in advertising will also be different. When determining the advertising techniques and marketing strategies for the health care facility, you must consider the patients seeking treatment as your **target audience** seeing the advertisement. The type of advertising should be timed appropriately according to the needs of your patient; for example, a primary care physician may advertise flu vaccinations around flu season for the surrounding area.

When reviewing advertising techniques you are considering, remember to keep in mind the purpose behind the advertising. There is an abundance of advertising, but knowing some key factors before deciding will allow for appropriate advertising techniques that will create a return on your investment. Realizing the positive and negatives of the advertising techniques will assist management in its decision.

Questions to ask about advertising that is available:

- Does the advertising company help with the design and setting up of the advertisement?
- How does it edit its written material?
- Is there a discount with a larger order or repeat business?
- Will it charge more for color advertising?
- Is anyone willing to join hands and advertise together to decrease expenses?
- Are we able to make changes to the advertising once we begin?
- If there is expiration, will there be an alert to let us renew the advertising if desired?

Consider the **bottom line**, which ultimately is the purpose of advertising for the health care facility, when you enter into a decision on the type of advertising. The appearance may be inexpensive, but spending money on something that will not work is quite expensive. It is not about what is going to save money but how it will generate revenue without losing the investment. Figure 13-1 shows the common marketing tools.

BROCHURES

Advertising within the health care facility can be done through a **brochure**, which is a written advertisement that provides information about the health care facility and its providers. Brochures should include some color and be easy to read in order to catch someone's attention and make him or her want to read it. Once attention has been grabbed, he or she will pick up the brochure to read the details. This should include the health care facility's information, such as office hours and locations, provider information, including credentials, and photos if possible. A careful approach should be taken when developing brochures because too much information can be overwhelming and too little information will be ineffective. When creating brochures to market your health care

Marketing	
Tool	**Potential Uses and Value**
Seminars	Can educate patients and provide good will in the community. All staff—administrative and clinical—can work as a team to organize, publicize, and deliver the seminars.
Brochures	Brochures are typically of two types: patient education brochures and brochures on office services. Can be simple 8-1/2" x 11" fact sheets, with text only, or more elaborate brochures folded to 4" x 9" that incorporate both text and graphics or photos. Both types of brochures are informative for patients and present a professional image of the ambulatory care setting.
Practice Web Site and E-zines	The practice Web site is an excellent means of promoting the practice. Personnel can be introduced, and procedures and technologies can be discussed. The E-zine approach is rapidly catching on as a promotional tool. It can be e-mailed to patients so it saves time and money. The patient may choose to view, delete, or save to read at a later time.
Newsletters	Newsletters can be produced on a biannual or quarterly basis and can form the nucleus of a marketing program. Because they are versatile tools, they can include a wide range of information from health-related articles to staff introductions to insurance updates. They should be sent to individuals on the office's mailing list and be available in the reception area.
Press Releases	Periodic press releases on new equipment, new staff, and expanded or remodeled office space can be a vital link to the local community.
Special Events	Special events are an effective way to join with other community organizations to promote wellness. They can include participation in health fairs, cosponsorship of a charity event, or an open house on the premises to acquaint the community with new services or equipment.

FIGURE 13-1 Marketing Tools

facility, network with others and review brochure information to get feedback on the success of their advertisements.

When a decision is made to use a brochure, the next step is to determine the type of brochure you want to use. With a brochure being used at your health care facility for existing patient, the information provided is usually more detailed information about the providers' credentials and background. However, if you are advertising to an outside market, then including more information about the health care facility is appropriate. With internal marketing, the patient already knows who you are and is searching for more information, whereas identifying the location and availability is better for external marketing.

Brochures can be developed in several ways: Here are a few examples:

- Three-fold
- Full sheet, 8x10
- Half sheet, 5x7
- Mailer

Some of the benefits to creating a brochure include the ability to create a brochure in your own facility, thereby saving on design costs, having the option to print on your own (which allows for immediate reproduction), and being able to edit often. Brochures are usually done as a permanent type of advertising and are only changed when necessary. Outside advertising agencies can also generate brochures and are also able to make changes. Using a brochure as a form of advertisement can be considered long-term advertising if management continues with the changes. They are a great source of information for your patients to learn more about the health care facility that is treating them. Figure 13-2 shows an example of brochures accessible to patients in the waiting area.

ONLINE

Another consideration for management when it comes to advertising is to use the computer to go online. With technology advancements, many businesses are utilizing the Internet due to low-cost or no-cost advertising. As with any advertising opportunities, there are positive and negative aspects. Some positive aspects include setup and monitoring for free if done by the health care

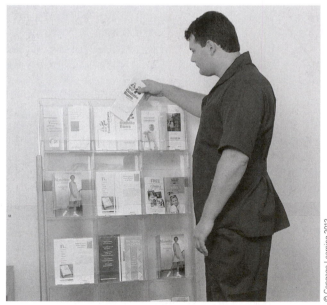

FIGURE 13-2 Brochures Accessible to Patients

© Cengage Learning 2013

facility, an easier way to reach larger target audiences, changes made easily by management, and termination of advertising in an instant. The negative aspects include the need for management to constantly monitor advertising and feedback, difficulty in getting to an appropriate target audience without assistance, and having to pay a lot of money to be at the top of the search engine's results.

Researching the online programs should be done ahead of time to ensure this is the direction to proceed, as there are many avenues to investigate. Many advertising companies have entered into the online advertising forum and developed criteria that will help businesses advertise online. Regardless of the type of advertising done, the health care facility must always remember the target audience and be sure it is reaching the appropriate people.

Questions to consider include:

- What is involved in setting up the initial online programs?
- Is someone monitoring feedback?
- How much time is needed to set up and monitor the online programs?
- Will there be reminders in place to remember what needs to be done?
- How many people will you reach when sending advertisements online?
- How many people will find the health care facility when searching online?

These questions are a good start to defining whether online advertising will work for your health care facility. The type of health care facility you are managing will determine whether online programs will work for you. For example, if you work in the field of geriatrics, your patients tend to be older and are not online as much; therefore, paying for advertisement online would not be cost effective. With every type of advertising, your target audience plays a role, and if management determines online is appropriate, then consideration should be given to e-mail and online advertisement.

E-Mail Lists

Due to the fact that e-mailing is free, many companies have developed **e-mail lists** of addresses in order to reach out to their clients in an effort to advertise. When you use an e-mail list, advertising can be done more frequently at no cost. If an event, free clinic, or health information seminar is being held, e-mail lists make it easier to get the information to your patients. Although patients may not be interested in the events you are advertising, your e-mail may be a reminder about an appointment they need to make. E-mail lists make it easier to stay in contact with patients on an ongoing basis. When dealing with e-mail lists as an advertising tool, the health care facility can purchase e-mail lists for a fee and reach a larger target audience or it can decide to only use its own patients at no cost.

In the health care facility, you would be required to gather e-mail addresses during the registration process. An approval to use e-mail as a form of communication would also be needed. Although this is not common in most health care facilities, some health care providers have taken this path with patients, and many are understanding and welcome the idea. In some instances, patients are able to use e-mail to address questions to the health care facility or provider, making it easier to get a response. If the health care facility is using e-mail for treatment purposes, it must also get approval to use the e-mail address for advertising. Figure 13-3 shows an example of an E-mail consent form. When working in a health care facility that uses e-mail as advertising, be sure to have an e-mail policy in place for alerting your patients in advance.

Internet Advertising

Internet-based advertising has grown tremendously over the last couple of years, and health care facilities are beginning to venture in this direction. There are many opportunities for Internet advertising, and research must be done to determine the most appropriate method. With

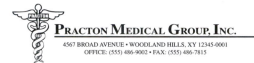

PRACTON MEDICAL GROUP, INC.

4567 BROAD AVENUE • WOODLAND HILLS, XY 12345-0001
OFFICE: (555) 486-9002 • FAX: (555) 486-7815

Fran Practon, M.D.
Gerald Practon, M.D.

CONDITIONS FOR THE USE OF E-MAIL

Provider will use reasonable means to protect the security and confidentiality of electronic mail (e-mail) information sent and received. Provider cannot guarantee the security and confidentiality of e-mail communication, and will not be liable for improper disclosure of confidential information that is not caused by provider's intentional misconduct. Therefore, patients must consent to the use of e-mail for patient information. Consent to the use of e-mail includes agreement with the following conditions:

1. All e-mail messages to or from the patient concerning diagnosis or treatment will be printed and made part of the patient's medical record. Because they are a part of the medical record, other individuals authorized to access the medical record, such as staff and billing personnel, will have access to those e-mail messages.
2. Provider will not forward e-mail messages to independent third parties without the patient's prior written consent, except as authorized or required by law.
3. Provider cannot guarantee that any particular e-mail message will be read and responded to within any particular period of time. The patient shall not use e-mail for medical emergencies or other time-sensitive matters.
4. It is the patient's responsibility to follow up and/or schedule an appointment if warranted.

ACKNOWLEDGMENT AND AGREEMENT

I acknowledge that I have read and fully understand the risks associated with the communication of e-mail between the provider and me, and consent to the conditions outlined herein. I agree to the instructions outlined herein and any other instructions that the provider may impose to communicate with patients by e-mail. Any questions I may have had were answered.

_____   _____
Patient's Signature   Date
Patient name:

_____
Patient address:

_____
Patient e-mail address:

_____

FIGURE 13-3 E-mail Consent Form

advancements in software and an attempt to make things easier, Internet advertising is becoming more user friendly. Health care facility managers can choose to enroll in Internet advertising at little or no cost if they monitor the process themselves. However, if they choose to have assistance, they can hire an Internet-based advertiser to enroll them and monitor their accounts.

The target audience will determine whether free or low-cost advertising monitored by the manager is sufficient for his or her needs. Some of the advertising forums that are used for free advertising include Facebook, Twitter, LinkedIn, and other social networks. Managers must be cautious about the way they portray themselves when choosing a social network because patients will be viewing their postings. One way to use social networks in a positive manner is to post event information that patients may be interested in, such as the cancer walk or flu vaccine clinic. Once a health care facility decides to enter a social network, you should keep the information up to date for patients.

Another Internet advertising tool is using pop-up ads, such as Google AdWords, Facebook Ads, and Microsoft Advertising. There is a cost involved when deciding to create ads online, and management must ensure the advertisements will reach the target audience. Monitoring the process can be challenging because you will have to determine whether the advertising is successful or not. If the manager is not familiar with the process, he or she may consider hiring an Internet advertiser to assist.

MEDIA

One of the most popular methods of advertising is **media advertising** that uses newspaper, radio, or television outlets. Many people are familiar with this form of advertising and tend to reference these options first. Whatever type of media the health care facility chooses, there is a fee involved, and management must be cautious in its decisions. When using media, there are a few options available, and management must be aware in order to make appropriate choices.

Questions to ask before advertising in media:

- What are the different options and costs?
- Is it more money for a color advertisement?
- Will the advertising company assist with the setup and development of the advertisement?
- What is the deadline for submitting the advertisement?
- How long will the advertisement run?
- What is the location of the advertisement?
- What is the timing of the advertisement?
- Is the advertisement reaching the target audience?

Television or radio advertising can be very effective if done appropriately; however, it can also be very costly. When you advertise on television or radio, determining the time of day to advertise is most important to reach the target audience and should be the first step in deciding to use television or radio advertising. Although the health care facility is involved in choosing the commercial, most of the acting is done by someone else. Developing the idea for the television or radio commercial is done by the advertising company in conjunction with the health care facility.

When using media as a form of advertisement, management must work directly with the advertising company to achieve an appropriate advertisement. Although the advertising company is familiar with the job at hand, it is not necessarily familiar with your needs, and management must be certain that it works together during the process to ensure appropriate advertising.

LOCAL FACILITIES

In the health care industry, working with other facilities is common practice. Referring patients among each other is something that is done on a daily basis. When using local facilities to advertise your services or procedures, they become advocates for you. Within the health care industry, there are many types of providers with specific qualifications to treat patients. Due to the nature of the business, advertising at a local facility is a great way to promote business. For example, a physical therapy clinic will advertise at the orthopedic surgeon's office by bringing information about its facility to the provider's office. Because orthopedic surgeon patients are in need of physical therapy, the facility welcomes your advertisement. As you research local facilities for advertising opportunities, the target audience must be considered during the process.

Advertising Board

One approach to local facility advertising is to inquire about an advertising board. By using an advertising board to post your brochure for information, you are ensuring the information is visible to patients and providers. In addition, when you visit the facility with more brochures, it will be easier for you to check the success of your advertising with them. The opportunity to maintain up-to-date advertising is also an advantage, and the manager must ensure this occurs.

On-Site Visits

Introducing yourself at an on-site visit is one of the most promising ways to advertise. When a provider and the employees at a health care facility are able to visit with you, the information you present will be more memorable. Making an appointment with the provider and staff for an on-site visit is most appropriate to be sure there is time for you to present your information. Depending on the circumstances, there may also be questions that will be easier to answer during the appointment. In addition, an on-site visit will allow them to realize the type of person you are and that you are there to help them. Although there is an advantage to an on-site visit, be sure you are welcome, as some locations do not allow visitors.

INVESTMENT

Deciding which type of advertising to approach is determined by how much you want to invest in the process. Investing in advertising is not all about money; your personal investment of time and stress should also be considered. When approached about doing advertising for the health care facility, you should review three key factors prior to proceeding: the **labor hours** necessary to accomplish the research involved in initiating appropriate advertising; the advertising expense (whether done internal or external), and whether hiring an advertising designer will be necessary.

Advertising and marketing may appear to be easy to work with, but when researching the options available for the health care facility, there are many factors to consider. An office manager working with advertising can be overwhelmed due to the many options, setup work, and deadlines that have to be met. Understanding the work involved and the need to use appropriate advertising for a return on your investment should be included in the final decision for investing in advertising.

LABOR HOURS

When you began to work on advertising for the health care facility, the labor hours must be determined. The labor hours will begin with the research you conduct on the different advertising techniques and costs. Finding appropriate advertising is an involved process, and the search will take you away from your current job. In addition, if you choose to do internal advertising to save costs—whether done by you or a staff—consider the need for labor hours. Time calculations should include setup, designing, telephone calls, changes, and deadlines that have to be met. Advertising to market the health care facility should be appropriate and return a profit, especially if labor hours are being paid out.

As discussed previously, some advertising is free if you do it yourself; however, if you are unfamiliar with the process or it is time consuming, you could be costing the company more money in labor hours. When management is making the decision to use internal staff or outside advertising agencies, they need to include labor hours in its market analysis.

ADVERTISING EXPENSE

Prior to initiating advertising, management should be aware of the expected advertising budget. Advertising can be inexpensive or costly, but when investing money, you should find appropriate advertising. The manager should also consider the type of advertising and the likelihood of it being successful. Spending money on advertising is a difficult decision because not all advertising works. For this reason, management must contribute labor hours in researching advertising options and expenses as well as the history of success.

Finding appropriate advertising should be based on previous years of advertising and success rates—whether with your health care facility or someone else's. Spending money for advertising can be disheartening when the advertisement does not return business. Understanding advertising and the time and energy it takes can sometimes be difficult, especially when it is expensive. Sometimes, advertising takes some time to work and must be initiated for long period of time, increasing the advertising expense. Whatever situation you find yourself in, be sure that your decision is intended on meeting the bottom line and returning a profit.

Outside Agencies

When researching advertising, managers should consider the possibility of using an outside agency. Inquiring about an outside agency could be cost effective in some cases. Although the initial expense may seem higher than what you expected, the advertising agency is knowledgeable and can accomplish better results for the health care facility. It has more resources for developing an advertisement, a better understanding of the target audience, and has staff available to accommodate your needs. In some cases, it may consider doing a portion of the advertising, allowing you to participate in the process to save money. Advertising agencies will work with the manager to get the best results possible, as they want to be sure you use them again. During your search for advertising, be sure to consider contacting someone and getting more information to make an informed decision.

Internal Advertising

Internal advertising can be very effective if done appropriately. If you or your staff have previous experience with advertising, then working with internal brochures and online or e-mail can decrease your advertising expense. While researching advertising techniques, notate whether the advertising can be done internally or needs to be done by external agencies. The labor hours need to be considered when deciding on this direction. In the event you choose the external advertising, internal advertising can also still be done, including e-mail lists and brochures or event announcements. Internal advertising can be less expensive as long as the labor hours are not overwhelming and the advertising is effective fort the health care facility.

DESIGN ELEMENTS

After the decision to advertise is made, the next step is to consider the design of the advertisement. Many labor hours can be put into designing, and in some situations, a graphic designer should be considered. The detail of the advertisement will be the deciding factor in using a graphic designer. Although graphic designers may be another advertising expense, they are qualified to develop an appropriate advertisement in a timely manner. The expense of creating a design internally can be more expensive in labor hours, resulting in higher expenses in the end.

Questions that can help in choosing a graphic designer include:

- Has the graphic designer done work for a health care facility before?
- Can this graphic design be used again for future advertising?
- Can you have a digital copy of the advertisement to recreate it later?
- Will the design be copyrighted by the graphic designer?

Designing should be eye-catching at first but not overwhelming. You want the reader to notice the advertisement and want to read further for more information. Sometimes, too much design or information will be distracting. Whether working with a graphic designer or having it created internally, understanding the purpose of the design and the advertisement is important. In addition, management will be responsible for the decision on **design elements,** which are the items included in the advertisement to attract the target audience.

Design elements for advertising:

- Color scheme
- Font size
- Font style
- Position of advertisement
- Photographs of facility
- Photographs of providers
- Other photographs (such as medical pictures)
- Information to include (such as address)
- Overall appearance

One method of creating a design quickly is to use previous advertisements or view advertisements of similar health care facilities for comparison. Using existing items such as appointment cards would be an option by including additional information about the office. Figure 13-4 shows a sample appointment card that can be used. With the amount of time spent on designing an advertisement, you want to be sure it is appropriate for what you need.

NETWORKING

One of the most effective ways of advertising for the health care facility is through **networking**, which involves sharing information and services among groups. Networking with other health care facilities and groups allows for a personal approach when sharing your information, and you are able to gain more respect. By attending meetings, social gatherings, or informational presentations, you can network with other attendees, allowing you to be a personal advocate.

By presenting at local events, you are able to represent the health care facility and network with local facilities in a social environment. There is a great advantage to being present and participating in discussions in person. Even if you are not in need of the education an event has to offer, attending can be a great networking tool. In addition, the other attendees are also networking with you to promote their services or businesses in the health care industry. Consider some of the following approaches to networking with local facilities at events where attendees may have an interest in your services.

Some of the venues to attend include:

- Hospital meetings
- Professional organization meetings
- Workshops
- Seminars
- Health care clinics
- Charitable events
- Professional organization meetings
- Local health groups

Mrs. Mary Woolsey

has an appointment with

GERALD PRACTON, MD

PRACTON MEDICAL GROUP, INC.

4567 Broad Avenue
Woodland Hills, XY 12345
Tel. 555/486-9002
Fax No. 555/488-7815

for

Mon.	_____	at _____
Tues.	_____	at _____
Wed.	*Oct. 29*_____	at *2:30 pm.*_____
Thurs	_____	at _____
Fri.	_____	at _____
Sat.	_____	at _____

If unable to keep this appointment kindly give
24-hours notice.

© Cengage Learning 2013

FIGURE 13-4 Appointment Card

Although networking can be more time consuming, the return of business is usually worth the time. Your presence and discussion with other attendees will allow you to represent the facility and communicate vital information appropriately. In addition, you are able to give more information and answer questions if necessary. Offering a free health clinic and inviting other professionals would allow networking. Figure 13-5 shows a sample promotional advertisement you could utilize to attract others. Networking with others in the same field tends to be more welcoming and rewarding when everyone is employed in the health care industry.

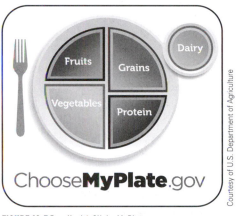

Courtesy of U.S. Department of Agriculture

FIGURE 13-5 Free Health Clinic: MyPlate

PROFESSIONAL ORGANIZATIONS

Joining professional organizations affiliated with your type of work and health care facility is a great approach to networking with people who have the same interests. **Professional organizations** are nonprofit groups of people with the same educational background that network to promote their field of expertise and hold continuing education meetings. Hosting informational meetings is a requirement for them as a nonprofit organization, and many of the topics are helpful. Enrolling in a professional organization allows you to get up-to-date information regarding the organization as well as their meeting topics, dates, and times.

Another approach to networking with professional organization without a commitment is to attend as a guest if possible. Even if you are not in that profession but wish to attend, some professional organizations will allow you to attend as a guest on your own or with another member who has invited you. Networking with other health care facilities is one approach to finding out about professional organizations and their attendance policies. Be proactive and get information, as this can be another way to advertise.

Some of the professional organizations affiliated with the health care field include:

- American Management Association (AMA)
- American Association of Medical Assistants (AAMA)
- The Joint Commission
- American Academy of Professional Coders (AAPC)
- American Health Information Management Association (AHIMA)
- American College of Surgeons (ACOS)
- Medical Group Management Association (MGMA)

Professional organizations have rules and regulations, so before attending an event or spending money to sign up, research the policies and decide whether this is the direction you wish to pursue. Respect the policies, and call someone in charge if you are unsure and need clarification. Some of the exceptions to the rules may not be listed in the policies, and contacting a representative can help clarify the information. When reaching out to professional organizations, remember to represent the health care facility with the utmost respect. Figure 13-6 lists professional organizations affiliated with the health care field.

Title and Abbreviation	Description to Obtain Certification or Registration	Professional Association Mailing Address and Telephone Number	Web Site and E-Mail Addresses
Certified Bookkeeper (CB)	Self-study program and employment experience; pass three tests	American Institute of Professional Bookkeepers 6001 Montrose Road, Suite 207 Rockville, MD 20852 (800) 622-0121	http://www.aipb.org info@aipb.org
Certified Coding Associate (CCA); Certified Coding Specialist (CCS); Certified Coding Specialist—Physician based (CCS-P)	Self-study program; pass certification examination	American Health Information Management Association PO Box 97349 Chicago, IL 60690-7349 (800) 335-5535	http://www.ahima. orginfo@ahima.mhs. compuserve.com

FIGURE 13-6 Professional Organizations

Title and Abbreviation	Description to Obtain Certification or Registration	Professional Association Mailing Address and Telephone Number	Web Site and E-Mail Addresses
Certified Electronic Claims Professional (CECP)	Self-study program; pass certification examination	Alliance of Claims Assistance Professionals 873 Brentwood Drive West Chicago, IL 60185 (877) 275-8765	http://www.claims.org askus@claims.org
Certified Healthcare Billing and Management Executive (CHBME)	Complete comprehensive program; pass proficiency test	Healthcare Billing and Management Association 1550 South Coast Highway, Suite 201 Laguna Beach, CA 92651 (877) 640-4262	http://www.hbma.com info@hbma.com
Certified Medical Assistant (CMA)	Graduate from accredited medical assisting program; apply to take national certifying examination	American Association of Medical Assistants 20 North Wacker Drive Chicago, IL 60606 (800) 228-2262	http://www.aama-ntl.org visit Web site
Certified Medical Billing Specialist (CMBS)	Complete six courses and provide evaluation of billing performance by supervisor	Medical Association of Billers 2441 Tech Center Court, Suite 108 Las Vegas, NV 89128 (702) 240-8519 Fax: (702) 243-0359	http://www.physicians websites.com mailroom@ physicians websites.com
Certified Medical Office Manager (CMOM)	Examination for supervisors or managers of small-group and solo practices	Professional Association of Health Care Office Managers 461 East Ten Mile Road Pensacola, FL 32534-9712 (800) 451-9311	http://www.pahcom.com pahcom@pahcom.com
Certified Medical Practice Executive (CMPE) •Nominee (1st level) •Certification (2nd level) •Fellow (3rd level)	1st level: Eligible group managers join; membership/nominee 2nd level: Complete six- to seven-hour examination 3rd level: Mentoring project or thesis	Medical Group Management Association, American College of Medical Practice Executives (affiliate) 104 Inverness Terrace East Englewood, CO 80112 (303) 397-7869	http://www.mgma.com/acmpe acmpe@mgma.com
Certified Medical Reimbursement Specialist (CMRS)	Self-study program; successfully pass 18 sections of examination	American Medical Billing Association 4297 Forrest Drive Sulphur, OK 73086 (580) 622-2624	http://www.ambanet.net/ cmrs.htm

FIGURE 13-6 continued

Title and Abbreviation	Description to Obtain Certification or Registration	Professional Association Mailing Address and Telephone Number	Web Site and E-Mail Addresses
Certified Medical Transcriptionist (CMT)	Self-study program and successfully pass written and practical examinations offered by Medical Transcription Certification Commission (MTCC)	American Association for Medical Transcription 100 Sycamore Avenue Modesto, CA 95354-0550 (800) 982-2182	http://www.aamt.org visit Web site
Certified Patient Account Technician (CPAT); Certified Clinic Account Technician (CCAT); Certified Clinic Account Manager (CCAM)	Complete self-study course; pass standard examination administered twice yearly	American Association of Healthcare Administrative Management National Certification Examination Program 11240 Waples Mill Road, Suite 200 Fairfax, VA 22030 (703) 281-4043	http://www.aaham.org debra@statmarketing.com
Certified Professional Coder (CPC); Certified Professional Coder— Apprentice (CPC-A); Certified Professional Coder— Hospital (CPC-H)	Independent study program; examination approximately five hours (CPC) and eight hours (CPC-H) in length. No practical experience for CPC-A. Two years experience for CPC.	American Academy of Professional Coders 309 West 700 South Salt Lake City, UT 84101 (800) 626-CODE	http://www.aapcnatl.org aapc@worldnet.att.net
Certified Claims Assistance Professional (CCAP)	Self-study program; pass certification examination	Alliance of Claims Assistance Professionals 873 Brentwood Drive West Chicago, IL 60185 (877) 275-8765	http://www.claims.org askus@claims.org
Healthcare Reimbursement Specialist (HRS)	Successfully complete open-book examination	National Electronic Biller's Alliance 2226-A Westborough Blvd. #504 South San Francisco, CA 94080 (650) 359-4419 Fax: (650) 989-6727	http://www.nebazone.com mmedical@aol.com

FIGURE 13-6 continued

Title and Abbreviation	Description to Obtain Certification or Registration	Professional Association Mailing Address and Telephone Number	Web Site and E-Mail Addresses
National Certified Insurance and Coding Specialist (NCICS)	Graduate from an insurance program; sit for certification examination given by independent testing agency at many school sites across the nation	National Center for Competency Testing 7007 College Blvd., Suite 250 Overland Park, KS 66211 (800) 875-4404 Fax: (913) 498-1243	http://www.ncctinc.com visit Web site
Registered Medical Assistant (RMA)	Take certification offered by the American Medical Technologist (AMT)	Registered Medical Assistant (AMT) 710 Higgins Road Park Ridge, IL 60068-5765 (847) 823-5169	http://www.amt1.com amtmail@aol.com
Registered Medical Coder (RMC)	Yearly correspondence program governed by the National Coding Standards Committee and pass an examination	Medical Management Institute 1125 Cambridge Square Alpharetta, GA 30004-5724 (800) 334-5724	http://www.the-institute.com bobby.carvell@ipractice.md

© Cengage Learning 2013

FIGURE 13-6 continued

ONLINE SOCIAL NETWORKS

Online social networks are a creative way to engage in free networking and advertising while sitting in your office. The time involved is less than attending events, and you can post upcoming information about your health care facility regularly. Some of the networks that allow you to join at no cost are Facebook, Twitter, LinkedIn, and Ning.

As with anything else, there are advantages and disadvantages to using this free form of networking. Management must be familiar with the process and ensure that appropriate information is posted on the social network.

Some social networking advantages and disadvantages include:

Advantages

- Free networking
- Daily presence for audience
- Can answer questions without telephone calls
- Others can post positive comments
- Can update information regularly
- Posting of events are easy
- Sending messages to members

(Continues)

Disadvantages:

- May not be your target audience
- Words can get misinterpreted
- Others can post negative comments
- Lack of presence can appear ignorant
- Creating a page that is appropriate
- Inviting people to become members

When posting on an online social network, remember that there are many things that can be interpreted incorrectly in addition to your posting. Written words cannot be taken back and may be misinterpreted. Always keep a positive outlook on your postings, and be sure to answer questions on a daily basis. Forgetting to answer a question or not posting can also create a negative view of the health care facility. A continued presence and constant monitoring by management is required to be sure the online social networking is creating a form of positive advertisement.

MARKETING SUCCESS

After all the planning, research, and networking, the final decision is made based on the potential for success of marketing the health care facility in the area. Taking the results of available advertising techniques, networking opportunities, the initial investment expense, and the opportunity for free advertising, the next step is to create a market plan. The marketing plan should identify the possibility of increasing revenue, the time frame needed to achieve the goal, and the bottom line of how much profit or new business will be generated. If the market plan demonstrates increased revenue over a short amount of time, there is a market need and advertising will be successful. However, if the area is saturated with other health care facilities and the advertising expense is too high to increase revenue, then the market is not appropriate. Advertising and networking opportunities are available in every area; therefore, you must also determine a need for your services. Without the market need, the advertising and networking will not be successful.

INCREASED REVENUE

The ultimate goal of your facility is to increase revenue by bringing in more patients. Revenue is generated from patient and insurance payments, and there must be a need for your services in the area. The health care facility will have the option of advertising and networking wherever they go, but you do not want to initiate advertising expenses if the market is not appropriate. Determining the potential for increased revenue should be done prior to your decision to choose a location.

In the event you are employed in a health care facility in a poor market area, be cautious about how you spend your advertising budget. Free advertising may be the best approach; use online or social networking if the area is not marketable through advertising. Another approach may be to offer free clinics with your advertising budget in order to generate patients to your facility. As discussed earlier, there are many opportunities to increase revenue, even with networking, websites, and local facilities. Whatever type of market you are in as a manager, determining appropriate advertising for the health care facility is important. By analyzing the market need and researching the options, you will be able to determine the most appropriate advertising for increasing revenue.

TIME FRAME

Timing is important when discussing the potential for advertising. Understanding the time variations can help your decision. Rushing to advertise because there is a discount on advertising is not conducive if the advertising is not appropriate at that time. Keep in mind that advertising can sometimes take awhile and may need to be repeated before results are seen. If there is an outside agency, ask for their advice based on past experiences. When working with the advertisement, notice the time frame and ask yourself if this is an appropriate time for what you are trying to accomplish.

Time factors include:

- Waiting for the appropriate time to advertise
- Giving a time frame before discontinuing
- Advertising a service when there is a market need
- Timing promotional advertisements accordingly
- Advertising at the time of day in the event of a television or radio commercial
- Giving enough advanced notice when advertising an event

BOTTOM LINE

With many factors involved in the decision process, the culmination of all the work is the bottom line. Managers are responsible for understanding the process as they approach marketing and advertising as part of their job. They should also be aware of the expectations of the health care facility as they make decisions. A profit or loss statement should be created to address these questions. See figure 13-7.

Some of the questions to ask when estimating the bottom line include:

1. What will be the overall income as a result of the planning, marketing, and advertising for the health care facility?
2. Will the increased revenue be more than the advertising expenses?
3. Is the time frame for success a short-term goal under 12 months?
4. Is the time frame for success a long term goal of 1-5 years?
5. Can the company handle a decrease in revenue if the goal is long term?
6. Will the long-term bottom line be significant enough to wait?

There are long-term and short-terms goals to reach, and although increasing revenue is great, the bottom line shows whether the overall investment to advertise was worth it.

In the end, when all is said and done, the bottom line is what it is all about!

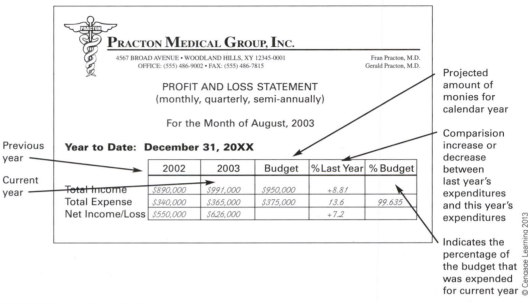

FIGURE 13-7 Example of Profit or Loss Statement

SUMMARY

- No-cost, low-cost, and expensive advertising are available for health care facilities to participate, and examining the options should be done with the target audience in mind.

- Investing in advertising can be costly, and researching appropriate advertising is necessary for a return on your investment.

- Networking with other health care facilities or professional organizations creates a positive approach to advertising if done on a regular basis.

- Advertising is a way to market your business and must be done efficiently and in a timely manner to accomplish a positive outcome and improve your bottom line.

REVIEW EXERCISES

TRUE OR FALSE

1. _____ All online advertising is free, including e-mail lists.

2. _____ You should reach a large target audience when advertising.

3. _____ Brochures are required to include the location of the facility.

4. _____ The final decision on design elements is ultimately the manager's responsibility.

5. _____ All television advertising for health care facilities should be presented during the daytime.

6. _____ Investing in advertising is not all about money; it also includes investing time.

7. _____ Advertising does not always increase revenue and could lose the company money if not done appropriately.

8. _____ Professional organizations do not allow outside members to belong, and you must have the credentials to participate.

9. _____ Other health care facilities will never advertise for you because you are their competition.

10. _____ The bottom line for advertising and marketing is increasing revenue.

MATCHING

A Revenue

B Online Social Networks

C Internal Advertising

D Design Element

E Labor Hours

F Advertising Board

G Brochure

H Advertising

I Networking

J Media

1. _____ Determining the font size and color of the advertisement is part of deciding this feature.

2. _____ When you advertise at local facilities, this is one place to include an advertisement.

3. _____ The internal hours that must be considered in the cost of advertising.

4. _____ The process of using employees in the office to advertise.

5. _____ A mailer that is sent out to include information about the facility and any upcoming event.

6. _____ Involves sharing information and services among groups.

7. _____ A way to generate information regarding the health care facility in order to promote future business.

8. _____ LinkedIn and Facebook are examples of this type of advertising.

9. _____ Advertising in the newspaper, radio, or television is considered this type of advertising.

10. _____ Increasing this is the concept behind successful advertising.

CRITICAL THINKING ACTIVITIES

ACTIVITY 1

Research local facilities in the area in which you can make an appointment for an on-site visit. Create a list of 10 local facilities in which it may be appropriate for you to advertise. Include the name, providers, type of facility, location(s), office manager, and contact information.

Name: _____

Providers: _____

Type of Facility: _____

Addresses: _____

Contact _____

Manager: _____

ACTIVITY 2

Identify the following with an O if there is potential to do online marketing.

_____ Local facilities   _____ Google AdWords

_____ Advertising boards   _____ Facebook Ads

_____ Radio   _____ Professional organizations

_____ Ning   _____ Television

_____ Twitter   _____ Brochure

ACTIVITY 3

Develop steps to creating a market plan of success for determining whether you would use an outside agency or do internal advertising.

Include steps to calculate revenue based on patient flow and expenses based on staff:

1. _____

2. _____

3. _____

4. _____

5. _____

6. _____

7. _____

8. _____

9. _____

10. _____

11. _____

12. _____

13. _____

14. _____

15. _____

ACTIVITY 4

Mark an X next to the following questions that should be asked to determine whether advertising is appropriate for the health care facility and will satisfy the bottom line.

1. _____ If the advertising fails, can you run it again for free?

2. _____ What will be the overall income as a result of the planning, marketing, and advertising for the health care facility?

3. _____ Will the increased revenue be more than the advertising expenses?

4. _____ Will the manager include his or her advertising experience in his or her résumé?

5. _____ Is the time frame for success a short-term goal under 12 months?

6. _____ Is the time frame for success a long-term goal of 1–5 years?

7. _____ Can the company handle a decrease in revenue if the goal is long term?

8. _____ Should the advertising agency be affiliated with the hospital to use it?

9. _____ Can employees expect a raise if the advertising is successful?

10. _____ Will the long-term bottom line be significant enough to wait?

CRITICAL THINKING QUESTIONS

1. Explain the relationship between marketing and advertising. Relate them to the revenue cycle and how the bottom line is to make money.

2. Debate the pros and cons of using labor hours to do internal marketing, including the staff or manager.

3. Discuss the process of using an e-mail list for your advertising. Include the steps involved as well as the need for permission and answering questions.

4. Identify the cautions of advertising with a company whom you never used. Refer to online and local advertising techniques.

WEB ACTIVITIES

1. Research three advertising companies to compare what they offer. Include their time frame, the target audience that would be interested, and the pricing.

2. Search online for advertising with Microsoft (http://www.advertising.microsoft.com), Google (http://www.google.com/ads/adwords), and Facebook (http://www.facebook.com/advertising/). Compare these to the research you did in question 1.

3. Go online to research free advertising and then create a list of online advertising or networking websites you can utilize to advertise a seminar for "Free Blood Pressure Checks." Then, create an advertisement with the date, time, location, and any pertinent information for all those websites. Remember: If it is free, take advantage!

CHAPTER 14

ADVERTISING AND MARKETING

MANAGING

Chapter 14 will discuss the approach to advertising as the manager attempts to market the health care facility. Identifying the type of target audience prior to determining the advertising techniques will be reviewed. The market area and the need for advertising as a cost-effective approach will be discussed. In addition, an overview will be given on how management can create successful advertisements for particular needs in order to generate revenue as expected.

KEY TERMS

- Closed questions
- Cost effective
- Internal patients
- Marketable
- Market analysis
- Market analysis survey
- Open-ended
- Outside market
- Patient surveys

OBJECTIVES

Upon completion of this chapter, the student will be able to:

- Discuss the need for a target audience for advertising and marketing purposes.
- Understand different types of advertising and their costs.
- Evaluate the market and determine cost-effective advertising.
- Understand the need for a market analysis prior to advertising.
- Create effective advertising for the health care facility.

INTRODUCTION

The success of the health care facility is a result of the market area and the need for the services it provides. Once a location is determined as a marketable area for your services, management must examine the advertising needs. Many opportunities are available for advertising, including advertising agencies, networking, and online advertising. The decision for management to move forward with advertising is involved, and all aspects must be considered with caution as it journeys toward successful advertising.

DETERMINING THE TARGET AUDIENCE

When management approaches advertising options, the first step is to consider the target audience it wants to reach. When you advertise services, there must be a need for the services you are presenting. Advertising is specific and is usually for a certain audience, but if this is not determined ahead of time, then advertising may be done for nothing. You should develop a checklist of questions to use when determining your target audience to be sure this necessary step is taken.

Some questions that may help you identify your target audience include:

- Is there an age for the service being offered?
- Is the service gender specific?
- Is the service seasonal, such as the flu vaccine?
- What is the cost of the service being offered?
- Is the service covered under insurance?
- Are there other health care facilities offering the same service?
- Do clinics offer the same service, such as flu vaccines?
- What is the patient cost at other facilities?
- Does the potential patient watch daytime television?
- Does the potential patient watch children's television?
- Does the potential patient read the newspaper?
- Does the potential patient go online?

By understanding the target audience, you can more easily identify the advertising techniques and details. Decisions to advertise can be made if you have outlined the answers to the aforementioned questions. Knowing who you are reaching and what type of advertising may work is the way to make appropriate choices. If the target audience is the working adult who does not watch television, then online advertising may be more successful. However, if the patient is a child or parent who watches daytime television and children's shows, then these types of advertising will be successful. Realizing the need to reach the target audience can promote successful advertising for management.

INTERNAL PATIENTS

Advertising for **internal patients** as the target audience is usually easier. They are already presenting to the facility, and advertising can be done to provide a background on the health care facility and providers. When the patients are already aware of where you are, the brochure in the waiting room may be a way to give them more information that helps promote you further. Developing an advertisement that identifies facility information, such as location, contact information, and providers, is easier for management because they are looking to attract a new audience or present an appealing opportunity. Figure 14-1 shows patients in a waiting room, reading brochures.

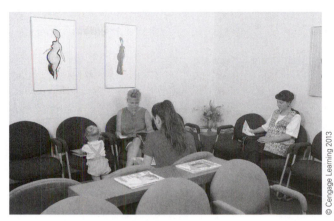

FIGURE 14-1 Patients in Waiting Room with Brochures

OUTSIDE MARKET

When a manager decides he or she has to reach an **outside market** or external target audience, the advertising process is more involved and requires some decision making. Depending on the service being offered, the advertising has to stand out yet not be overwhelming. Timing is also a factor if the service is time sensitive, such as physical examinations being advertised just before students go back to school. If the service being offered is physical examinations, then the larger target audience is children returning to school or attending summer camps.

Careful consideration must be given as the advertising options are reviewed and the investment opportunity is determined. Discussing costs as well as the use of advertising agencies and graphic designers will be determined based on the size of the target audience. Advertising should be done using media, networking, or online outlets to appropriately reach the external target audience.

OTHER FACILITIES

If the target audience you are trying to reach is patients of another practice, especially a different specialty, then using a referral system will help reach the target audience. By delivering advertisements to the health care facility, you are creating a personal connection. Advertising with other facilities is usually done through brochures in a facility that works in conjunction with you, such as a dermatologist advertising for a plastic surgeon.

Some other professional relationships that exist amongst health care providers include:

- Orthopedic and physical therapy
- Cardiology and cardiovascular surgeon
- Pediatrician and otorhinolaryngologist (ENT)
- Neurologist and pain management
- Obstetrician and pediatrician

Networking with health care facilities that can complement your services is a great way to help each other out with referrals. Networking is a personal touch, and the target audience is more likely to trust the provider in its opinion to refer them to your facility. Figure 14-2 represents a list of potential department that will network with your facility in order to improve patient care and increase business. This type of advertising should be done on a regular basis with hospitals, other physician offices, and clinics.

Hospital Adjunct Departments

Dietetic/Nutrition Department

Furnishes:

- Dietitian
- Nutritional assessment
- Therapy
- Diet preparation
- Nutritional education

Emergency Department

Physician and staff on duty 24 hours a day to handle trauma and emergencies and observe and monitor patients while collecting data to make decisions regarding admissions. Sections include:

- Casting room
- Examination room
- Observation room
- Trauma room

Gastrointestinal Laboratory (GI Lab)

Performs endoscopic procedures such as:

- Colonoscopy
- Proctoscopy
- Sigmoidoscopy

Laboratory Department

Offers inpatient and outpatient services such as:

- Blood bank
- Chemistry
- Cytology
- Hematology
- Histopathology
- Microbiology
- Organ bank
- Pathology
- Urinalysis

Magnetic Resonance Imaging Department (MRI)

Performs:

- MRI scans with and without contrast material

Nuclear Medicine Department

Handles radioactive materials used in tests such as:

- Bone scans
- Liver scans
- Radioimmunoassays
- Thyroid testing

One-Day Surgery Department

Takes care of patients who do not require overnight stay for procedures such as:

- Angiography
- Blood transfusion
- Heart catheterization
- Myelogram

Pharmacy Department

Supplies medication to inpatients such as:

- Injectable medications
- Intravenous solutions
- Oral medications
- Topicals, suppositories, inhalers, and so on

Physical Therapy Department

Provides:

- Inpatient physical therapy
- Outpatient physical therapy
- Occupational therapy
- Speech therapy

Physiology Department

Offers a variety of services such as:

- Cardiology (ECG, treadmill, 2-D echocardiogram)
- Electrophysiology (EMG, EEG, nerve conduction studies)
- Vascular medicine (deep vein Doppler)
- Myelogram

Radiology Department

Performs the following procedures:

- Barium enema
- Barium swallow
- Computed tomography
- Diagnostic x-ray
- Mammography
- Therapeutic radiation
- Ultrasound

FIGURE 14-2 Hospital Adjunct Departments

Respiratory Care Department

Provides diagnostic and therapeutic services including the administration of:

- Bronchodilators
- Oxygen

Performs:

- Arterial blood gases
- Pulmonary function studies
- Spirometry

Sets up and assists with:

- Cardiopulmonary resuscitation
- Mechanical ventilators

Social Services Department

Employs medical and psychiatric social workers to work with patients and families regarding:

- Economic factors
- Emotional situations
- Social issues
- Discharge planning
- Community services
- Medical resources

© Cengage Learning 2013

FIGURE 14-2 continued

IDENTIFYING ADVERTISING OPTIONS

Researching advertising options can be time consuming, but the information is necessary to determine the appropriate technique for your facility. After deciding who the target audience will be, you can make a more informed decision about the type of advertising preferred and view options that may be eye catching to them. If there is more than one target audience, consider analyzing the advertising separately. Advertising options are specific to the audience, and doing the same advertising for different people may be unproductive.

Use the Internet or past advertising to assist in your research as you compile the information. With the online forum, researching advertising cost is much easier and more information is provided in one place. Consider locating costs of printing out advertisements, such as brochures, mailers, or business cards; ordering promotional products, such as pens, pencils, or magnets; or advertising online with streaming advertising. Most of these advertising options can be found easily; however, options that need further research would be television, radio, or newspaper. Contacting local businesses to inquire about pricing, length, and advertisement preparation is usually very easy to obtain because they want advertisers in their publications. Generate a list of appropriate options and then compare them in a spreadsheet with pricing, time involved, length of advertising necessary, and estimated return on investment. Be sure to include web addresses and contact information for reaching them in the future. Once everything you research is outlined, your decision will be easier.

Questions to ask prior to choosing an advertising option include:

- Who is the target audience?
- What type of health care services and procedures are being offered?
- Will the patients be willing to give feedback through a survey or questionnaire?

(Continues)

- Are other health care facilities advertising for this service or procedure or is it exclusive to your health care facility?
- How long will the anticipated advertisement be effective?
- Will the type of advertising reach a large audience?
- Is it reaching new patients or existing patients?
- Does the type of advertising present as cost effective?

Focus should be on the reason for advertising at all times. When advertising is within the budget and affordable for the health care facility and also generates increased revenue, then consider the advertisement **cost effective**. Making the decision to maintain cost-effective advertising can sometimes be difficult because we are not sure what will happen in the end. With advertising options and a target audience, the best decision is one that returns an investment and shows increased revenue—either short term or long term.

LENGTH OF ADVERTISING

After determining what type of advertising option you want, looking at the time involved is the next step. Advertising is not always successful, and sending an advertisement one time may not reach the target audience. The estimated time for someone to remember is three times, and depending on what services you are advertising, you can determine the length of time needed. If the services are not time sensitive, then the length may be decided by the need for revenue, the cost, the advertising budget, and the potential for return on your investment. Many factors are considered when deciding the length of placing an advertisement or how often something should be sent.

In addition, the target audience may not have a need for your services at the time you advertise but may decide at a later date the services are more appropriate. For example, people may not think they need the flu vaccination, but when they hear that others have received one, they may change their minds. In this case, repetitive advertising would work to reach a larger target audience over a period of time. Keep in mind that advertising length can always be changed; when short term is decided, an extension can be granted if the advertising is effective. However, canceling advertising may still cost the company, and lengthy advertising can also have a negative effect. Deciding on a perfect length is challenging for management but necessary for successful advertising.

Long Term

A health care facility that decides to initiate long-term advertising typically wants to advertise the location and providers on a regular basis. If the health care facility is new to the area, this type of advertisement would be appropriate to ensure longer exposure. Using long-term advertising can be costly, but the consistent presence to the target audience will be more memorable. If management uses an outside advertising agency and it is encouraging long-term advertising, be sure to investigate the reason for long term, the cost, and the expected return on investment to be sure the agency is guiding you appropriately. If the services will continue to reach the target audience over the extended period of time and generate new business, then the long-term advertising is feasible.

Short Term

Short-term advertising is usually directed toward a promotional service or event the health care facility wants to advertise. A short-term advertisement is usually less expensive and can be done quickly. The information is generated for a specific service or event, and the development of the advertisement is straightforward and easier to create. The target audience for this type of advertising is typically done for the external outside market in order to encourage new business. Although internal patients are welcomed, the current promotion or event is a way to bring in new patients and introduce them to the health care facility for the first time. Once they are aware of your location and you are able to advertise your health care facility and providers, the patients become long-term patients that the short-term advertising helped initiate. If you decide to offer short-term advertising, a particular service or event is a great way to catch the eye of the target audience quickly because interest in the service or event will get people's attention to look further and learn more about your facility.

COST INCURRED

Expenses are always a key factor when managing a health care facility. Prior to spending money on advertising, the manager must consider the target audience and determine if the cost incurred will reach a small or large target audience and for how long. Free advertising is always an option—whether you do low cost or expensive—as long as you have the labor hours for someone to accomplish. Creating a cost-effective approach to advertising is required to meet your bottom line; therefore, all three scenarios need to be reviewed for potential advertising opportunities prior to making a final decision.

Free Advertising

If there is someone who has the time to assist, then using free advertising should be done on a regular basis. Consider the cost of the labor hours as you determine whether you or a staff member has time. Consider setting aside a small amount of time per day to take advantage of the free advertisings, such as one hour, as long as the time is not affecting patient care or collections.

Some of the ideas for free advertising include:

- Online advertising
- Professional organizations
- Local meetings
- Free clinics
- Local facilities
- Charity events
- Networking

In the event that the free advertising is ongoing, taking advantage will help promote the health care facility. Having a constant presence in free advertising will help promote the business. Figure 14-3 shows an example of a way to help advertise for a free scoliosis clinic. Also, networking with people in the industry is a great way to create a word-of-mouth advertising or referral system. Try to take advantage of the opportunities; it will make a difference.

Low Cost

Low-cost advertising can be very successful if done with appropriate advertising. When advertising for a long period of time, low cost is appropriate because the long-term expense is ongoing. In addition, low cost can be beneficial when you are not sure of the target audience or the success rate of the advertising you want to accomplish. An announcement of special events can also be done as a low cost, especially if the target audience is small and you know where to focus the advertising.

Some of the ideas for low-cost advertising include:

- Brochures
- Appointment cards
- Business cards

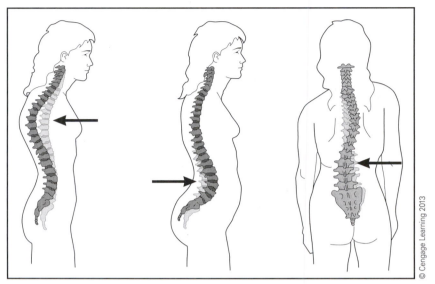

FIGURE 14-3 Free Scoliosis Clinic

- Mailers
- Postcards
- Promotional products
- Flyers
- Questionnaires

Using this method can assist in keeping the costs low and allow for a longer advertising period. Figure 14-4 shows an appointment reminder card, which is another way patients will know who you are and remember his or her appointment. When you are attempting new advertising, this is the best option to avoid using your entire advertising budget. For health care facilities, low cost is usually the most economical way to advertise and still get a return on your investment.

High Cost

Larger health care facilities will usually use expensive advertising if their budget is higher and they have a larger target audience to reach. Small scale health care facilities may find it necessary to also use expensive advertising, especially if the advertisement is geared toward the target audience with regards to timing, need for the service, and appeal.

Some of the ideas for expensive advertising include:

- Television
- Radio
- Newspaper
- Billboard
- Movie theaters
- Professional games

If you operate a large facility with several departments, the need for patients is greater and the variety of patients is also different. Advertising becomes a necessity, and the cost-effective approach sometimes does not bring in revenue. For smaller health care facilities, the advertising budget needs to be considered as well as the return on investment. Expensive advertising is not always effective, so ensure research is done ahead of time when making a decision.

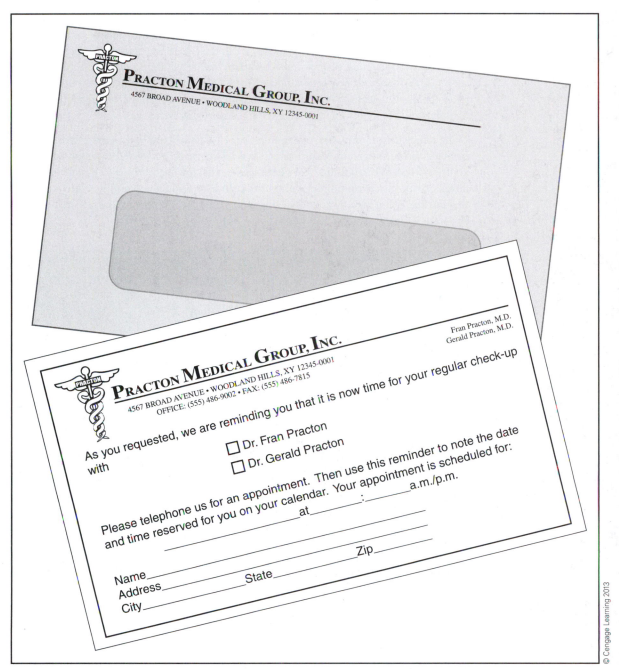

FIGURE 14-4 Appointment Card Reminder

PERFORMING MARKET ANALYSIS

The process for performing a detailed market analysis is extensive but necessary when finding a location for a health care facility or determining how much advertising is necessary to return a profit. A **market analysis** will take a look at the potential for growth in the area based on the industry by looking at market size, trends, costs, profits, and the potential for new clients. It should be performed for any type of health care facility—whether small, large, or a satellite facility—because a market need should be identified in advance.

Surveying the local residents and businesses can assist in gathering information needed. A **market analysis survey** would include questions that pertain to potential patient care and services you offer at the health care facility or plan to offer in the future. When creating questions, keep them short, easy to read, and easy to answer so patients are willing to take the time to complete the survey. Questions may be worded to allow for a "Yes" or "No" definitive answer or open-ended to allow for an explanation. When questions are returned, ensure they are all read in detail and information is used to determine your market and advertising needs.

Using templates and statistics for the area can be helpful as you look at the trends. Acquiring data from local government offices or businesses is an option if you are able to set up meetings with the appropriate staff. In addition, real estate agencies are another avenue to pursue because they are familiar with the surrounding neighborhood and are usually welcoming to anyone interested in the moving. Being proactive in retrieving information is best because the research is complex and you want your results to be accurate.

Market analysis information includes:

- Market size
- Current growth rate
- Future potential growth rate
- Industry trends
- Market profitability
- Health care facility cost
- Medical industry cost
- Appeal to new patients
- Potential for success

The primary focus is to review everything and determine whether the area is **marketable** in terms of meeting the needs of the target audience and having a successful response to advertising. Advertising depends on the market analysis because the target audience can be identified through the information obtained. Marketing and advertising work together because without a market need, the advertising is unsuccessful.

NETWORKING WITH LOCAL FACILITIES

An effective method in determining the market need is to perform a market analysis of local health care facilities that have had experience in the market already. Networking with similar businesses in the area is another way to approach the market analysis and obtain information about their past and current market need. Figure 14-5 represents a list of hospital departments that would be great resources to network with in the area before and after you approach advertising. This will assist you in determining whether the area is also appropriate and marketable for you.

In addition, the information obtained will be more focused toward the information you need. When discussing the potential for marketing and advertising in the area, you can get an idea of

---

Hospital Administrative Departments

Administration Department

- Oversees the management and operations of the hospital.
- The Chief Executive Officer (CEO) or President works in this department.
- The Board of Directors establishes bylaws outlining duties and responsibilities for the governing body, administrator, and all hospital committees.

Admitting Department

Handles:

- Admittance/discharge of patients
- Insurance verification
- Precertification of insurance
- Preauthorization for hospitalization and procedures

Business Department

- Provides cashiers and patient statements (bills)
- Submits insurance claims
- Collects accounts receivable

Financial Department

Oversees and controls:

- Business department
- Accounts receivable/payable
- Budgets and financial reports
- Insurance contracts
- Payroll

Medical Records Department

Manages:

- Coding diagnoses and procedures
- In- and outpatient medical records
- Medical transcription
- Registries

Medical Staff Department

- Processes credentialing of all allied health professionals
- Schedules and monitors department meetings

Nursing Administration Department

Supervises:

- Nursing care, staffing, and education
- Nursing care of patients in specialized medical care units
- Utilization review nurses who may report to this department

FIGURE 14-5 Hospital Administrative Departments

---

what type of advertising has worked in the market as well as how much it may cost. Discussion about the return on investment and length of advertising can also be beneficial. If given the opportunity to network with local facilities, you would be able to ask questions and access firsthand information, which is more valuable to your research.

REVIEWING PREVIOUS ADVERTISING

A helpful way to determine the market need is to review previous advertising that was done in the area by other health care facilities. Advertising agencies would have this information available if you are working with someone. Contacting the health care facility and networking with it is another way to get information. With the use of the Internet, searching for services that are being advertised or were advertised is feasible. In addition, you may be successful contacting the newspaper, radio, or television to ask about its experience with previous advertisers with the same needs. Being proactive with advertising results is one approach to ensuring your advertising will be successful and worth the investment.

CONDUCTING PATIENT SURVEYS

An excellent way to help with the market analysis is by conducting **patient surveys** or questionnaires on a regular basis. Be cautious as to what you ask because they may respond with something you do not like or ask for changes that you disagree with. Have an open mind and be ready to make appropriate changes or address staff when asking them to complete a survey. Keep in mind that the purpose of the survey is to determine the need for the services in the area in addition to making improvements that will better assist patients during their visits.

Timing is crucial when conducting surveys with patients. Two areas to consider when deciding on time is the best time to present surveys and how often they should be conducted. The best approach in presenting surveys is to provide them at the end of the visit; however, some patients are anxious to leave. Presenting the survey at the visit is more productive because the survey is done immediately and you do not have to try to reach the patient at a later time; however, keeping it short will be more conducive to patients' time. In addition, this is also the least expensive because there is no need for stamps or envelopes and the questions can easily be printed by the office. A schedule should be developed to assist in the survey process. Keep track of when the surveys are administered and only give to patients who have not completed them. Quarterly or yearly surveys are usually successful and can allow for different patient responses at a later date. If you are looking at conducting future surveys, be sure they are spread out and patients are not overwhelmed.

Deciding on questions to ask in a patient survey can be challenging because you want to accomplish results for your market analysis without presenting a negative outlook on the health care facility. Questions with negative connotations can lead patients to believe they need to find something negative. Keep the questions positive, and design the questions according to the answers you are looking for. When you are looking for an explanation from patients about how their visit was, then provide them with **open-ended** surveys that allow them to explain their answers. Remember that what they write in an open-ended question must be read and taken seriously. Addressing their concerns is part of conducting a patient survey, and as a manager, you will be responsible for follow-up on their answers. On the other hand, **closed questions**—those with a "Yes" or "No" answer—can also provide the information you are searching for if you have appropriate questions. Designing the questions around the information you need is best when using "Yes" or "No" questions because this will allow for a straightforward answer and follow-up directed toward the information you desire. Both types are appropriate for a patient survey, and deciding which approach to use is based on the information you need and the time you have to address the answers.

Closed questions for patient survey include:

1. Is this your first visit to our health care facility?
2. Was the purpose of your visit a sickness or routine?
3. Were you able to get an appointment in a satisfying amount of time?
4. Did the staff meet your needs during the appointment?
5. Was the discharge process timely?

(Continues)

6. Do you need to follow up with us?

7. Do you typically get vaccines every year for seasonal illness?

8. Do you routinely have physical exams every year?

9. Was your overall experience a positive one?

10. Would you return to the facility again for future needs?

Open-ended questions for patient survey include:

1. What was your history with the health care facility before today?

2. Describe your experience scheduling your appointment at the office today.

3. Explain the purpose of your visit today.

4. Describe your wait time in the facility with regards to the waiting room, examination room, and discharge.

5. Evaluate the clinical staff and their attention to you during your visit.

6. Rate your experience at the office as bad, good, or excellent and explain why.

7. Indicate your last physical examination.

8. Indicate any other physicians in the area that you see.

9. Indicate any vaccinations you received to prevent illness and diseases.

10. List the reasons you would return to the facility in the future.

Conducting patient surveys can give you wonderful feedback that can assist you in your market analysis for the health care facility. You should include appropriate questions when conducting patient surveys because your current patients are the best referrals for advertising your facility. However, if negative feedback is given, remember to approach the situation positively and be sure the information is accurate. Focus on the reason for the patient survey as being a market analysis for advertising, and deal with the issues appropriately as a way to improve the quality of the health care facility for future patients.

CREATING ADVERTISEMENTS

Management should always be involved in the creation of advertisements because it knows the target audience and the health care facility requirements the best. When you create advertising, there is a skill to knowing just what needs to be included. The information provided must be informative yet not overwhelming. If you are unfamiliar with advertising, be sure to get some advice from others who have experienced advertising previously. The idea may seem easy, but to create exactly what you need without having too much information takes talent.

The option chosen for advertising will determine the information on the advertisement based on the target audience and what you want them to know about your health care facility. The advertising space will affect the arrangement and how much information is allowed. For promotional products, you are limited to the name and contact information; however, a mailer will allow for a larger announcement with contact information but may be time sensitive. Be aware of the requirements regarding information, timing, and reaching the target audience successfully because this all has to come together in the end.

Whichever option you choose, expect that several design options may be necessary for the advertisement, including the possibility of deleting information. Inquire about the expectations of your advertising, and keep a calendar of deadlines in order to stay on schedule, especially when you are promoting a service or an event. Be prepared ahead of time in order to make the design process easier, especially if working with an advertising agency and a deadline. Lastly, participate in the authorization of the final draft prior to the printing to ensure the advertisement is what you anticipated so mistakes can be corrected beforehand.

INFORMATIONAL BROCHURE

In an attempt to provide people with a background about your facility, including the location and hours, a brochure is an appropriate way to advertise. When creating a brochure, the initial appearance should be attractive to the audience, making people have an interest in more information. The office location(s), hours, and contact numbers should be clearly visible. If possible, the provider's information should also be included in the brochure to give the patient a background and credentials. However, if there are too many providers, then a picture of the health care facility or some features of the facility should be included.

Once the brochure is opened, you want to be sure the information inside is understandable. Keep in mind that the patient or potential patient does not understand medical terms, so be sure to use wording that is familiar to everyone. Be informative about the services you have, but do not make promises, such as same-day appointments, if you cannot fulfill them. Be sure that what you include in your brochure is also going to reflect positively on the health care facility.

When the brochure is completed, as manager, you should have the final approval and read it carefully. Be sure everything is accurate, including numbers, addresses, hours, and information, in order to avoid any miscommunication with patients. Also, consider yourself a patient and view as if you have not seen the brochure before. Ask yourself if you would be interested in picking it up to read more. Finally, once you approved them, always keep the brochures available to patients because this is a great way to advertise for your facility. Figure 14-6 shows a sample brochure that may be utilized in the facility.

SERVICE OR PRODUCT SPECIFIC

Advertising for a specific service or product is probably the easiest way to advertise. When there is particular service or event, the target audience is easier to identify due to the patient's age, gender, or health status. Back-to-school physical exams are focused on the students in grade school or college, whereas the heart health clinic is typically for older patients. Each of these groups views advertising differently and at different times; therefore, advertising is accomplished with different methods, times, and approaches. These are a couple of the presumptions we can make about target audiences in almost all areas; however, this should not be done on a regular basis.

In the situation where you are attempting to attract new patients and you are offering services or products, you may need multiple promotions to get in different target audiences. Unless, of course, you offer a discount on services, then the promotion is more generalized to attract various

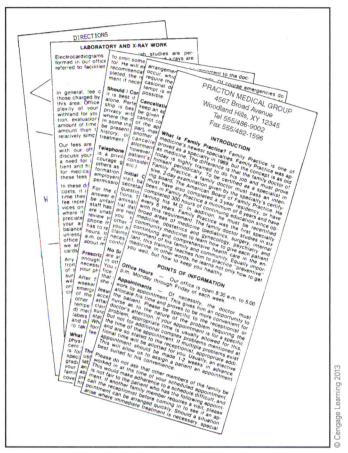

FIGURE 14-6 Sample Brochure

patients. Under certain circumstances, you may realize you want to attract a certain type of patient and decide to create a promotion or event that appeals to them. With specific services being offered, advertising can be a result of knowing your promotion or service and discovering the audience or vice versa. Figure 14-7 shows a sample brochure that may be utilized during advertising for such events. Whichever method you are leaning toward, you also need to be concerned with timing.

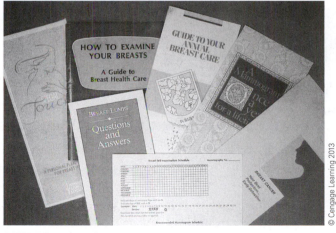

FIGURE 14-7 Information Brochures

TIME-SENSITIVE ADVERTISEMENT

When advertising time-sensitive material, deadlines have to be followed carefully. As soon as you know you are promoting a service or event, create a calendar of dates that you can use as a guide. Consider the option of some advertisements being run twice if there is not enough feedback on the first run. The date should be included immediately, along with the day of the week—for example, Friday, September 23—as most people can relate to the day of the week quickly when considering their schedules. With the time, be sure to include morning or night as well as start and end times. Including the option for appointments may be necessary depending on the event, and if there is no appointment necessary, it can be stated as such.

Lastly, be sure to include whether you want a response from the advertising due to the nature of the event. If there is a limit for attendance, give contact information that is easy to read so no one misses this vital information. A deadline for responding should also be listed in an obvious location so it is not confused with the date of the event.

With regards to advertising, time-sensitive advertisements should be a priority. If you find the need, engage help by approaching staff or outside agencies for assistance. Remember to contribute to the final approval process if you are not involved throughout. As a manager, you are a reflection of what you distribute, and your advertising should be delivered with confidence.

SUMMARY

- Determining the target audience you want to reach is the first step in the advertising process.

- When researching advertising options, management should consider the length of advertising and the cost incurred for the entire process.

- Before deciding which option of advertising to choose, the manager should conduct a market analysis to determine the potential for success of the desired advertisement.

- Advertising expense and market need should be analyzed thoroughly before decisions are made.

- Management should be involved in creating the advertisements—whether they are internally or externally developed—to ensure the advertising is appropriate and reaches the target audience in a timely manner.

REVIEW EXERCISES

TRUE OR FALSE

1. _____ Another health care facility can be considered a target audience for advertising.

2. _____ Timing of the advertisement can be important if advertising specifies services.

3. _____ Management is always given a budget for advertising and should follow it.

4. _____ Brochures are a great advertising tool for internal advertising to existing patients.

5. _____ When attempting to reach a new target audience, advertising can be more complicated.

6. _____ Patient surveys do not help when trying to conduct a marketing analysis.

7. _____ Searching online for advertising options is more time consuming for managers.

8. _____ Long-term advertising is more appropriate for a new health care facility.

9. _____ Management should be involved in the creation of advertising.

10. _____ Health care facilities cannot refer patients to each other because it is a conflict of interest.

MATCHING

A   Closed

B   Market Analysis

C   Streaming Advertising

D   Long Term

E   Outside Market

F   Open-Ended

G   Labor Hours

H   Short Term

I   Low Cost

J   Mailer

1. _____ Taking advantage of free advertising can cost the health care facility a lot if it does not pay attention to this.

2. _____ Determines potential for growth in the area based on the industry by looking at market size, trends, costs, profits, and potential for new clients.

3. _____ Questions on a patient survey that allow for an explanation to the question.

4. _____ The type of announcement that allows for more information but is time sensitive for promotions and events.

5. _____ Advertising a promotion or event is better when done with this length of time for advertising.

6. _____ Promotional products—such as pens, pencils, and magnets—are this type of advertising, which keeps the advertising budget minimal.

7. _____ Patient surveys that present "Yes" or "No" questions have this type of question.

8. _____ An advertising option that can be done online with advertisements passing across the screen.

9. _____ When the target audience is considered an external target.

10. _____ The length of advertising time that is used when advertising your location and providers, especially for new health care facilities.

CRITICAL THINKING ACTIVITIES

ACTIVITY 1

Identify the following for the target audience. Put a C for children, A for adult, and S for senior. More than one answer may be appropriate in some cases.

1. _____ Tetanus vaccination

2. _____ Free hearing test

3. _____ Scoliosis screening

4. _____ Hepatitis vaccination

5. _____ Free mammogram

6. _____ Free EKG

7. _____ Stress clinic

8. _____ Back-to-school physical exam

9. _____ Cholesterol screening

10. _____ Free nutrition clinic

ACTIVITY 2

Some advertisements are long term and some are short term depending on the need for the advertising. Next to the type of advertisement, write your opinion of what you think the advertisement time length should be by using ST for short term and LT for long term. Then, explain why you would make this choice.

1. _____ Mailer or postcard

_____

_____

2. _____ Movie theatre

_____

_____

3. _____ Promotional products, including pens and pencils

_____

_____

4. _____ Online streaming advertising

_____

_____

5. _____ Brochures

_____

_____

6. _____ Patient survey or questionnaire

_____

_____

7. _____ Online social networks

_____

_____

8. _____ Advertising boards/local facilities

_____

_____

9. _____ Media: newspaper, television, or radio

_____

_____

10. _____ Networking: professional organizations or local meetings

_____

_____

ACTIVITY 3

Identify potential problems in the following advertisement. The mistakes can be misspellings, design issues, or missing information. Discuss the errors and explain what you would do differently.

Free Clinic for Blood Pressure Checks

FRIDAY

TIME: 8:00

Location: The Hospital

Sponsored by: Medical Health

11 Stone Street

ACTIVITY 4

Mark an X next to the advertising that is time sensitive, indicating that the advertisement needs to be sent within a reasonable amount of time due to the nature of the advertising.

1. _____ Seasonal flu vaccination

2. _____ Discount for new patients

3. _____ Scoliosis screening for under 18 years of age

4. _____ Seasonal pneumonia vaccination

5. _____ Free glucose test for diabetes over age 50

6. _____ Free EKG on Saturday only

7. _____ Stress clinic on Friday only

8. _____ Meningitis vaccination

9. _____ Free psychiatric screening on Sunday only

10. _____ Free mammogram for new patients

CRITICAL THINKING QUESTIONS

1. Explain what approach you would take if an advertising agency was supposed to run an advertisement and did not meet the deadline. Consider time-sensitive and also other advertisements.

2. Debate pros and cons of Free clinics and health screenings at your health care facility. Include information based on diabetes, heart, and cholesterol screenings.

3. Discuss ideas in which the search for advertising options can be narrowed down and not take so long. Review online and local advertising.

4. Identify the target audience for a scoliosis screening at a pediatrician's office. Include the time-sensitive nature for running this clinic.

WEB ACTIVITIES

1. Go online to research advertising that uses promotional products and then create a list of 10 online companies. Get pricing for pens, pencils, magnets, and appointment calendars to give to patients during their visit. Research turnaround time and write it next to each company.

2. Research online for at least five advertising options of your choice. Use ideas from this chapter if you are unsure. Generate a list of appropriate options and then compare them in a spreadsheet, with pricing, time involved, length of advertising necessary, and estimated return on investment. Be sure to include web addresses and contact information for reaching them in the future.

3. Search online for advertising templates, including purchasable and free templates. Choose an advertisement layout that fits your needs and then save it for future use.

THINK LIKE A MANAGER
CREATE YOUR PRACTICE

Using the templates found in Appendix B and the information presented in this unit, complete the following interactive exercises:

1. Write an **open-ended** patient survey about your office. Include at least 10 items you may ask a patient with regards to your facility. Also, include the time frame in which you will administer the patient survey.

2. Write a **close-ended** market analysis survey about patients' preferences when it comes to health care. Include at least 10 items that you may ask with regards to your facility that will help you determine the need for your services in the area.

3. Write an advertisement for a health clinic that offers a free health screening. Include the target audience, advertising time frame, and amount of time.

4. Write a schedule for when an advertisement needs to begin and when it should end according to the schedule of the event.

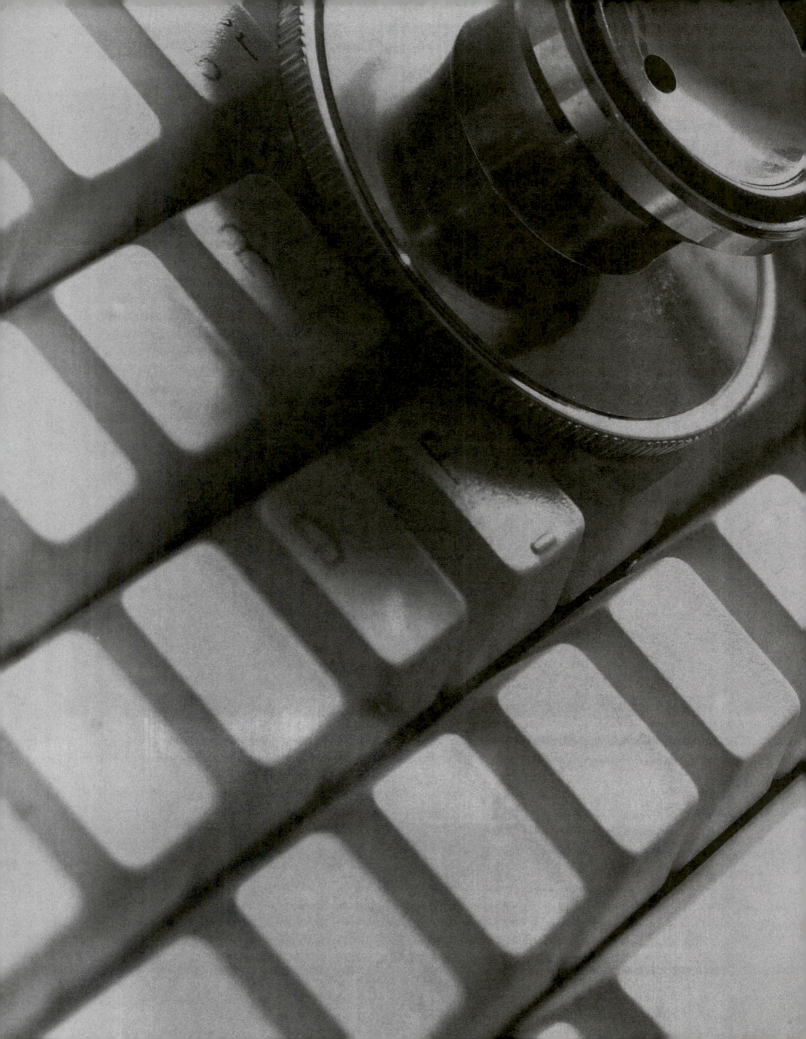

APPENDIX A:
Create Your Practice

INTRODUCTION TO THE CREATE YOUR PRACTICE PROJECT AND ACTIVITIES

Starting with chapter 2, you will first create the dynamics of your practice by using the worksheet in this appendix. In each of the management activities, you will be asked to perform management functions that pertain to each of the chapter topics. It will be a good idea to create a cover for your practice by using the practice information in this appendix and then add each of the activities to it. It creates a great visual tool when you are on an interview and seeking that management job!

Name your facility: _____

Your setting:

City: ☐

40% of patients are Medicaid

25% of patients are Medicare

20% of patients are considered charity care

15% of patients have commercial insurance

Suburbs: ☐

30% of patients have Medicare

30% of patients have commercial insurance

25% of patients have government insurance

15% of patients have other types of insurance

Insert one of the following:

Two-physician practice:

           Dr. _____

           Dr. _____   ☐

Four-physician practice:

           Dr. _____

           Dr. _____   ☐

           Dr. _____

           Dr. _____

Outpatient facility: Dr. _____   ☐

Specialties (choose how many providers your practice will have):

Internal medicine   ☐

Cardiology   ☐

Family practice   ☐

Pediatrics   ☐

Obstetrics   ☐

Other: _____ ☐

Insert your name as manager: _____

Pick and insert your personnel and how many your practice will need.

Receptionist(s)   ☐ ☐

Biller(s)   ☐ ☐

Nurse(s)   ☐ ☐

Lab personnel   ☐ ☐

Radiology personnel   ☐ ☐

Respiratory therapist   ☐ ☐

Physical therapist   ☐ ☐

Other positions   ☐ ☐

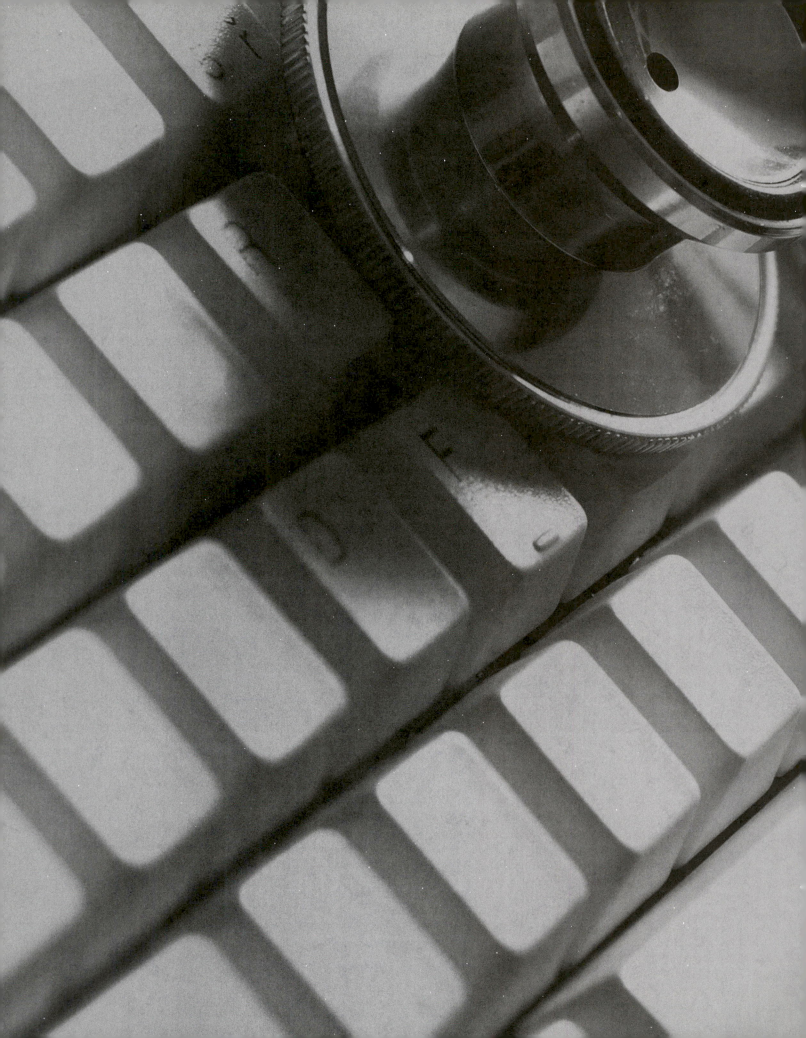

APPENDIX B:
Templates for create your own practice activities

Unit 1: Chapter 2, Question 1

Template for Creating a Policy and Procedure

Write a policy and procedure for the use of advanced beneficiary notices (ABNs).

Name of policy: Advanced Beneficiary Notices

Department: Medical Administration

Date enacted: Jan. 2012   Revised:

Purpose of policy: The purpose of this policy and procedure is to guide the administrative personnel as to when to have a patient sign an ABN.

Procedure:

1. Recognize when a patient needs to sign an ABN.

2. Review the ABN with the patient.

3.

4.

Attachments:

Unit 1: Chapter 2, Question 2

Template for Creating a Policy and Procedure

Write a policy and procedure for when to use an MSP (Medicare as a secondary payer) questionnaire.

Name of policy: Completing the MSP Questionnaire

Department: Medical Administration

Date enacted: Jan. 2012   Revised:

Purpose of policy: The purpose of this policy and procedure is to guide the frontline medical administrative personnel as well as others in this role as to when to complete a MSP questionnaire.

Procedure:
1. Identify situations in which an MSP form needs to be completed:

      a.

      b.

      c.

2.

etc.

Attachments:

Unit 1: Chapter 2, Question 3

Template for Creating a Policy and Procedure

Write a policy and procedure for triaging or screening phone calls.

Name of policy: Triaging Telephone Calls

Department: Medical Administration

Date enacted: Jan. 2012   Revised:

Purpose of Policy: The purpose of this policy is to establish guidelines for triaging phone calls to the correct personnel in the health care facility.

Procedure:
1. Identify the type of call.

2.

3.

etc.

Attachments:

Unit 1: Chapter 2, Question 4

Template for Creating a Policy and Procedure

Write a policy and procedure for collecting copayments.

Name of policy: Collecting Copayments

Department: Medical Administration

Date enacted: Jan. 2012   Revised:

Purpose of policy: The purpose of this policy and procedure is to establish a consistent policy and procedure to collect copayments at the time of visit.

Procedure:
1. Identify the patient and the patient's insurance.

2.

3.

etc.

Attachments:

Unit 2: Chapter 4, Question 1

Template for Creating a Policy and Procedure

Write a policy and procedure for the hiring process.

Name of policy: The Hiring Process

Department: Human Resources

Date enacted: 2012   Revised:

Purpose of policy: To have a uniform policy in the hiring process that incorporates the scope of practice for all personnel and includes all related licensing, certification, and knowledge of applicable regulations.

Procedure:
1. Determine what job openings the health care facility has.

2. Know the responsibilities for each position.

3.

4.

5.

Attachments: Job description

Unit 2: Chapter 4, Question 2

Template for Creating a Policy and Procedure

Write a policy and procedure for conducting a background check.

Name of policy: Conducting a Background Check

Department: Human Resources

Date enacted: 2012   Revised:

Purpose of policy: To have a uniform procedure in place for conducting a background check on affected personnel.

Procedure:
1. Complete the hiring process.

2. Offer applicant the position, indicating that employment will depend on results from a background check.

3. Give the applicant the background check form to complete, with instructions.

4.

5.

Attachments: Background check form

Unit 2: Chapter 4, Question 3

Template for Creating a Policy and Procedure

Write a policy and procedure for terminating employment

Name of policy: Termination of Employment

Department: Human Resources

Date enacted: 2012   Revised:

Purpose of policy: This policy is to follow a uniform procedure when an employee is terminated from a position, ensuring consistency with documentation.

Procedure:
1. Perform an exit interview.

2.

3.

4.

Attachments:

Unit 2: Chapter 4, Question 4

Template for Creating an Employment Advertisement

Write an employment advertisement to place in the classifieds of the local newspaper for a medical assistant. Include the role, responsibilities, education, and salary.

Employment job type: Medical Assistant

Practice name:

Full-time or part-time position:

Hours:

Qualifications:

Other points:

Respond to you (the manager): _____

Telephone/fax number: _____

E-mail: _____

Unit 2: Chapter 4, Question 5

Template for Creating Job Descriptions

Write a job description for the medical assistant for your practice. Information about this job is located on the Department of Labor's Occupational Outlook Handbook website (http://stats.bls.gov/oco). (See website activities.)

Job title:

Department:

Reports to:

Qualifications (education, licenses, certifications, etc.):

Summary of responsibilities:

1.

2.

3.

4.

5.

6.

7.

8.

9.

10.

etc.

Unit 2: Chapter 4, Question 6

Template for Writing an Offer Letter

Write an offer letter for a prospective hire.

Date:

Dear _____,

Sincerely,

_____

Office Manager

Unit 3: Chapter 6, Question 1

Template for Creating a Policy and Procedure

Write a policy and procedure for determining eligibility for charity care.

Name of policy: Determining Eligibility for Charity Care

Departments: Billing and Insurance

Date enacted: 2007   Revised: 2012

Purpose of policy: This policy will determine who meets the requirements for charity care.

Procedure:
1. Patient makes an appointment.

2.

3.

4.

Attachments:

Unit 3: Chapter 6, Question 2

Template for Creating a Policy and Procedure

Write a policy and procedure for taking action based on the aging report.

Name of policy: Collection activity action

Departments: Billing and Insurance

Date enacted: 2007   Revised: 2012

Purpose of policy: This policy outlines the steps to take in the process of collection based on the accounts aging report.

Procedure:
1. At the 30-day mark . . .

2. At the 60-day mark . . .

3.

4.

Attachments: Sample letters

Unit 3: Chapter 6, Question 3

Template for Creating a Policy and Procedure

Write a policy and procedure for whose responsibility it is for collection activities.

Name of policy:

Department: _____

Date enacted: _____   Revised: _____

Purpose of policy: _____

Procedure:

1. _____

2. _____

3. _____

etc.

Attachments:

Unit 3: Chapter 6, Question 4

Template for Developing a Teaching Session or In-Service Training

You want to teach your new employees about accounts aging reports and collection activities. Plan a teaching session:

- *Create an outline of content to be discussed.*
- *Create a sign-in sheet.*
- *Review the policies and procedures you created for your practice.*

Topic:

Departments or positions included in session:

Outline:

How this topic pertains to your department or job title:

Why it needs to be discussed today:

Brief description of the history of this topic:

Situations that apply to this setting:

Discussions:

Questions and answers:

Handouts to be distributed:

1. Sign-in sheet to be created, including date and topic.

2.

Unit 4: Chapter 8, Question 1

Template for Creating a Policy and Procedure

Write a policy and procedure for developing a consistent review of a medical record.

Name of policy: Reviewing Medical Records

Department: Medical Records

Date enacted: 2/14/2012   Revised:

Purpose of policy: To create a consistent procedure in reviewing the medical record.

Procedure: Each medical record component needs to be reviewed for completeness. Each medical record must contain:
1. Patient name

Attachments:

Approved by:

Date:

Unit 4: Chapter 8, Question 2

Template for Creating a Policy and Procedure

Write a policy and procedure for ensuring the consistency within a medical record. Include documenting, necessary requirements, and organization.

Name of policy:

Department : _____

Date enacted: _____   Revised: _____

Purpose of policy: _____

Procedure:

1. _____

2. _____

3. _____

etc.

Attachments:

Unit 4: Chapter 8, Question 3

Template for Developing a Teaching Session or In-Service Training

You have found when auditing a medical record that it is incomplete. Prepare a teaching session on what goes in the medical record and how to ensure its consistency. Create an outline, a sign-in sheet, and a handout.

Topic:

Departments or positions included in session:

Outline:

How this topic pertains to your department or job title:

Why it needs to be discussed today:

Brief description of the history of this topic:

Situations that apply to this setting:

Discussions:

Questions and answers:

Handouts to be distributed:

1. Sign-in sheet to be created, including date and topic.

2.

Unit 4: Chapter 8, Question 4

Template for Creating a Policy and Procedure

Write a policy and procedure for maintaining consistency in a medical record with regards to an abbreviation policy, including approved abbreviations.

Name of policy:

Department: _____

Date enacted: _____   Revised: _____

Purpose of policy: _____

Procedure:

1. _____

2. _____

3. _____

etc.

Attachments:

Unit 4: Chapter 8, Question 5

Template for Developing a Teaching Session or In-Service Training

You have found when auditing a medical record that the use of abbreviations is inconsistent and impacting patient care negatively. Prepare a teaching session on how to ensure their consistency. Create an outline, a sign-in sheet, and a handout.

Topic:

Departments or positions included in session:

Outline:

How this topic pertains to your department or job title:

Why it needs to be discussed today:

Brief description of the history of this topic:

Situations that apply to this setting:

Discussions:

Questions and answers:

Handouts to be distributed:

1. Sign-in sheet to be created, including date and topic.

2.

Unit 5: Chapter 10, Question 1

Template for Creating a Policy and Procedure

Write a policy and procedure for auditing a hospital record.

Name of policy: Auditing the Chart of a Hospitalized Patient

Department: Management

Date enacted: Revised:

Purpose of policy: Ensure compliance and continuity in the chart of a hospitalized patient.

Procedure:

1. Review chart components for the patient's name, record number, and date consistency.

2. Obtain the claim form to compare documentation to the claim form.

3.

4.

Attachments:

Unit 5: Chapter 10, Question 2

Template for Creating a Policy and Procedure

Write a policy and procedure for auditing a surgical chart.

Name of policy: Auditing the Chart of the Patient Who Has Had Surgery

Department:

Date enacted: Revised:

Purpose of policy: To review the medical chart for compliance and consistency.

Procedure:
1. Review the chart for consistency in patient name, medical record number, and dates.

2. Preoperative review:

3.

4.

Attachments:

Unit 5: Chapter 10, Question 3

Template for Developing a Teaching Session or In-Service Training
Write an in-service training session to teach your billing department how to recognize situations and prevent denials by an insurance company.

Topic:

Departments or positions included in session:

Outline:

How this topic pertains to your department or job title:

Why it needs to be discussed today:

Brief description of the history of this topic:

Situations that apply to this setting:

Discussions:

Questions and answers:

Handouts to be distributed:

1. Sign-in sheet to be created, including date and topic.

2.

Unit 5: Chapter 10, Question 4

Template for Creating an Employment Advertisement

Write an employment advertisement to place in the classifieds of the local newspaper for an on-site medical auditor. Include the role, responsibilities, education, and salary.

Employment job type: Medical Auditor

Practice name:

Full-time or part-time position:

Hours:

Qualifications:

Other points:

Respond to you (the manager): _____

Telephone/fax number: _____

E-mail: _____

Unit 6: Chapter 12, Question 1

Template for Creating a Policy and Procedure

Write a policy and procedure for employee exposure control for compliance with OSHA standards.

Name of policy:

Department: _____

Date enacted: _____   Revised: _____

Purpose of policy: _____

Procedure:

1. _____

2. _____

3. _____

etc.

Attachments:

Unit 6: Chapter 12, Question 2

Template for Developing a Teaching Session or In-Service Training

Perform in-service training for a medical assistant to cover the OSHA exposure control requirements. Include clinical and administrative standards for your state.

Topic:

Departments or positions included in session:

Outline:

How this topic pertains to your department or job title:

Why it needs to be discussed today:

Brief description of the history of this topic:

Situations that apply to this setting:

Discussions:

Questions and answers:

Handouts to be distributed:

1. Sign-in sheet to be created, including date and topic.

2.

Unit 6: Chapter 12, Question 3

Template for Creating a Policy and Procedure

Write a policy and procedure for effective communication when recording critical test results.

Name of Policy:

Department: _____

Date enacted:_____   Revised: _____

Purpose of policy: _____

Procedure:

1. _____

2. _____

3. _____

etc.

Attachments:

Unit 6: Chapter 12, Question 4

Template for Developing a Teaching Session or In-Service Training

Perform in-service training for all employees on effective communication when recording critical test results.

Topic:

Departments or positions included in session:

Outline:

How this topic pertains to your department or job title:

Why it needs to be discussed today:

Brief description of the history of this topic:

Situations that apply to this setting:

Discussions:

Questions and answers:

Handouts to be distributed:

1. Sign-in sheet to be created, including date and topic.

2.

Unit 6: Chapter 12, Question 5

Template for Creating a Policy and Procedure

Write a policy and procedure for developing an action plan after a sentinel event (such as a patient falling).

Name of policy:

Department: _____

Date enacted: _____   Revised: _____

Purpose of policy: _____

Procedure:

1. _____

2. _____

3. _____

etc.

Attachments:

Unit 6: Chapter 12, Question 6

Template for Creating an Exposure Plan

Write an exposure plan for protecting clinical employees from blood-borne pathogens. Include information necessary to keep employees safe from patient's blood or body fluids.

Exposure Plan

Prevention techniques: _____

_____

_____

Engineering controls: _____

_____

_____

Workplace controls: _____

_____

_____

Additional comments: _____

_____

_____

Unit 7: Chapter 14, Question 1

Template for Patient Survey

Write an open-ended patient survey about your office. Include at least 10 items you may ask a patient with regards to your facility. Also, include the time frame in which you will administer the patient survey.

Patient Survey

1. _____
2. _____
3. _____
4. _____
5. _____
6. _____
7. _____
8. _____
9. _____
10. _____

Unit 7: Chapter 14, Question 2

Template for Market Analysis Survey

Write a close-ended market analysis survey about patients' preferences when it comes to health care. Include at least 10 items that you may ask with regards to your facility that will help you determine the need for your services in the area.

Market Analysis Questionnaire
Create questions that have "Yes" or "No" answers.

1. _____
2. _____
3. _____
4. _____
5. _____
6. _____
7. _____
8. _____
9. _____
10. _____

Unit 7: Chapter 14, Question 3

Template for a Marketing Advertisement

Write an advertisement for a health clinic that offers a free health screening. Include the target audience, advertising time frame, and amount of time.

Advertising type:

Practice name:

Address:

Date:

Time frame:

Target audience:

Advertisement:

Other points:

Respond to you (the manager): _____

Telephone/fax number: _____

E-mail: _____

Unit 7: Chapter 14, Question 4

Template for an Advertising Schedule

Write a schedule for when an advertisement needs to begin and when it should end according to the schedule of the event.

	Monday	Tuesday	Wednesday	Thursday	Friday		
Week 1	Monday	Tuesday	Wednesday	Thursday	Friday	Notes	Due
Week 2	Monday	Tuesday	Wednesday	Thursday	Friday		
Week 3	Monday	Tuesday	Wednesday	Thursday	Friday		
Week 4	Monday	Tuesday	Wednesday	Thursday	Friday		
Week 5	Monday	Tuesday	Wednesday	Thursday	Friday		
Week 6	Monday	Tuesday	Wednesday	Thursday	Friday		
Week 7	Monday	Tuesday	Wednesday	Thursday	Friday		
Week 8	Monday	Tuesday	Wednesday	Thursday	Friday		

Extra Templates
Template for Creating Policies and Procedures

Name of Policy: _____

Department: _____

Date enacted: _____   Revised: _____

Purpose of policy: _____

Procedure:

1. _____

2. _____

3. _____

etc.

Attachments:

Template for Creating Job Descriptions

Job title: _____

Department: _____

Reports to: _____

Qualifications (education, licenses, certifications, etc.): _____

Summary of responsibilities:

1.

2.

3.

4.

5.

6.

7.

8.

9.

10.

etc.

Template for Creating an Employment Advertisement

Employment job type: _____

Practice name: _____

Full-time or part-time position: _____

Hours: _____

Qualifications: _____

Other points: _____

Respond to you (the manager): _____

Telephone/fax number: _____

E-mail: _____

Template for Writing an Offer Letter

Date: _____

Dear_____,

Sincerely,

_____
Office Manager

Template for Developing a Teaching Session or In-Service Training

Topic: _____

Departments or positions included in session: _____

Outline

How this topic pertains to your department or job title

Why it needs to be discussed today

Brief description of the history of this topic

Situations that apply to this setting

Discussions

Questions and answers

Handouts to be distributed:
1. Sign-in sheet to be created, including date and topic

2.

Template of Creating an Exposure Plan

Exposure Plan

Prevention techniques: _____

_____

_____

Engineering controls: _____

_____

_____

Workplace controls: _____

_____

_____

Additional comments: _____

_____

_____

Template for Patient Survey

Patient Survey

1. _____

2. _____

3. _____

4. _____

5. _____

6. _____

7. _____

8. _____

9. _____

10. _____

Template for Market Analysis Survey

Market Analysis Questionnaire

Create questions that can have "Yes" or "No" answers.

1. _____

2. _____

3. _____

4. _____

5. _____

6. _____

7. _____

8. _____

9. _____

10. _____

Template for a Marketing Advertisement

Advertising type: _____

Practice name: _____

Address: _____

Date: _____

Time frame: _____

Target audience: _____

Advertisement:

Other points:

Respond to you (the manager): _____

Telephone/fax number: _____

E-mail: _____

Template for an Advertising Schedule

	Monday	Tuesday	Wednesday	Thursday	Friday		
Week 1	Monday	Tuesday	Wednesday	Thursday	Friday	Notes	Due
Week 2	Monday	Tuesday	Wednesday	Thursday	Friday		
Week 3	Monday	Tuesday	Wednesday	Thursday	Friday		
Week 4	Monday	Tuesday	Wednesday	Thursday	Friday		
Week 5	Monday	Tuesday	Wednesday	Thursday	Friday		
Week 6	Monday	Tuesday	Wednesday	Thursday	Friday		
Week 7	Monday	Tuesday	Wednesday	Thursday	Friday		
Week 8	Monday	Tuesday	Wednesday	Thursday	Friday		

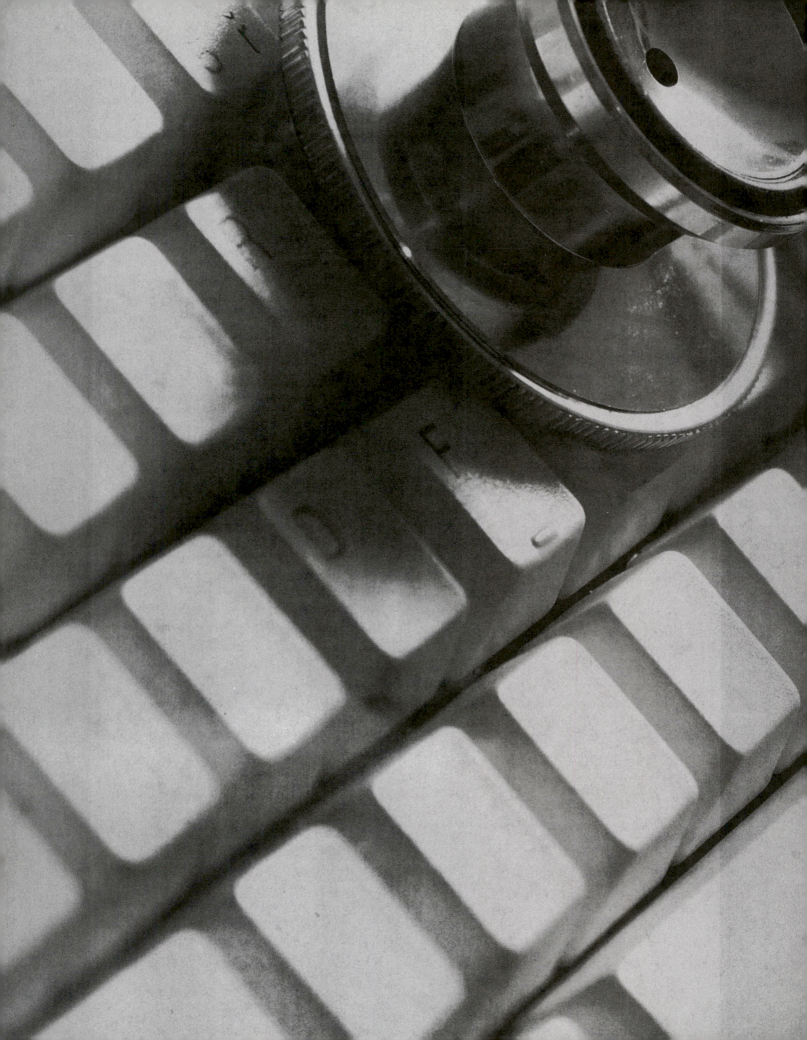

APPENDIX C: Common Medical Abbreviations

TABLE APP C1-1: Health Care Professionals and Their Abbreviations

Position	Abbreviation	Position	Abbreviation
Certified Bookkeeper	CB	Certified Medical Transcriptionist	CMT
Certified Claims Assistance Professional	CCAP	Certified Nurse Midwife	CNM
Certified Clinic Account Technician	CCAT	Certified Patient Account Technician	CPAT
Certified Clinic Account Manager	CCAM	Certified Professional Coder	CPC
Certified Coding Specialist	CCS	Certified Professional Coder— Hospital	CPC-H
Certified Coding Specialist— Physician based	CCS-P	Certified Registered Nurse Anesthetist	CRNA
Certified Electronic Claims Professional	CECP	Certified Surgical Technician (2nd surgical asst.)	CST
Certified First Assistant (surgical)	CFA	Doctor of Chiropractic	DC
Certified Laboratory Assistant; certified by Registry of American Society of Clinical Pathologists	CLA (ASCP)	Doctor of Dental Surgery	DDS
		Doctor of Dental Science	DD Sc
Certified Medical Assistant	CMA	Doctor of Emergency Medicine	DEM
Certified Medical Biller; certified by the Certified Medical Billing Association	CMB	Doctor of Hygiene	D Hy
		Doctor of Medical Dentistry	DMD
Certified Medical Billing Specialist	CMBS	Doctor of Osteopathy	DO
Certified Medical Office Manager	CMOM	Doctor of Public Health	DPH
Certified Medical Practice Executive	CMPE	Doctor of Podiatry	DPM
Certified Medical Reimbursement Specialist	CMRS	Doctor of Tropical Medicine	DTM

(continued)

TABLE APP C1-1: Health Care Professionals and Their Abbreviations (continued)

Position	Abbreviation	Position	Abbreviation
Doctor of Veterinary Medicine	DVM	Doctor of Ophthalmology	OphD
Doctor of Veterinary Surgery	DVS	Doctor of Optometry	OD
Emergency Medical Technician	EMT	Physician's Assistant—Certified	PA-C
Fellow of the American Academy of Pediatrics	FAAP	Doctor of Pharmacy	Pharm D
		Public Health Nurse	PHN
Fellow of the American College of Obstetricians and Gynecologists	FACOG	Registered Dietitian	RD
		Registered Medical Assistant	RMA
Fellow of the American College of Surgery	FACS	Registered Medical Coder	RMC
		Registered Nurse	RN
Health Care Reimbursement Specialist	HRS	Registered Nurse First Assistant (surgical)	RNFA
Health Information Management	HIM		
Inhalation Therapist	IT	Registered Nurse Practitioner	RNP
Licensed Practical Nurse	LPN	Registered Occupational Therapist	ROT
Laboratory Technical Assistant	LTA	Registered Physical Therapist	RPT
Licensed Vocational Nurse	LVN	Registered Respiratory Therapist	RRT
Doctor of Medicine	MD	Registered Technologist (Radiology)	RT(R)
Master of Public Health	MPH	Registered Technologist (Therapy)	RT(T)
Medical Technologist	MT (ASCP)	Senior Fellow	SF
National Certified Insurance and Coding Specialist	NCICS	Visiting Nurse	VN

TABLE APP C1-2: Appointment Abbreviations Used in Patient Scheduling

Abbreviation	Medical term	Abbreviation	Medical term
abd, abdom	abdominal	stat	immediately
accid	accident	inf	infection
an ck	annual check	flu syn	influenza syndrome
an PX	annual physical examination	inj, INJ	injection
AP	antepartum care	IUD	intrauterine device
BP	blood pressure check	Lab FU, Lab F/U	laboratory follow-up
breast ck	breast check	lac	laceration
canc	cancel, canceled	LBP	low back pain
cast ck	cast check	MMR	measles, mumps, rubella
check	ck, ✓	(N), N/P, NP	new patient
CXR, PA chest, AP chest	chest x-ray	New OB	new obstetric patient
		NFA	no future appointment
CBC	complete blood count	N/S, NS	no-show
CPX, CPE	complete physical examination	NTRA	no telephone requests for antibiotics
consult, cons, CON	consultation		
cysto	cystoscopy	OB	obstetric patient
DX, dx, dg, diag.	diagnosis	OV	office visit
DNKA	did not keep appointment	Pap	Papanicolaou smear
DNS	did not show	PE, PX, ph ex, phys	physical examination
DSHA	does she have appointment	PO, Post-op	postoperative check
dr, drsg	dressing	PP	postpartum care
DC	dressing change	PC	pregnancy confirmation
EKG, ECG	electrocardiogram	OB	prenatal care
EMG	electromyogram, electromyelogram	Pre-op, preop	preoperative office visit
E	emergency	procto	proctoscopic examination
ER	emergency room	REF, ref	referral
FU	follow-up visit	RTC	return to clinic
FX, Fx	fracture	RTO	return to office
GTT	glucose tolerance test	RV, ret, retn	return visit
Gyn ck, GYN	gynecological check	SIG, sigmoido	sigmoidoscopy
HA	headache	SR	suture removal
HC	house call	WI, W/I	walk-in, work-in
		WT	weight

TABLE APP C1-3: Patient Care Abbreviations

A	allergy; abortion	Brev	Brevital
AB	antibiotic	BUN	blood urea nitrogen
abdom	abdomen	Bx, BX	biopsy
abt	about	C	cervical; centigrade; celsius
Acc, acc	accommodation	C & S	culture and sensitivity
AD, a.d.	right ear	Ca, CA	cancer, carcinoma
adm	admit; admission; admitted	Cauc	Caucasian
adv	advice	CBC	complete blood count
aet.	at the age of	cc	cubic centimeter
AgNO$_3$	silver nitrate	CC	chief complaint
AIDS	acquired immune deficiency syndrome	CDC	calculated date of confinement
alb	albumin	chem	chemistry
ALL	allergy	CHF	congestive heart failure
a.m., AM	before noon	chr	chronic
AMA	American Medical Association	CI	color index
ant	anterior	cm	centimeter
ante	before	CNS	central nervous system
A & P	auscultation and percussion	CO, C/O	complains of
AP	anterior posterior; anteroposterior	CO$_2$, CO2	carbon dioxide
		comp	comprehensive
AP & L	anteroposterior and lateral	compl	complete
approx	approximate	Con, CON, Cons	consultation
apt	apartment	Cont.	continue
ASA	acetylsalicylic acid	COPD	chronic obstructive pulmonary disease
asap, ASAP	as soon as possible		
ASCVD	arteriosclerotic cardiovascular disease	CPX, CPE	complete physical examination
		C section	cesarean section
ASHD	arteriosclerotic heart disease	CT	computerized tomography
asst	assistant	CV	cardiovascular
auto	automobile	CVA	costovertebral angle; cardiovascular accident; cerebrovascular accident
Ba	barium		
BI	biopsy		
BM	bowel movement	CXR	chest x-ray
BMR	basal metabolic rate	Cysto	cystoscopy
BP, B/P	blood pressure	D & C	dilatation and curettage

TABLE APP C1-3: Patient Care Abbreviations (continued)

dc	discontinue	exc.	excision
DC	discharge	ext	external
del	delivery	F	Fahrenheit; French (catheter)
Dg, Dx, dx	diagnosis	FACP	Fellow, American College of Physicians
diag.	diagnosis, diagnostic	FACS	Fellow, American College of Surgeons
diam.	diameter	FH	family history
diff.	differential	FHS	fetal heart sounds
dilat	dilate	fluor	fluoroscopy
disch.	discharged	ft	foot; feet
DNA	does not apply	FU	follow-up
DNS	did not show	Fx	fracture
DOB	date of birth	G	gravida (number of pregnancies)
DPM	Doctor of Podiatric Medicine	g, gm	gram
DPT	diphtheria, pertussis, tetanus (vaccine)	GA	gastric analysis
Dr.	Doctor	GB	gallbladder
drsg	dressing	GC	gonorrhea
Dx, Dg, dx	diagnosis	GGE	generalized glandular enlargement
E	emergency	GI	gastrointestinal
ECG	electrocardiogram; electrocardiograph	GU	genitourinary
		Gyn, GYN	gynecology
ED	emergency department	H	hospital call
EDC	estimated date of confinement; due date for baby	HA	headache
		HBP	high blood pressure
EEG	electroencephalogram; electroencephalograph	HC	hospital call; hospital consultation
		HCD	house call, day
EENT	eye, ear, nose, and throat	HCl	hydrochloric acid
EKG	electrocardiogram; electrocardiograph	HCN	house call, night
epith.	epithelial	hct	hematocrit
ER	emergency room	HCVD	hypertensive cardiovascular disease
ESR	erythrocyte sedimentation rate	HEENT	head, eyes, ears, nose, and throat
est.	established; estimated	Hgb, Hb	hemoglobin
etiol.	etiology	hist	history
EU	etiology unknown	H_2O, H2O	water
Ex, exam.	examination	hosp	hospital

(continued)

TABLE APP C1-3: Patient Care Abbreviations (continued)

H & P	history and physical	lbs	pounds
HPI	history of present illness	LLL	left lower lobe
hr, hrs	hour, hours	LLQ	left lower quadrant
HS	hospital surgery	LMP	last menstrual period
Ht, ht	height	lt., LT	left
HV	hospital visit	ltd.	limited
HX	history	LUQ	left upper quadrant
HX PX	history and physical examination	M	medication; married
I	injection	MA	mental age
I&D	incision and drainage	med., MED	medicine
IC	initial consultation	mg	milligram(s)
i.e.	that is	MH	marital history
IM	intramuscular	ml	milliliter(s)
imp., IMP	impression	mm	millimeter(s)
inc	include	MM	mucous membrane
inf, INF	infected	mo	month(s)
inflam., INFL	inflammation	N	negative
init	initial	NA, N/A	not applicable
inj., INJ	injection	NaCl	sodium chloride
int, INT	internal	NAD	no appreciable disease
intermed	intermediate	neg.	negative
interpret	interpretation	NP	new patient
IPPB	intermittent positive pressure breathing	NPN	nonprotein nitrogen
		N&V	nausea and vomiting
IQ	intelligence quotient	NYD	not yet diagnosed
IV, I.V.	intravenous	O_2, O2	oxygen
IVP	intravenous pyelogram	OB	obstetrical, obstetrics
JVD	jugulovenous distention	OC	office call
K35	Kollmann (dilator)	occ	occasional
KUB	kidneys, ureters, bladder	O.D., o.d.	right eye
L	left; laboratory; living children; liter	ofc	office
lab., LAB	laboratory	OH	occupational history
L&A, l/a	light and accommodation	O.L.	left eye
L&W	living and well	OP, op.	operation, operative, outpatient
lat, LAT	lateral	OPD	outpatient department

TABLE APP C1-3: Patient Care Abbreviations (continued)

OR	operating room	prog	prognosis
orig.	original	P&S	permanent and stationary
O.S., o.s.	office surgery; left eye	PSP	phenolsulfonphthalein
OT	occupational therapy	Pt, pt	patient
OTC	over the counter	PT	physical therapy
OV	office visit	PTR	patient to return
P	pulse; preterm parity or deliveries before term	PX	physical examination
		R	right; residence call; report
PA	posterior anterior, posteroanterior	RBC, rbc	red blood cell
P&A	percussion and auscultation	rec	recommend
PAP, Pap	Papanicolaou (test)	re ch	recheck
Para I	woman having borne one child (Para II, two children, and so on)	re-exam, reex	reexamination
		reg.	regular
PBI	protein-bound iodine	ret, retn	return
PC	present complaint	rev	review
PD	permanent disability	Rh-	Rhesus negative (blood)
PE	physical examination	RHD	rheumatic heart disease
perf.	performed	RLQ	right lower quadrant
PERRLA, PERLA	pupils equal, round, react to light and to accommodation	RO, R/O	rule out
pH	hydrogen ion concentration	ROS	review of systems
PH	past history	rt.	right
Ph ex	physical examination	RT	respiratory therapy
phys.	physical	RTC	return to clinic
PI	present illness	RTO	return to office
PID	pelvic inflammatory disease	RUQ	right upper quadrant
p.m., PM	after noon	Rx, RX, R_x	prescription; any medication or treatment ordered
PMH	past medical history		
PND	postnasal drip	S	surgery
PO, P Op	postoperative; phone order	SD	state disability
pos.	positive	SE	special examination
post.	posterior	sed rate	sedimentation rate
postop	postoperative	Sep.	separated
preop	preoperative	SH	social history
prep	prepare, prepared	SLR	straight leg raising
PRN, p.r.n.	as necessary	slt	slight

(continued)

TABLE APP C1-3: Patient Care Abbreviations (continued)

Smr, sm.	smear	UTI	urinary tract infection
SMWD	single, married, widowed, divorced	vac	vaccine
SOB	shortness of breath	VD	venereal disease
sp gr	specific gravity	VDRL	Venereal Disease Research Laboratory (test for syphilis)
SQ	subcutaneous		
SR	suture removal; sedimentation rate	W	work; white
STAT, stat.	immediately	WBC, wbc	white blood cell or count; well baby care
STD	sexually transmitted disease		
strab	strabismus	WF	white female
surg.	surgery	wk.	week; work
Sx.	symptoms	wks	weeks
T	temperature; term parity or deliveries at term	WM, W/M	white male
		WNL	within normal limits
T&A	tonsillectomy and adenoidectomy	WR	Wassermann reaction
Tb, tbc, TB	tuberculosis	Wt, wt	weight
TD	temporary disability	X	x-ray(s); multiplied by
temp.	temperature	XR	x-ray(s)
TIA	transient ischemic attack	yr	year
TMs	tympanic membranes	Symbols	
TPR	temperature, pulse, respiration	*	birth
Tr.	treatment	$\bar{c}$, /c, w/	with
TTD	total temporary disability	$\bar{P}$	after
TURB	transurethral resection of bladder	$\bar{s}$, /s, w/o	without
		$\bar{cc}$, $\bar{c}/c$	with correction (eyeglasses)
TURP	transurethral resection of prostate	$\bar{sc}$, $\bar{s}/c$	without correction (eyeglasses)
TX, Tx	treatment	+	positive
U	unit	$\bar{-}$, $\bar{0}$,	negative
UA, U/A	urinalysis	±	negative or positive; indefinite
UCHD	usual childhood diseases	Ⓛ	left
UCR	usual, customary, and reasonable	ⓜ	murmur
UGI	upper gastrointestinal	Ⓡ	right
UPJ	ureteropelvic junction or joint	♂	male
UR, ur	urine	♀	female
URI	upper respiratory infection	μ	micron

TABLE APP C1-4: Common Prescription Abbreviations* and Symbols

$\overline{a}$	before	ID	intradermal
$\overline{aa}$	of each	IM	intramuscular
a.c.	before meals	inj.	injection; to be injected
ad lib.	As much as needed	IV or I.V.	intravenous
a.d. or AD	right ear	kg	kilogram
a.m. or AM	morning	liq	liquid
ante	before	M or m.	mix
aq.	aqueous/water	mcg	microgram
a.s. or AS	left ear	mg or mgm	milligram
a.u. or AU	both ears	ml	milliliter
b.i.d.	two times a day	N.E. or ne	negative
caps	capsule	noct.	night
$\overline{c}$	with	NPO or n.p.o.	nothing by mouth
$\overline{cc}$	with meals	O_2	oxygen
cc	cubic centimeter	OD or O.D.	right eye
comp. or comp	compound	o.d.	once a day
d	day	o.h.	every hour
DC or D/C	discontinue	oint	ointment
dos.	doses	o.m.	every morning
DSD	double starting dose	o.n.	every night
elix.	elixir	OS or O.S.	left eye
emul.	emulsion	OTC	over-the-counter (drugs)
et	and	OU or O.U.	both eyes
ext.	extract	oz	ounce
garg.	gargle	$\overline{p}$	after
gm or g	gram	p.c.	after meals
gr	grain	p.o.	by mouth (per os)
gt.	drop	p.r.	per rectum
gtt.	drops	p.r.n. or PRN	whenever necessary
h.	hour	q.	every
h.s.	before bedtime (hour of sleep)	q.a.m.	every morning

Many of these abbreviations are derived from Latin; they are usually typed in lowercase and with periods. Periods are especially important, if without periods an abbreviation would spell a word; for example, b.i.d. without periods is bid.

(continued)

TABLE APP C1-4: Common Prescription Abbreviations* and Symbols (continued)

q.d.	one time daily; every day	ss	one-half
q.h.	every hour	stat or STAT	immediately
q.h.s.	every night	syr.	syrup
q.i.d.	four times a day (not at night)	tab.	tablet
q. n.	every night	t.i.d.	three times a day
q.o.d.	every other day	top	topically
q.p.m.	every night	Tr. or tinct.	tincture
q.2 h.	every two hours	tsp	teaspoon
q.3 h.	every three hours	U	unit
q.4 h.	every 4 hours	vag.	vagina
rep, REP	let it be repeated; Latin repeto	X or x	times (X10d/times ten days)
Rx	take (recipe), prescription	i, ii, iii, iv, viii, etc.	1, 2, 3, 4, 8, etc.
$\bar{s}$	without	5″, 10″, 15″	5 , 10 , 15 minutes, etc.
SC or subq sat.	subcutaneous saturated	5°, 10°, 15°, or 5′, 10′, 15′, etc.	5 hours, 10 hours, 15 hours, etc.
Sig.	write on label; give directions on prescription		
SL	sublingual	3 or dr.	dram (drachm)
sol.	solution	3 or oz.	ounce

*Many of these abbreviations are derived from Latin; they are usually typed in lowercase and with periods. Periods are especially important, if without periods an abbreviation would spell a word; for example, b.i.d. without periods is bid.

TABLE APP C1-5: Common Errors and Dangerous Abbreviations to Avoid

When Penmanship Is Poor, This . . .	. . .Can Be Misread As This . . .	. . . So Write This Instead or Use This Guideline
1.0 mg	10 mg	"1 mg"
.3 mg	3 mg	"0.3 mg"
10000	100000	Insert comma (10,000)
6 units regular insulin/ 20 units NPH insulin	120 units of NPH	Never use a slash
BT (bedtime)	BID (twice daily)	"h.s." (before bedtime)
cc	U (units)	"ml"
D/C	Discharge or discontinue	Discharge or discontinue
DPT	Demerol-Phenergan-Thorazine or diphtheria-pertussis-tetanus	Completely spell out drug names
Every 3–4 hours	Every 3/4 hour	"every 3 to 4 hours"
HCl	KCl	Completely spell out drug names (hydrochloric)
HCT	Hydrocortisone or hydrochlorothiazide	Completely spell out drug names
IU	International unit	"unit"
MgSO4	Magnesium sulfate or morphine	Complete spell out
o.d. or OD (every day)	OD "right eye" (oculus dexter)	"daily"
per OS	OS (left eye)	"by mouth"
q.d. or QD	q.i.d. (4 times a day)	"daily" or "every day"
qn	qh (every hour)	"nightly"
qhs	Every hour	"nightly"
q6PM	Every six hours	"6 p.m. nightly"
q.o.d. or Q.O.D.	q.d. (daily) or q.i.d. (four times daily)	"every other day"
SC	SL (sublingual)	"subcut" or "subcutaneous"
sub q	Every	"subcut" or "subcutaneous"
TIW or tiw	Three times a day	Do not use this abbreviation
U or u	Zero (0), 6, cc, or a four (4), causing a 10-fold overdose or greater (e.g., 4U seen as "40" or 4u seen as "44")	"unit" (Do not abbreviate)
ug	microgram	"mcg"
x3d	three doses	"for three days"
1.0 Zero after a decimal point	10 mg (if the decimal point is not seen)	Do not use terminal zeros for doses expressed in whole numbers
.5 mg No zero before decimal dose	5 mg	Always use zero before a decimal when the dose is less than a whole unit

TABLE APP C1-6: Collection Abbreviations

B	Bankrupt	NSF	Not sufficient funds (check)
BLG	Belligerent	NSN	No such number
EOM	End of month	OOT	Out of town
EOW	End of week	OOW	Out of work
FN	Final notice	Ph/Dsc	Phone disconnected
H	He or husband	POW	Payment on way
HHCO	Have husband call office	PP	Promise to pay
HTO	He telephoned office	S	She or wife
L1, L2	Letter one, letter two (sent)	SEP	Separated
LB	Line busy	SK	Skip or skipped
LD	Long distance	SOS	Same old story
LMCO	Left message, call office	STO	She telephoned office
LMVM	Left message voice mail	T	Telephoned
N1, N2	Note one, note two (sent)	TB	Telephoned business
NA	No answer	TR	Telephoned residence
NF/A	No forwarding address	U/Emp	Unemployed
NI	Not in	UTC	Unable to contact
NLE	No longer employed	Vfd/E	Verified employment
NR	No record	Vfd/I	Verified insurance

TABLE APP C1-7: Bookkeeping Codes and Their Meanings, Used in Posting to Ledger Cards

AC or acct	account	J/A	joint account
A/C	account current	MO	money order
adj	adjustment	mo	month
A/P	accounts payable	NC, N/C	no charge
A/R	accounts receivable	NF	no funds
B/B	bank balance	NSF	not sufficient funds
Bal fwd, B/F	balance forward	PD	paid
c/a, CS	cash on account	PVT CK	private check
ck	check	recd	received
Cr	credit	ROA	received on account
def	charge deferred	TB	trial balance
disc	discount	UCR	usual, customary, and
Dr	debit		reasonable
EC, ER	error corrected	-	charge already made
Ex MO	express money order	0	no balance due (zero balance)
fwd	forward	✓	posted
I/f	in full	($0.00)	credit
ins, INS	insurance		
inv	invoice		

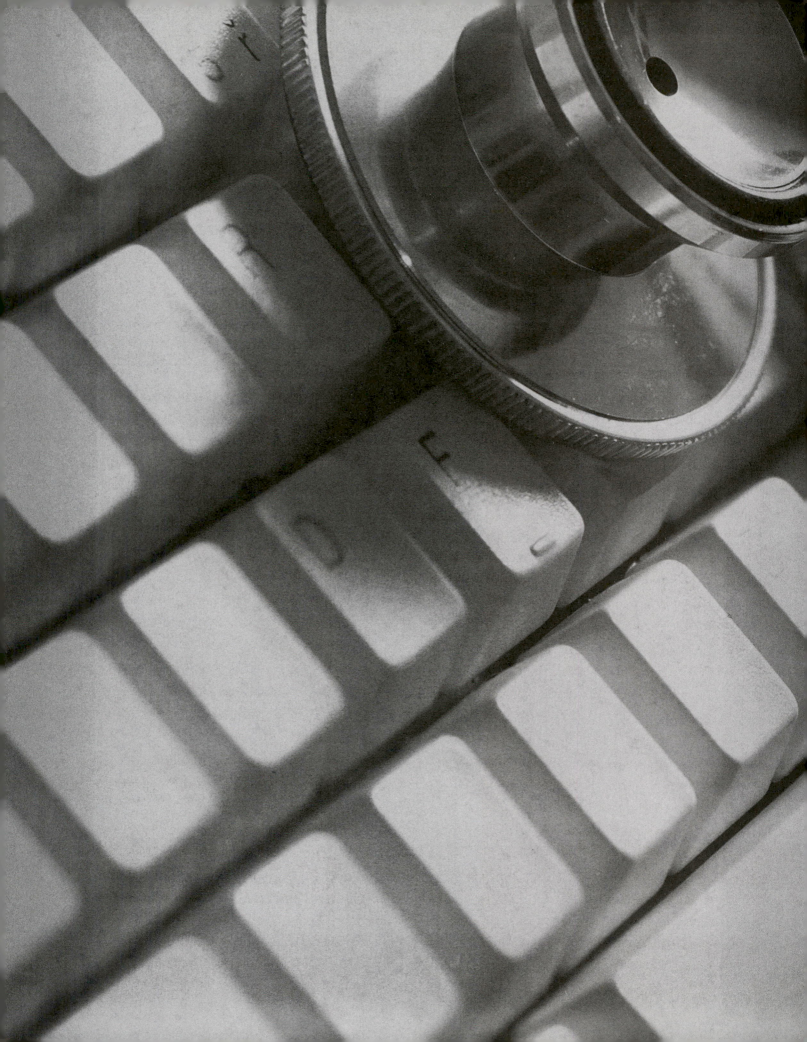

APPENDIX D:
Medical Specialties and Specialists

TABLE APP D1-1: Physician Specialties

Specialty	Title of Practitioner	Area of Specialization	Types of Patients Seen
Allergy	Allergist	Diagnosing and treating conditions of altered immunologic reactivity (allergic reactions)	Adults of all ages, children, both sexes
Anesthesiology	Anesthesiologist	Administering anesthetic agents before and during surgery	Adults of all ages, children, both sexes
Cardiology	Cardiologist	Diagnosing and treating abnormalities, diseases, and disorders of the heart	Adults of all ages, children, both sexes
Dermatology	Dermatologist	Diagnosing and treating disorders of the skin	Adults of all ages, children, both sexes
Endocrinology	Endocrinologist	Diagnosing and treating diseases and malfunctions of the glands of internal secretion	Adults of all ages, children, both sexes
Family practice	Family practitioner	Similar to general practice in nature, but centering around the family unit	Adults of all ages, infants and children of all ages, both sexes
Gastroenterology	Gastroenterologist	Diagnosing and treating diseases and disorders of the stomach and intestines	Adults of all ages, children, both sexes
Geriatrics	Gerontologist or geriatrician	Diagnosing and treating diseases, disorders, and problems associated with aging	Older adults, both sexes
Gynecology	Gynecologist	Diagnosing and treating diseases and disorders of the female reproductive tract; strong emphasis on preventive measures	Female adolescents and adults
Hematology	Hematologist	Diagnosing and treating diseases and disorders of the blood and blood-forming tissues	Adults of all ages, infants and children, both sexes
Infertility	Infertility specialist	Diagnosing and treating problems in conceiving and maintaining pregnancy	Couples who desire to have children but cannot

(continued)

TABLE APP D1-1: Physician Specialties (continued)

Specialty	Title of Practitioner	Area of Specialization	Types of Patients Seen
Internal medicine	Internist	Diagnosing and treating diseases and disorders of the internal organs	Adults of all ages, children, both sexes
Nephrology	Nephrologist	Diagnosing and treating diseases and disorders of the kidney	Adults, children, both sexes
Neurology	Neurologist	Diagnosing and treating diseases and disorders of the central nervous system	Adults, children, both sexes
Nuclear medicine	Nuclear medicine specialist	Diagnosing and treating diseases with the use of radionuclides	Adults, both sexes
Obstetrics	Obstetrician	Providing direct care to women during pregnancy, childbirth, and immediately thereafter	Pregnant women
Occupational Medicine	Occupational medicine specialist	Diagnosing and treating diseases or conditions arising from occupational circumstances (e.g., chemicals, dust, or gases)	Adults of all ages, both sexes
Oncology	Oncologist	Diagnosing and treating tumors and cancer	Adults of all ages, children, both sexes
Ophthalmology	Ophthalmologist	Diagnosing and treating diseases and disorders of the eye	Adults of all ages, children, both sexes
Orthopedics	Orthopedist	Diagnosing and treating disorders and diseases of the bones, muscles, ligaments, and tendons and fractures of the bones	Adults of all ages, children, both sexes
Otorhinolaryngology	Otorhinolaryngologist, commonly referred to as an ENT (ear, nose, and throat) specialist	Diagnosing and treating disorders and diseases of the ear, nose, and throat	Adults of all ages, children, both sexes
Pathology	Pathologist	Analysis of tissue samples to confirm diagnosis	Usually has no direct contact with patients
Pediatrics	Pediatrician	Diagnosing and treating diseases and disorders of children; strong emphasis on preventive measures	Infants, children, and adolescents
Physical medicine	Physical medicine specialist	Diagnosing and treating diseases and disorders with physical agents (physical therapy)	Adults, children, both sexes
Plastic surgery	Plastic surgeon	Evaluates and improves appearance of scars, deformities, and birth defects; also provides elective procedures that patients desire for aesthetic purposes	Adults of all ages, children, both sexes
Psychiatry	Psychiatrist	Diagnosing and treating pronounced manifestations of emotional problems or mental illness that may have an organic causative factor	Adults of all ages, children, both sexes. (Note: Child psychiatry is a further specialized field dealing exclusively with children and adolescents.)

(continued)

TABLE APP D1-1: Physician Specialties (continued)

Specialty	Title of Practitioner	Area of Specialization	Types of Patients Seen
Pulmonary specialties	Pulmonary, thoracic, or cardiovascular specialist	Diagnosing and treating diseases and disorders of the chest, lungs, heart, and blood vessels	Adults, both sexes
Radiology	Radiologist	Diagnosing and treating diseases and disorders with Roentgen rays (x-rays) and other forms of radiant energy	Adults of all ages, children, both sexes
Sports medicine	Sports medicine specialist	Diagnosing and treating injuries sustained in athletic events	Adults, especially young adults (athletes), both sexes
Surgery	Surgeon	Diagnosing and treating diseases, injuries, and deformities by manual or operative methods	Adults of all ages, infants, children, both sexes
Trauma medicine	Emergency physician (commonly referred to as ER or trauma physician since most work in hospital emergency rooms)	Diagnosing and treating acute illnesses and traumatic injuries	Adults of all ages, infants, children, both sexes
Urology	Urologist	Diagnosing and treating diseases and disorders of the urinary system of females and genitourinary system of males	Adults of all ages, infants, children, both sexes

TABLE APP D1-2: Nonphysician Specialties

Specialty	Title of Practitioner	Degree	Area of Specialization	Types of Patients Seen
Chiropractic	Chiropractor	DC, or Doctor of Chiropractic	Manipulative treatment of disorders originating from misalignment of the spinal vertebrae	Adults of all ages, children, both sexes
Dentistry	Dentist	DDS, or Doctor of Dental Surgery	Diagnosing and treating diseases and disorders of the teeth and gums	Adults of all ages, children, both sexes
Optometry	Optometrist	OD, or Doctor of Optometry	Measuring the accuracy of vision to determine whether corrective lenses are needed	Adults of all ages, children, both sexes
Podiatry	Podiatrist	DPM, or Doctor of Podiatric Medicine	Diagnosing and treating diseases and disorders of the feet	Adults of all ages, children, both sexes
Psychology	Psychologist	PhD, or Doctor of Philosophy	Evaluating and treating emotional problems; these professionals give counseling to individuals, families, and groups	Adults of all ages, children, both sexes

TABLE APP D1-3: The Cardiovascular System

Combining Form	Definition	Example
aden/o	Gland	*Lymphadenopathy* is often found with viral illnesses such as infectious mononucleosis.
angi/o, vas/o	Vessel	*Angioplasty* may be performed when a blockage is found in a blood vessel to repair or remove the blockage.
aort/o	Aorta	An *aortic* aneurysm is a ballooning out of this major vessel and is frequently life-threatening.
arteri/o	Artery	*Temporal arteritis* is an inflammation of the temporal artery.
ather/o	Yellow, fatty plaque	*Atherosclerosis* is hardening of the arteries due to deposits of yellow, fatty plaque.
atri/o	Atrium (atria), upper chambers of the heart	The *atrioventricular* node is located between the atrium and ventricle of the heart and provides stimulation for the heart's beat.
cardi/o	Heart	*Cardiac* surgery pertains to surgery on the heart.
erythr/o	Red	*Erythrocytes* are the red blood cells, which are responsible for transporting oxygen.
hem/o, hemat/o	Blood	*Hemodialysis* is cleansing of the blood by a machine; a *hematologist* is one who specializes in blood disorders.
leuc/o, leuk/o	White	*Leukocytes* are the white cells that help to protect the body from infections.
lymph/o	Lymph	*Lymphoma* is a tumor found in the lymph system.
phleb/o, ven/o	Vein	A *phlebotomist* or *venipuncturist* is a person that draws a patient's blood for diagnostic testing.
splen/o	Spleen	When a person's spleen becomes overactive and removes too many blood cells, a *splenectomy*, removal of the spleen, may have to be performed.
thromb/o	Clot	*Thrombophlebitis* is an inflammation of a vein due to a blood clot.
ventricul/o	Ventricle, lower chambers of the heart	*Ventricular* bigeminy is an abnormal heart rhythm involving the ventricles of the heart.

TABLE APP D1-4: The Integumentary System—Dermatology

Combining Form	Definition	Example
adip/o, lip/o	Fat	*Adipose* tissue is the layer just below the skin, consisting primarily of fat cells. A *lipoma* is a benign, fatty tumor.
albin/o, leuk/o	White, without color	*Albinism* is a condition in which there are no melanocytes to provide color to the skin, giving the person a white appearance. *Leukoderma* is abnormal patches of white skin.
cutane/o, derm/o, dermat/o, integument/o	Skin	A *subcutaneous* injection is given beneath the skin's layers; a *dermatologist* is one who specializes in disorders of the skin.
cyan/o	Blue	*Cyanosis* of the nail beds or lips is a bluish tint due to the lack of oxygen.
erythem/o	Red	*Systemic lupus erythematosus* is an autoimmune disease often characterized by a red butterfly rash on the face.
melan/o	Black	*Malignant melanoma* is a black tumor of the skin.
onych/o	Nail	*Onychomycosis* is an abnormal fungal infection of the nails.
scler/o	Hard, hardening	*Scleroderma* is a condition of hardened skin.
xanth/o, icter/o	Yellow	*Xanthoderma* is yellowish appearing skin. A patient described as being *icteric* has a yellow discoloration of the skin from a liver disorder. Sometimes the word "jaundice" is used for the same condition.
xer/o	Dry	*Xeroderma* is a condition of extremely dry skin.

TABLE APP D1-5: The Gastrointestinal System—Gastroenterology

Combining Form	Definition	Example
abdomin/o	Abdomen	*Abdominal* pain is pain felt pertaining to the abdomen.
aden/o	Gland	*Sialadenitis* is inflammation of the salivary glands.
aliment/o	Nourishment, food	*Hyperalimentation* is the process of providing more or additional nourishment.
amyl/o	Starch	*Amylase* is an enzyme secreted by the pancreas that breaks down starches into simple sugars.
an/o	Anus	An *anal* fissure is a tear in the anus, the terminal portion of the digestive (GI) tract.
append/o, appendic/o	Appendix	An *appendectomy* is the surgical removal of the appendix, a small projection off the cecum; *appendicitis* is the condition that most frequently leads to this operation.
bucc/o	Cheek	Dentists frequently administer local anesthetic into the *buccal* (cheek) area.
cec/o	Cecum (first segment of the large intestine)	The ileocecal junction is where the small intestine merges with the large intestine.
cheil/o	Lip(s)	*Cheilitis* is an inflammation of the lip.
cholecyst/o	Gallbladder	*Cholecystolithiasis* is the condition most commonly referred to as gallstones.
choled/o	Common bile duct	*Choledolithotomy* is the process of removing stones from the common bile duct.
col/o, colon/o	(Large) intestine, colon	A *colostomy* is the formation of a new opening into the colon; a *colonoscopy* is the process of using a lighted instrument to visualize the colon.

(continued)

TABLE APP D1-5: The Gastrointestinal System—Gastroenterology (continued)

Combining Form	Definition	Example
dent/i, dent/o odont/o	Tooth (teeth)	A *dentist* is a tooth specialist.
duoden/o	Duodenum (first section of the small intestine)	*Duodenal* ulcers develop as a result of too much stomach acid passing from the stomach into the duodenum.
enter/o	(Small) intestine	*Enteral* stasis is a condition that occurs when digestion fails to take place in the small intestine.
epiglott/o	Epiglottis	*Epiglottitis* is an inflammation of the epiglottis, the structure that closes over the trachea to prevent food from passing into the respiratory system.
esophag/o	Esophagus (food tube)	*Esophageal* ulcers can occur when a patient has gastroesophageal reflux disease (GERD) and acid backs up into the esophagus.
gastr/o	Stomach	A *gastrectomy* is partial surgical removal of the stomach.
gloss/o, lingu/o	Tongue	*Ankyloglossia* is a condition of being "tongue tied."
hepat/o	Liver	*Hepatitis* is a viral inflammation of the liver; there are at least five different viruses that can cause hepatitis.
ile/o	Ileum (last section of the small intestine)	The *ileocecal* junction is where the ileum joins with the first section of the large intestine, the cecum.
intestin/o	Intestine	*Gastrointestinal* pertains to the stomach and intestines.
jejun/o	Jejunum (second section of the small intestine)	A *jejunectomy* is the surgical removal of the jejunum.
lith/o	Stone, calculus	Sialolithectomy is the surgical removal of salivary stones.
or/o, stomat/o	Mouth	*Oral* means pertaining to the mouth.
pancreat/o	Pancreas	*Pancreatitis* is an inflammation of the pancreas that causes the patient a good deal of pain; *pancreatic* secretions include amylase, lipase, and insulin.
periton/o	Peritoneum	The *peritoneal* cavity is lined by the peritoneum and houses the viscera.
pharyng/o	Pharynx (throat)	*Oropharyngeal* means "pertaining to the mouth and the throat."
proct/o, rect/o	Rectum	A *rectal* examination involves digital examination of the rectum; a *proctologist* is a specialist in rectal diseases.
sial/o	Saliva	*Sialolithiasis* is a condition of having stones in a salivary (gland).
sigmoid/o	Sigmoid colon	A *sigmoidectomy* is the surgical removal of the sigmoid colon, part of the large intestine.
Suffix	Meaning	Example
-ase	Enzyme	*Amylase, protease,* and *lipase* are all enzymes that break down food products for assimilation into the body

TABLE APP D1-6: The Special Senses—Pediatrics

Combining Form	Definition	Example
audi/o	Sound, hearing	An *audiogram* is a record of how well a patient is able to hear various pitches of sound.
aur/o, ot/o	Ear	*Aural* and *otic* drops are used in the ear to soften ear wax. *Microtia* is a condition of very small ears.
blephar/o	Eyelid	*Blepharoptosis* is a sagging (drooping) eyelid.
conjunctiv/o	Conjunctiva(e)	*Conjunctivitis* is an inflammation of the mucous membrane lining of the eye, commonly referred to as "pink-eye."
corne/o	Cornea	A *corneal* abrasion is a scratch on the cornea of the eye.
myring/o, tympan/o	Ear drum	A *myringotomy* is often performed on children to relieve pressure on the ear drum; a *tympanic* thermometer is one inserted into the ear canal to measure temperature.
ocul/o, ophthalm/o	Eye	*Ocular* implants are placed in the eye; an *ophthalmologist* is a specialist in the eye and associated diseases.
olfact/o	Smell	The *olfactory* nerve endings in the nose provide the sense of smell.
retin/o	Retina	*Retinal* surgery would be performed to repair a detached retina.
Prefix		
presby-	Aging, elderly	*Presbyopia* and *presbycusis* are medical terms given to diminished vision and hearing associated with the aging process.
Suffix		
-cusis	Hearing	*Presbycusis* is the medical term given to hearing loss that occurs as a result of the aging process.
-ptosis	Sagging or drooping	*Blepharoptosis* is a sagging (drooping) eyelid.

TABLE APP D1-7: The Reproductive System—Gynecology and Obstetrics

Combining Form	Definition	Example
amni/o	Amnion	*Amniocentesis* is a surgical puncture of the amnion (amniotic sac) for diagnostic testing for birth defects.
cervic/o	Neck, cervix (neck) of the uterus	*Cervical* cancer may be revealed with the use of a Pap smear.
colp/o, vagin/o	Vagina	A *colposcopy* is examination of the vagina with a lighted instrument; *vaginitis* is inflammation of the vagina, usually bacterial or fungal.
embry/o	Embryo	*Embryology* is the study of human development through the eighth week after conception.
gravida	Pregnancy	The terms *nulli gravida* indicates a woman has never been pregnant.
gyn/o, gynec/o	Female, woman	A *gynecologist* is a specialist in the anatomy of the female reproductive system.
hyster/o, metr/o, uter/o	Uterus	A *hysterectomy* is the surgical removal of the uterus; a *uteroscopy* may be performed prior to the surgery. *Metrorrhagia* is uterine bleeding at a time other than the monthly cycle.
lact/o	Milk	*Prolactin* is a hormone secreted by the pituitary gland so a mother can nurse her baby by producing milk.
mamm/o, mast/o	Breast	A *mammogram* is a common radiologic test for detection of breast cancer; a *mastopexy* may be done to correct sagging breasts.
men/o	Month, menstruation	*Menopause* is when a woman no longer has monthly periods.
nat/o	Birth	A *neonate* is a newborn; the *prenatal* period pertains to the months prior to the baby's birth.
oophor/o, ovari/o	Ovary	An *oophorectomy*, surgical removal of an ovary, may be performed in the case of an *ovarian* cyst.
orch/o, orchi/o, orchid/o, test/o	Testes	*Cryptorchidism* is a condition in which one or both testes (testicles) have not descended in the male and may require an *orchiopexy* to correct. *Testosterone* is the hormone produced by the testes in the male.
ov/o	Egg	*Oval* means "pertaining to an egg"; an oval is shaped like an egg.
prostat/o	Prostate	A *prostatectomy* is the surgical removal of the prostate.
salping/o	Tube (fallopian)	*Salpingitis* is an inflammation of the fallopian tube that may impede pregnancy.
sperm/o, spermat/o	Sperm	A *spermaticide* is used to kill sperm and prevent pregnancy.

TABLE APP D1-8: The Respiratory System—Pulmonology

Combining Form	Definition	Example
aer/o	Air	*Anaerobic* microorganisms prefer a lack of air for growth.
atel/o	Imperfect	*Atelectasis,* when taking the literal definition, means imperfect stretching. In premature infants, atelectasis indicates that the lungs cannot fully expand.
bronch/o, bronchi/o	Bronchus (bronchi)	*Bronchitis* is an inflammation of the bronchi found in upper respiratory tract infections; *bronchiectasis* is an abnormal stretching of the bronchi.
bronchiol/o	Bronchioles (little bronchi)	Toddlers are often diagnosed with *bronchiolitis,* an inflammation of the bronchioles.
laryng/o	Larynx (voice box)	A *laryngectomy* is the surgical removal of the larynx, usually due to cancer.
lob/o	Lobes	*Lobar* pneumonia indicates an infection in only one lobe of a lung. A *lobectomy* is the surgical removal of a lobe of a lung.
muc/o	Mucus	The *mucous* membranes are responsible for secreting mucus in the respiratory tract.
nas/o, rhin/o	Nose	*Nasal* sprays are used in the nose to alleviate symptoms of *rhinitis,* an inflammation of the nose and nasal passages.
ox/o	Oxygen	*Hypoxia* is a condition of below-normal oxygen levels.
pharyng/o	Pharynx (throat)	The *pharyngeal* tonsils are the lymph glands found in the back of the throat.
pleur/o	Pleura (membrane surrounding each lung)	*Pleurisy* is an inflammation of the pleura around one of the lungs.
pneum/o, pnemon/o	Lung, air	A *pneumothorax* is a collapsed lung from air rushing in; *pneumonitis* is an inflammation of a lung, more commonly known as *pneumonia.*
pulmon/o	Lung	Chronic obstructive *pulmonary* disease (COPD) is a disease that affects the lungs and the oxygen levels.
sinus/o	Sinus(es)	*Sinusitis* is an inflammation of the sinuses, often from an allergic reaction.
spir/o	To breathe	A *spirometer* is a device used to measure the amount of air a patient breathes in and out. *Respiratory* literally means "pertaining to repeat(ed) breathing."
tonsill/o	Tonsil(s)	In repeated cases of strep throat, a *tonsillectomy,* surgical removal of the tonsils, may be performed.
trache/o	Trachea (windpipe)	A *tracheotomy* is performed when a person is unable to breathe through the mouth or nose; this involves creating a new opening for air to pass.
Suffix		
-ptysis	To spit	*Hemoptysis* is spitting up blood.

TABLE APP D 1-9: The Urinary System—Urology

Combining Form	Definition	Example
bacteri/o	Bacteria	*Bacteriuria* indicates the presence of bacteria in the urine, usually from a urinary tract infection (UTI).
cyst/o	Bladder, sac	A *cystoscopy* is viewing the interior of the bladder with a lighted instrument.
glomerul/o	Glomerulus, filtering unit of a nephron	*Glomerulonephritis* is an inflammation of the glomerulus of the nephrons.
hemat/o	Blood	In some cases of nephrolithiasis, *hematuria,* or blood in the urine, is present.
lith/o	Stone, calculus	*Nephrolithiasis* is a condition of having kidney stones.
nephr/o, ren/o	Nephron, functional cell of the kidney, kidney	A *nephrectomy* is the removal of a kidney; the *renal* artery supplies blood to the kidney.
noct/o	Night	Older patients frequently complain of *nocturia,* a condition of having to get up during the night to void.
py/o	Pus	*Pyuria* is the presence of pus in the urine.
pyel/o	Renal pelvis	*Pyelolithotomy* is the surgical removal of kidney stones from the renal pelvis.
ur/o, urin/o	Urine	*Pyuria* is an abnormal condition of pus in the urine; a *urinometer* is an antiquated device that was used to measure the specific gravity of urine.
ureter/o	Ureter	An *ureteroscopy* is the procedure that is used to view the ureter(s) with a scope.
urethr/o	Urethra	A voiding *cystourethrogram* is an examination that is done while a patient is voiding that allows visualization of the bladder and the urethra.

TABLE APP D 1-10: Surgery – Musculosketal System—Orthopedics

Combining Form	Definition	Example
ankylos/o	Stiffening	*Ankylosing spondylitis* is an abnormal stiffening of the spine that results in a lack of mobility.
arthr/o	Joint	*Arthritis* is inflammation of a joint.
carp/o	Wrist (bones)	*Carpal tunnel syndrome* affects the nerves in the wrist.
cervic/o	Neck	The *cervical* spine is the vertebrae that compose the neck.
chondr/o	Cartilage	*Costochondritis* is an inflammation of the cartilage around the ribs that often mimics the pain of a heart attack.
cost/o	Ribs	When performing an electrocardiogram, the medical assistant needs to locate the *intercostal* spaces for proper electrode placement.
crani/o	Skull, head	The *cranial* cavity is located within the skull.
dactyl/o	Digit	*Dactylography* is the process of taking someone's fingerprints.
femor/o	Femur (thighbone)	The *femoral* artery is located near the femur in the upper part of the leg.
fibul/o	Fibula (smaller bone in the calf)	A *fibular* fracture would be a break of the fibula.
humer/o	Humerus (upper bone in the arm)	When one hits the *humeral* nerve, it is often described as hitting the "funny" bone.
ili/o	Ilium (pelvic bones)	The *iliac* crest of the pelvis is used as a landmark for administering intramuscular injections.
lamin/o	Lamina of a vertebra	A *laminectomy,* removing a portion of the vertebra, may be performed by a surgeon to relieve back pain.
mandibul/o	Mandible (lower jaw, only movable bone in the skull)	*Temporomandibular joint* (TMJ) pain occurs when the bone of the mandible does not align correctly with the temporal bone to which it is attached.
maxill/o	Maxilla (upper jaw)	*Maxillary* sinuses are located just above the maxilla of the face.
muscul/o, my/o	Muscle	*Muscular* pertains to muscles; the *myocardium* is the muscular portion of the heart.
orth/o	Straight, straighten	An *orthopedist* is one that specializes in straightening bones.
oste/o	Bone	*Osteitis* is inflammation of a bone.
patell/o	Patella (knee cap)	The *patellar* reflex is solicited when striking a patient's leg just below the knee cap.
pelv/i	Pelvis	The *pelvic* cavity is housed within the bony structure of the pelvis.
phalang/o	Fingers or toes	*Phalangitis* is inflammation of a finger or a toe.
rachi/o, spondyl/o, vertebr/o	Vertebra(e), spine	*Rachitis* and *spondylitis* are both inflammation of the vertebrae/spine. The *vertebral* column is composed of bones of the spine.
stern/o	Sternum (breastbone)	*Substernal* chest pain is pain described as being just below the breastbone, often indicating a heart attack.
ten/o, tend/o, tendin/o	Tendon	*Tendonitis* is inflammation of a tendon.
tibi/o	Tibia (shin)	A *tibial* contusion, caused by striking the shin, is quite painful.

TABLE APP D 1-11: Surgery – Nervous System - Neurology

Combining Form	Definition	Example
cerebell/o	Cerebellum	If there is an interruption in *cerebellar* nerve impulses, voluntary movements of the body become difficult.
electr/o	Electricity	An *electroencephalogram (EEG)* is a recording of the electrical impulses transmitted by the brain.
encephal/o, cerebr/o	Brain, cerebrum	Viral *encephalitis* is an inflammation of the brain by a virus; the *cerebral* part of the brain is what gives each individual unique personalities and thought processes.
mening/o	Meninges	*Meningococcal encephalitis* is an infection of the meninges resulting in inflammation of the brain.
neur/o	Nerve	*Neuralgia* is a generalized term meaning pain in a nerve.
phas/o	Speech	Occasionally when a patient has a stroke, *aphasia,* or inability to speak, may occur.

TABLE APP D 1-12: Surgery—Endocrine System—Endocrinology

Combining Form	Definition	Example
gluc/o, glyc/o	Sugar, sweet	*Glucosuria* and *glycosuria* both mean "sugar in the urine." *Hyperparathyroidism* is
parathyroid/o	Parathyroid glands	a condition of excessive parathyroid activity.
thym/o	Thymus gland	*Thymosin* is a hormone secreted by the thymus gland.
thyr/o	Thyroid gland, shield	*Thyrotoxicosis* is a serious condition of the thyroid being "poisoned."
toxic/o	Poison, toxin	See previous example.
Suffix		
-oid	Resembling	*Thyroid* means "resembling a shield."
-ose	Sugar	*Sucrose* and *lactose* are different types of sugars than *glucose*.

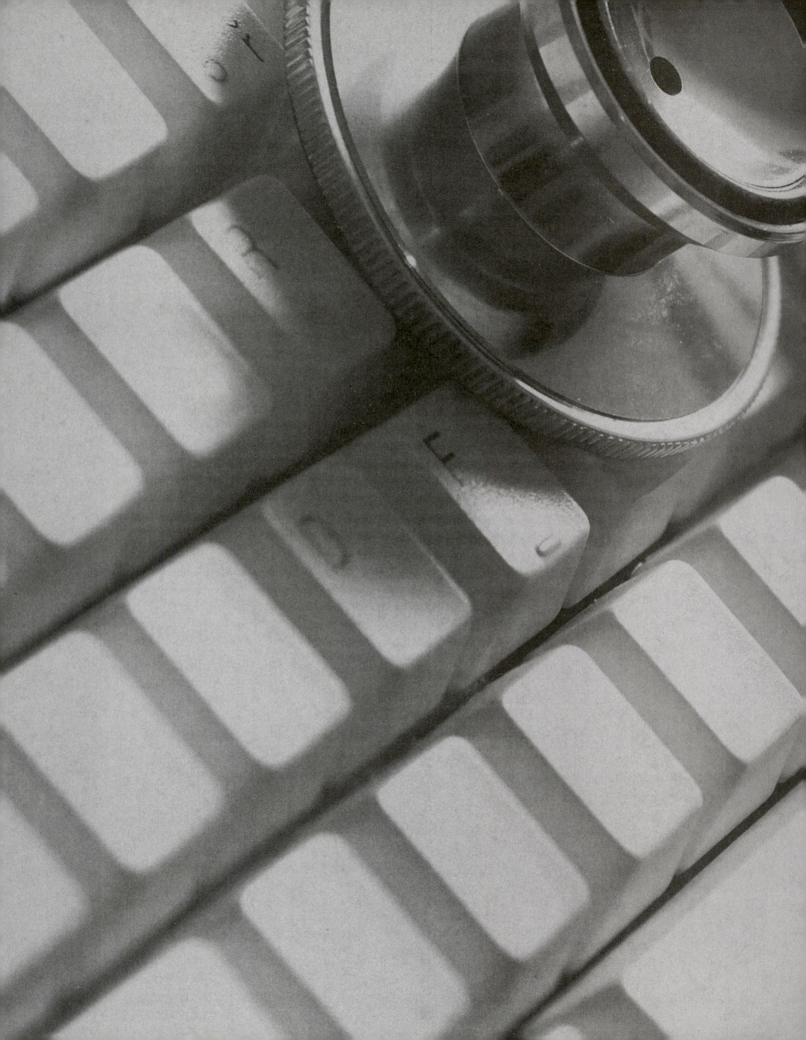

APPENDIX E:
Medical Websites

- *Advance* magazine: www.advanceweb.com
- American Academy of Professional Coders (AAPC): www.aapc.com
- American Association of Medical Assistants (AAMA): www.aama-ntl.org
- American Health Information Management Association (AHIMA): www.ahima.org
- American Medical Technologists (AMT): www.americanmedtech.org
- Americans With Disabilities Act (ADA): www.ada.gov
- Association for Healthcare Documentation Integrity (AHDI): www.ahdionline.org
- CareerBuilder: www.careerbuilder.com
- Centers for Disease Control and Prevention (CDC): www.cdc.gov
- Centers for Medicare & Medicaid Services (CMS): www.cms.hhs.gov
- Empire Medicare: www.medicaresolutions.com/Empire-Medicare.asp
- Facebook Ads: www.Facebook.com/Advertising
- Google AdWords: www.Google.com/Ads/Adwords
- Internet-Only Manuals (IOM): www.cms.gov/Manuals/IOM
- The Joint Commission: www.jointcommission.org
- Medicare Learning Network (MLN): www.cms.gov/MLNGenInfo
- Microsoft Advertising: www.advertising.Microsoft.com
- Monster: www.monster.com
- Nurse.com: www.nursingspectrum.com
- Occupational Health and Safety Act (OSHA): www.osha.gov
- Occupational Outlook Handbook: http://stats.bls.gov/oco
- Office of Civil Rights: HIPAA: www.hhs.gov/ocr/hipaa
- Office of Inspector General (OIG): www.oig.hhs.gov
- Professional Association of Health Care Management (PAHCOM): http://www.pahcom.com
- Society for Human Resource Management: www.shrm.org
- U.S. Bureau of Labor Statistics: http://www.bls.gov

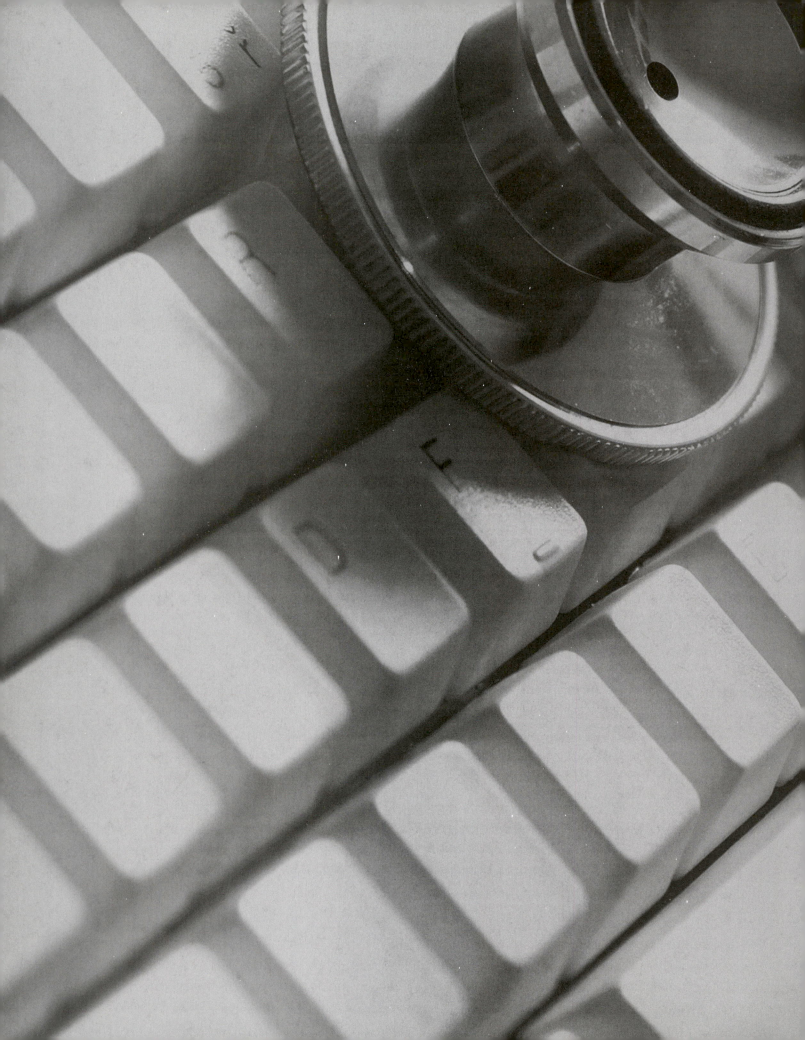

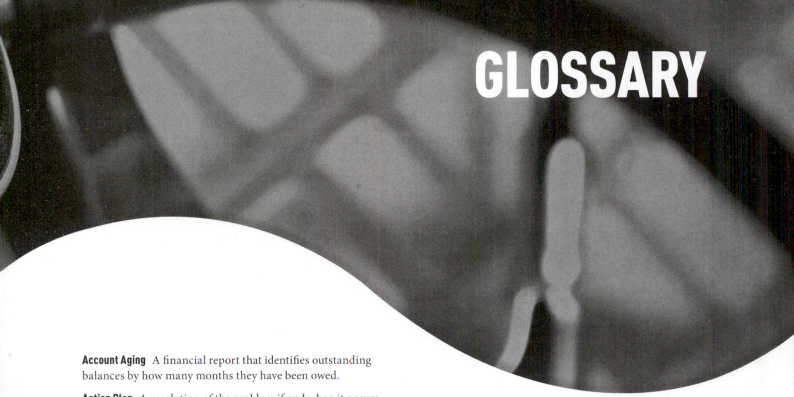

GLOSSARY

Account Aging A financial report that identifies outstanding balances by how many months they have been owed.

Action Plan A resolution of the problem if and when it occurs to ensure it will not happen again.

Advanced Beneficiary Notice (ABN) A notice signed by Medicare patients that provides a written notice when a service may not be covered or when it is believed not to be covered. This notice allows the patient to decide whether or not they still want the service.

Advanced Directive A form that gives the providers a written notice of the patient's wishes for end-of-life cases, including resuscitation.

Advertising A way to generate information regarding the health care facility in order to promote future business.

Ambulatory Surgical Centers (ASC) An outpatient center where physicians perform surgical procedures that can be done on a same-day schedule. The facility is not an overnight facility and patients need to be discharged the same day.

American Association of Medical Assistants (AAMA) An organization that certifies medical assistants and maintains their continuing education and membership.

American Association of Professional Coders (AAPC) An organization that certifies medical coders and maintains their continuing education and membership.

American Health Information Medical Association (AHIMA) An organization that certifies medical coders and maintains their continuing education and membership.

American Medical Association (AMA) Professional organization that publishes the CPT manual.

American Medical Technologists (AMT) An organization that certifies allied health professionals and maintains their continuing education and membership.

Americans With Disabilities Act (ADA) Regulation that strictly prohibits discrimination in hiring based on disabilities, marital status, children, sexual preference, gender, age, and race.

Anesthesia Procedure used to reduce the feeling of pain during a procedure.

Application for Employment A list of personal information which employees are asked to complete during or after an interview.

Asthma Disease that causes inflammation and narrowing of the lungs and airways.

Audit The process of reviewing what was billed to the insurance carrier for reimbursement and ensuring there is no fraud or abuse.

Authorization Approval for a medical service or procedure based on the medical necessity of the procedure to be performed.

Bad Debt Patients who have not paid their bills and even with the use of a collection agency have not or cannot pay.

Benchmarking Industry-standard tools to assess the effectiveness of practices in a health care facility.

Biohazards Containers Products used to seal up medical supplies and equipment to prevent the spread of disease or injury, such as sharps containers for dirty needles.

Bottom Line The amount of money that will be earned for a company after expenses have been subtracted from income and the company shows a profit or loss.

Brochure A notice that provides information about a company, including office information and services provided.

Bundled Codes Medical procedure codes that are included in a larger procedure when performed and are not allowed to be billed separately.

Cardiologist One who practices in the specialty of the heart and its structures.

Cardiology The study of the heart and its structures.

Centers for Disease Control and Prevention (CDC) A federal agency that assists health care facilities in providing safe conditions in order to prevent the spread of disease.

Centers for Medicare and Medicaid Services (CMS) Federal agency that has regulations that affect all aspects of medical care, providers, facilities, and services as well as medical records, billing, and reimbursement.

Certificate of Accreditation Laboratories can only perform tests under the waived category and those classified as PPMP—physician-performed testing.

Certificate of Compliance Certificate of accreditation allows a facility to perform tests that are considered moderate- or high-complexity tests as well as tests from the waived and PPMP categories. The last category requires that labs have a fully accredited laboratory that includes a physician/pathologist.

Certificate of Waiver Allows a medical facility to perform only those tests that are on the waived category list. A certificate of waiver is valid for two years. An updated list of tests can be found on the Internet.

Certified Registered Nurse Anesthetist (CRNA) Nurse who specializes in administering medication that reduces pain.

Charity Care Patients with no insurance and who fall below a certain income level.

Chief Complaint, History, Exam, Details, Drugs, Assessment & Return (CHEDDAR) A medical document with a particular format with the patient's problem, a brief description, exam, and expectations after the visit.

Chronic Obstructive Pulmonary Disease (COPD) Progressive disease of the lungs that makes it difficult to breathe due to blockage of the airways.

Clean Claim A medical claim that is sent to the insurance carrier with no errors and is paid upon the first submission.

Clinical Lab Improvement Act (CLIA) Congress passed this act in 1988 to establish standards for all laboratory testing done, including physician offices, to ensure accuracy, reliability, and timeliness of patient testing.

Closed Questions Provide a yes or no answer to obtain the appropriate answer.

CMS-1500 A medical claim form that is used to submit outpatient services to an insurance carrier. The form includes patient information, insurance information, diagnosis, and procedures as well as the provider information.

Collections The process of bringing revenue into the facility through insurance payments and patient payments.

Comprehensive The level of history and examination that requires an extensive description of a visit.

Continuing Education Units (CEU) Training hours that are completed after certification that are used to maintain up-to-date information and skills.

Continuity of Care In a continuum of care, a patient has a medical record—either in a paper or an electronic form—at his or her family physician's or primary care physician's office.

Contractual Adjustment A write-off after the allowance is determined because the provider is contracted under the insurance.

Coordination of Care The involvement of other agencies or health care professionals as they contribute to the patient's treatment plan at the request of the provider.

Cost Effective Advertising is within the budget and affordable for the health care facility and also generates increased revenue.

Counseling A discussion with the patient and/or family about the diagnosis, treatments, options, and risks. The information must be specific to the patient's presenting problem.

Cover Letter The cover letter introduces a résumé and should reference the source of the job posting and include a brief description of your qualifications, including how you would fit with the position available.

Credentialing A process that confirms that a physician is indeed who he or she says he or she is.

Credentials Demonstration of qualifications that a medical professional holds.

Current Procedural Terminology (CPT) A five-digit numeric or alphanumeric code to identify the procedure or service provided to the patient.

Curriculum Vitae (CV) Professional résumé; includes an objective statement and the education, experience, licenses, credentials, and professional organizations for the employee.

Date of Birth (DOB) The month, day, and year the patient was born.

Day Sheet A printout that details the days patient's, charges, and any payments that were made and amount still owed.

Denials Insurance claims that are not paid for a particular reason and may be a write-off or transferred to the patient.

Dermatologist One who practices in the field of the skin and its structures.

Dermatology The study of the skin and its structures.

Design Elements The items included in the advertisement to attract the right customers or patients.

Detailed The level of history and examination that requires more information but not complex.

Discharge Summary A medical document that lists all the information in relation to the patient's release from the inpatient or outpatient facility, including current condition and future plans.

Electronic Data Interchange (EDI) Transmission of medical documentation through an electronic process.

Electronic Health Record (EHR) The record will include all the administrative, medical, and clinical areas that the now traditional paper medical record does. This must comply with all HIPAA privacy standards.

E-Mail Lists Electronic addresses of customers and patients, which is used to forward advertising information.

Emergency Medical Treatment and Labor Act (EMTALA) The law was enacted by Congress to prevent emergency rooms or departments who participate in Medicare from turning away poor or uninsured patients or from transferring patients before they have been evaluated for emergency conditions and stabilized.

Engineering Controls The devices that are used to comply with the exposure plan. It can include sharps containers, needleless systems, and self-sheathing needles.

Evaluation and Management (E&M) Services that range from office exams, hospital visits, consultation visits, case management, and observation codes.

Examination A review of the affected body area or organ as well as other body systems that are affected by the current problem.

Expanded Problem Focused (EPF) A level of history and examination that deals with just the reason for the visit and no other body systems.

Explanation of Benefits (EOB) A statement that contains information on the service, date of service, CPT code, charges, deductible, coinsurance, copayments, and insurance payments. It may also contain information on payments reduced or denied if something was not covered or paid appropriately.

Exposure Plan A written plan that outlines the ways the employee facility protects their employees from exposure to blood-borne pathogens. The plan details what types of equipment is used and is updated yearly to reflect new and safer methods.

Eyewash Station In the event a staff member has an accident, the equipment is hooked directly to an existing faucet and should be visible and easily accessible. It is designed to aim water at both eyes in the event a hazardous substance gets in the eyes. The eyes should be flushed for 15–20 minutes and/or until the employee can get further help.

Federal Register Official daily publication from the government, which includes the OIG work plan.

Freedom of Information Act (FOIA) Allows for access to information that was prohibited from being released by the U.S. government.

Gastroenterologist The physician specialty is internal medicine, with additional training in the field of the stomach, small and large intestines, and mouth to anus.

Gastroenterology This specialty deals with the stomach, the small and large intestines, and mouth to anus.

Gerontologist The physician specialist will have additional training in the normal and abnormal process of aging.

Gerontology This specialty deals with the health of seniors and normal and abnormal conditions as one ages.

Health Information Technologist (HIT) Professional involved with data and electronic communication who also serves as a link between documentation and coding. Qualifications include training at the technical or college level, and the knowledge can be as diverse as knowledge of computers, coding, and medical records.

Health Insurance Portability and Accessibility Act (HIPAA) Compliance regulations that includes the privacy law to protect inappropriate release of PHI and keeps that release to a minimum. The patient indicates on the form about how the health care facility can communicate with the patient or other individuals.

Healthcare Common Procedural Coding System (HCPCS) A five-digit alphanumeric character that represents procedures or services provided to the patient.

Hepatitis B Vaccine A vaccine to prevent hepatitis B that must be made available to all employees within a given time period—usually about 10 days.

History The chief complaint, a description of the present problem, and a review of the patient's own background as well as their social and family history.

History and Physical (H&P) A medical document that lists all the information necessary for a patient upon arrival to admission or a procedure. This includes the patient's previous health information that relates to or can affect the current visit.

I-9 A form that documents information about your identity and citizenship.

Inpatient Patients who are admitted to the hospital.

Insurance Carrier Reimburses the provider for services and procedures.

Internal Patients People already presenting to the facility for treatment.

International Classification of Diseases 9th Revision, Clinical Modifications (ICD-9CM) Diagnostic code set is a numeric or alphanumeric three-, four-, or five-digit code with a decimal after the third digit. These codes identify signs, symptoms and diseases of patients and are submitted on the claim form to the insurance carrier.

Internet Online Manual (IOM) Changes that have recently been made to the HCPCS coding system and can be found on the Internet.

Job Description A written explanation of the responsibilities of an employee.

The Joint Commission An independent nonprofit organization that establishes standards in the practice for patient safety and accreditation of health care settings.

Labor Hours Requirement of the staff to work on the advertising—whether via internal or external methods.

Layered Process The steps involved in the claim form creation. The first step is patient registration, then the visit, and finally the claim submission with appropriate procedure and diagnostic codes.

Levels of E&M Visit code choices, in which one determines the history, the exam, and medical decision and chooses the appropriate code according to the work involved by the provider.

Licensure Permission to perform job duties; demonstrates proof of qualifications and the appropriate process followed.

Linking Showing the relationship and consistency of procedures, services, and POS on the claim form and justifying them as medically necessary with an appropriate diagnosis.

Long-Term Care (LTC) Health care facility where patients are admitted for an extended time for rehabilitation and recovery.

Market Analysis Looking at the potential for growth in the area based on the industry by reviewing market size, trends, costs, profits, and potential for new clients.

Market Analysis Survey A list of questions that pertain to potential patient care and services you offer at the health care facility or plan to offer in the future.

Marketable Advertising is meeting the needs of the target audience and having a successful response.

Marketing Determining if the health care facility will be successful in that area and how it can advertise to promote its services.

Material Safety Data Sheets (MSDS) Forms from companies and suppliers on items that could be hazardous if not used correctly, such as testing materials and even alcohol. The sheets provide descriptions of what is in the material and how to act if someone is affected.

Media Advertising Using newspapers, radio, or television to demonstrate what you offer and get customers or patients interested.

Medical Decision Making (MDM) The end result, which involves the number of diagnoses, the amount of tests and information to be reviewed, and the risk of morbidity or mortality.

Medically Necessary Diagnosis justifies the services and procedure in order for the insurance carrier to decide to pay.

Medicare Secondary Payer (MSP) When a patient has two insurance carriers, including Medicare, and the other insurance carrier is the first to pay.

Mission Statement Identifies the purpose of the company or organization and explains what direction it intends to move.

Modifier Two-digit codes added to a procedure code to change the meaning.

National Center for Competency Testing (NCCT) An organization that certifies allied health professionals and maintains their continuing education and membership.

National Coverage Determination (NCD) A unified policy from Medicare on whether a service or procedure will be covered under CMS.

National Patient Safety Goals (NPSG) Standards designed to help create a new method of changing something that can promote better patient care.

National Provider Identifier (NPI) Number for providers next to each procedure code to identify the health care provider. The NPI numbers demonstrate one number that providers can use to identify themselves for all carriers rather than each carrier issuing a separate provider number, as was previously done.

Nature of Presenting Problem The type of disease, illness, or condition the patient has presented to the facility with and the level of intensity required in treating the disease, illness, or condition.

Networking Joining or meeting with other facilities to share information and services among each other.

Nonparticipating A physician who has not signed an agreement with an insurance carrier to accept a set reimbursement fee.

Notice of Privacy Notifies patients of their rights and informs them about how their information is protected, who it is shared with, and how it is stored or destroyed.

Objective Included in a résumé and states the goal of the individual during his or her employment.

Occupational Safety and Health Administration (OSHA) A federal agency that details the types of protections that employers need to provide their employees to protect them from exposure to patients' fluids, such as blood and urine.

Office of Inspector General (OIG) A federal agency that develops projects each year in the area of program audits and program inspections, investigates potential areas of fraud or misconduct, and resolves fraud and abuse cases. Each year, the OIG publishes the proposed plan in the *Federal Register*.

Online Social Networks Groups that are created on the Internet and allow posting or blogging amongst each other.

Open Ended Survey questions that allow them to explain the answer and elaborate.

Orientation A meeting in which rules and regulations are given to the new employee.

Outpatient Patients who are not admitted but seek treatment and leave the same day.

Outpatient Prospective Payment System (OPPS) A bundled payment made to the hospital for services under CMS reimbursement.

Outside Market An external target audience and individuals who are not current patients.

Participating A physician who has signed an agreement with an insurance carrier to accept a set reimbursement fee.

Patient Surveys Questionnaires sent to find out what patients like and do not like about the health care facility in order to improve.

Pediatrician A physician who has trained in the specialty of children. They must be aware of all types of medical and surgical conditions for children.

Pediatrics The study and practice of growth and disorders for children—usually from newborn to adolescents.

Personal Protective Equipment (PPE) Covers the employee when treating patients and includes gloves, gowns, masks, and goggles. When bodily fluids are involved in patient care, the more covering the health care employee uses, the less chance for exposure.

Place of Service (POS) The location where procedures were performed.

Portfolio A visual picture of all education, credentials, accomplishments, awards, and skills possessed by the applicant.

Postexposure Follow-Up Given to any employee who has been in contact with hazardous materials, such as blood-borne pathogens or any other fluids. The health care employee is urged to seek medical attention—depending on the type of exposure—to be monitored.

Postoperative The time period after a procedure in which the provider has to care for the patient as part of the original procedure.

Preoperative The time period before a procedure in which a provider has to evaluate the patient to be sure he or she is ready for the procedure.

Primary Care Physician (PCP) Specialist who deals with the common disorders affecting all members of a family—from children to the elderly.

Problem Focused (PF) This level of history and examination only states one condition or disease for the visit.

Problem-Oriented Medical Record (POMR) Patient's health documentation in which the diagnoses are listed to identify what conditions are being treated.

Professional Organizations Nonprofit groups of people with the same educational background that network to promote their field of expertise and hold continuing education meetings.

Provider Health care facilities that are contracted with Medicare and are required to follow their regulations as well as accept assignment on claims.

Provider-Performed Microscopy Procedures (PPMP) CLIA authorization to perform laboratory tests that are of medium difficulty and require the use of a microscope by an approved provider.

Pulmonologist The physician who is a specialist in internal medicine and who has additional training in the area of the lungs and its disorders.

Pulmonology The study of diseases and disorders of the lungs.

Receptionists Employee who greets the patients and gets them registered and checked in for their appointment.

Recordkeeping Detailed documentation kept on employees, including training and reporting of injuries, such as a sharps injury log. It is the method by which OSHA justifies compliance and the health care facility can demonstrate compliance during an investigation.

Recovery Audit Contractor (RAC) CMS auditors that have been asked to audit health care facilities. They began their auditing at the hospitals and have moved to the physician's office, auditing all aspects of the Medicare patients and determining if fraud or abuse was involved, for which the provider or health care facility might receive penalties or jail time.

Referral The process of notifying the insurance company of planned procedures, services, and surgery and getting authorization for those services.

Registration A form that has a number of parts that need to be completed the first time a patient goes to a health care facility, including personal and insurance information.

Remittance Advice (RA) A statement that contains information on the service, date of service, CPT code, charges, deductible, coinsurance, copayments, and insurance payments. It may also contain information on payments reduced or denied if something was not covered or paid appropriately.

Résumé A summary of important information about a person that outlines their education, experience, and professional life in an attempt to apply for a position.

Scope of Practice Working within the qualifications of your job duties as specified by your training or license.

Security Regulations that are part of HIPAA regulations to keep patient information confidential.

Sentinel Event An error or action that can cause serious harm or death to a patient.

Sharps Container Products used to seal up needles and supplies that are dangerous to prevent injury or the spread of disease.

Skilled Nursing Facility (SNF) A 24-hour health care facility where patients are treated overnight but do not need hospital care.

Social Security Act Provides federal assistance for the elderly, poor, and unemployed by giving a steady income.

Specialist A physician who has additional education in a specific area.

Specialty A type of medical treatment that deals with diseases and disorders of a particular body system.

Subjective, Objective, Assessment & Plan (SOAP) Medical document that contains information about the patient's visit in a particular format, with the patient's complaint, exam results, and future expectations.

Subscriber Person who holds the insurance coverage.

Surgeon The physician who has had additional training in operative procedures under sterile conditions.

Surgery A specialty that removes all or part of an organ. There are many specialties within surgery dependent on body systems.

Target Audience The group of individuals who are seeing the advertisement.

Thank-You Letter A letter in which the interviewers should be thanked for their time and the applicant should reiterate why he or she is the best candidate for the job.

Third-Party Payers Type of insurance and the company with whom an individual may have an insurance plan. It will process claims for services submitted.

Time Face-to-face meeting during which the physician performs a history and an examination and counsels the patient and/or family regarding the presenting problem and treatment.

Timely Filing A period of time during which the insurance carrier requires the health care facility to submit a claim for processing.

Triage Telephone screening to prioritize the urgency of phone calls and make appropriate decisions.

Unbundled Codes Services or procedures within bundled codes that are separated and billed separately as individual CPT or HCPCS codes.

Urologist The physician who has had additional training in diseases and disorders of the urinary system.

Urology The study of the urinary system and its parts, including the bladder and kidney.

W-4 A form is needed for the employer so the correct federal income tax can be withheld from your pay.

Waived A designated category of laboratory tests that a facility can perform with an insignificant risk of error.

Work Plan A written plan published yearly by the OIG with regard to yearly audits, program inspections, and areas for fraud and misconduct by the health care facility.

Work Practice Controls Procedures used to reduce exposure to injury in the workplace. These controls include hand washing, sharps disposing, lab specimen packaging, laundry handling, and cleaning surfaces and materials.

Write-Off Debts that cannot be paid, as in the case of deceased patients with no estates. When a balance needs to be removed from a patient's account permanently.

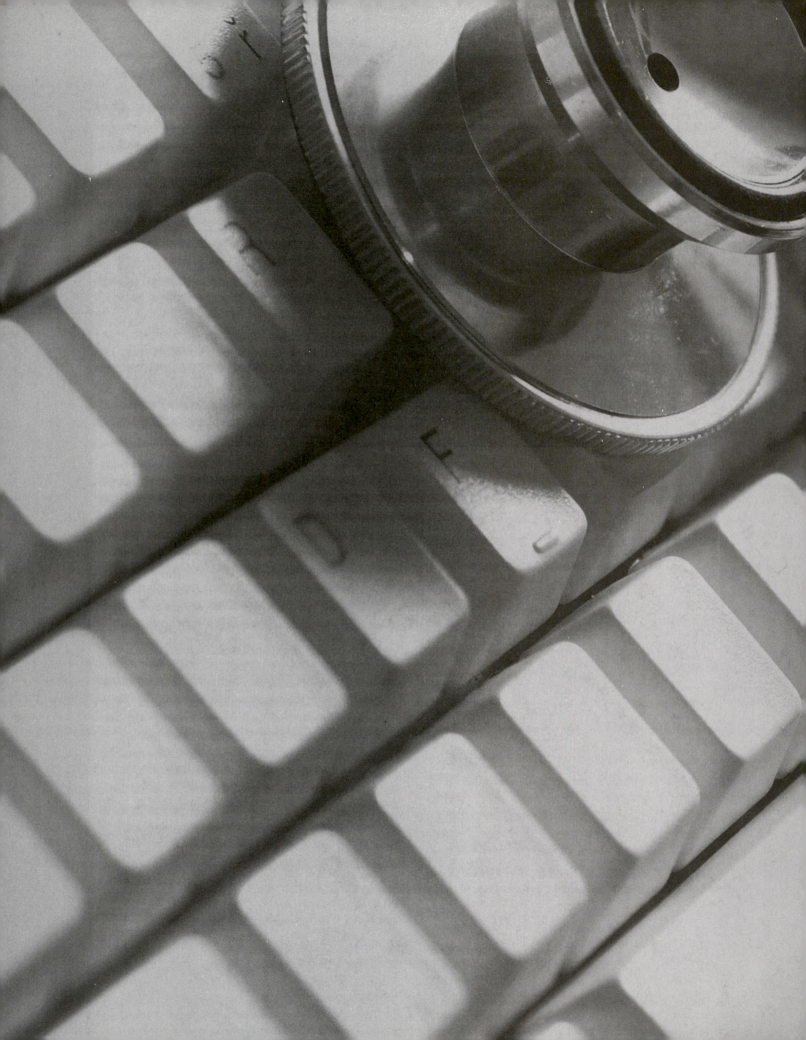

SPANISH GLOSSARY

Acreditación Proceso que confirma que un médico es quien dice ser.

Administración de seguridad y salud ocupacional (OSHA) Agencia federal que detalle los tipos de protecciones que los empleadores tienen que proveer a sus empleados expuestos a fluidos de pacientes, como sangre y orina, para protegerlos de la exposición.

Ajuste contractual Un valor cancelado después de la determinación del subsidio porque el proveedor está contratado con el asegurador.

Alcance de Práctica Trabajando dentro de las calificaciones de sus funciones de trabajo, según lo especificado por su formación o licencia.

Amplio enfocado al problema (EPF) Nivel de historia y examen que trata exclusivamente con la razón de la visita y ningunos otros sistemas de cuerpo.

Análisis de Mercado Examen del potencial para crecimiento local basado en el tamaño del mercado, tendencias, gastos, ganancias y potencial para nuevos clientes.

Anestesia Procedimiento para reducir el sentimiento de dolor durante un procedimiento.

Archivo de salud electrónica Archivo incluyendo la misma información administrativa, médica y clínica que el archivo tradicional de papel. Esto debe cumplir con todas las normas de privacidad HIPAA.

Archivo médico orientada al problema (POMR) Documentación de salud del paciente en el que se enumeran los diagnósticos para identificar qué condiciones están siendo tratadas.

Asesoramiento Una discusión con el paciente y su familia sobre el diagnósticos, tratamientos, opciones y riesgos. La información debe ser específica al problema presentado del paciente.

Asma Enfermedad que causa inflamación y estrechamiento de los pulmones y vías respiratorias.

Asociación americana de auxiliares médicos (AAMA) Organización que certifica a auxiliares médicos y mantiene su afiliación y educación continua.

Asociación americana de codificadores profesionales (AAPC) Organización que certifica a codificadores médicos y mantiene su afiliación y educación continua.

Asociación médica americana (AMA) Organización profesional que publica el manual CPT.

Asociación médica americana de la información sobre la salud (AHIMA) Organización que certifica a codificadores médicas y mantiene su afiliación y educación continua.

Auditoría El proceso de revisar lo que se facturó a la compañía de seguros para reembolso y asegurar que no hay fraude o abuso.

Autorización La aprobación de un servicio médico o procedimiento basado en la necesidad médica.

Aviso de Giro (RA) Declaración que contiene información sobre el servicio, fecha del servicio, código CPT, cargos, deducibles, coaseguros, copagos y pagos de seguros. También puede contener información sobre los pagos reducidos, o pagos negados si algo no estaba cubierto o pagado adecuadamente.

Aviso de privacidad Notificación al pacientes de sus derechos, informándoles como su información está protegida, con quién está compartida y como está almacenada o destruida.

Balance Resultado final del contabilización de gastos e ingresos de una empresa; se puede mostrar o una ganancia o una pérdida.

Caducidad de la cuenta Un informe financiero que identifica los saldos pendientes.

Cardiología El estudio del corazón y sus estructuras.

Cardiólogo Especialista del corazón y sus estructuras.

Carta de agradecimiento Carta en la que el solicitante debe dar las gracias a los entrevistadores para su tiempo y también debe reiterar por qué él o ella es el mejor candidato para el puesto.

Carta de presentación Introduzco un curriculum vitae. Debe dar referencia al fuente del oferto de empleo y comprimir una descripción breve de calificaciones, y incluso como el candidato cumplirá con los requisitos del puesto.

Cartera Una imagen visual de toda la educación, credenciales, logros, premios y habilidades del solicitante.

Centro de enfermería especializada (SNF) Centro de salud de 24 horas donde se tratan los pacientes que no necesitan atención hospitalaria por la noche.

Centro nacional de pruebas de habilidad (NCCT) Organización que certifica a profesionales de la salud aliada y mantiene su afiliación y educación continua.

Centros de cirugía ambulatoria (ASC) Donde practica procedimientos quirúrgicos el mismo día. No tiene comodidades para pasar la noche; necesita que dé de alta a los pacientes el mismo día.

Centros de medicare y medicaid (CMS) Agencia Federal que regula todos los aspectos de la asistencia médica, proveedores, instalaciones y servicios, así como archivos médicos, facturación y reembolsos.

Centros para el control y la prevención de enfermedades (CDC) Agencia federal que presta asistencia a centros de salud en proporcionar condiciones sanas y seguras a fin de evitar la propagación de la enfermedad.

Certificado de acreditación Permite a los laboratorios realizar las pruebas sometida baja la categoría renunciada y las que son clasificadas como PPMP—pruebas realizadas para médicos.

Certificado de cumplimiento Certificado de acreditación permite una facilidad a realizar las pruebas de medio o alta complejidad, y pruebas de las categorías renunciadas y PPMP. Esa última requiere que un laboratorio está plenamente acreditado, con un médico y patólogo.

Certificado de renuncia Permite al centro de salud realizar sólo pruebas baja la categoría renunciada. Un certificado de renuncia es vigente durante dos años. Una lista actualizada de pruebas puede ser encontrada en Internet.

Cirugía Especialidad para remover todo o parte de un órgano. Hay muchas especialidades dentro de la cirugía para los diferentes sistemas del cuerpo.

Cirujano Médico que ha tenido formación adicional en procedimientos quirúrgicos en condiciones estériles.

Clasificación Internacional de Enfermedades, 9ª revisión, Modificación Clínica (ICD-9CM) Conjunto de códigos diagnósticos. Puede ser o numérico o alfanumérico con 3, 4 o 5 caracteres, con un decimal después del tercer carácter.

CMS -1500 Un formulario de reclamaciones médicos usado para presentar servicios de consulta externa al aseguradora. El formulario recopila información personal, información de seguros, diagnósticos y procedimientos, así como la información de proveedor medico.

Códigos desagregadas Servicios o procedimientos en códigos incluidos que están separados y facturados por separado como códigos CPT o HCPCS individuales.

Códigos incluidos Códigos de procedimientos médicos que son incluidos en un procedimiento más grande, y no son permitidos ser facturados por separado.

Colecciones El proceso de conseguir ingresos al centro de salud, por pagos de seguros y pagos de pacientes.

Comisión conjunta Empresa independiente sin fines de lucro que establece estándares en la práctica y acreditación de lugares de cuidado de salud.

Compañía de Seguros Reembolsa al proveedor para los servicios y procedimientos.

Comprensivo Nivel de historia y exámenes que requiere una descripción extensiva de la visita.

Conexión de redes Juntar o reunir con otras instalaciones para compartir información y servicios entre sí.

Contenedor para objetos punzantes Producto utilizado para sellar agujas y materiales peligrosas, para evitar lesiones o la propagación de la enfermedad.

Contenedores de riesgos biológicos Los productos para cerrar medicamentos y equipaje para prevenir heridas o la propagación de la enfermedad, como contenedores de objetos punzantes (*sharps*) para agujas sucias.

Continuidad de cuidado En el contexto de cuidado continuando, el paciente tiene un registro médico, o en papel o en forma electrónica, a la oficina de su médico de familia.

Contratistas de recuperación de auditoría (RAC) Contadores de CMS cargados de auditar los centros de salud. Empezaron sus auditorías en los hospitales y se trasladaron a las oficinas de los médicos, auditando todos los aspectos de los pacientes de Medicare y determinar si habría fraude o abuso en la que el proveedor o centro de salud están involucrados: si hay, pueden llevar multas o penas de cárcel.

Controles de ingeniería Los dispositivos que se utilizan para cumplir con el plan de exposición. Puede incluir contenedores de objetos punzantes (*sharps*), sistemas sin agujas y agujas de auto aislamiento.

Controles de prácticas de trabajo Procedimientos utilizados para reducir riesgos de lesiones en el lugar de trabajo. Estos pueden incluir lavarse las manos, deshacerse de objetos punzantes, embalaje de muestras, servicio de lavandería y limpieza de las superficies y los materiales.

Coordinación de cuidado La participación de otros organismos o profesionales de la salud ya que contribuyen al plan de tratamiento del paciente, al pedido del proveedor de cuidado.

Credenciales Demostración de las calificaciones de un profesional médico.

Cuidado a largo plazo (LTC) Instalación de asistencia médica donde los pacientes son admitidos durante un tiempo ampliado para rehabilitación y recuperación.

Cuidado de caridad Pacientes sin seguros y abajo de un cierto nivel de ingresos.

Curriculum Vitae (CV) Currículum profesional: incluye una declaración objetiva y la educación, experiencia, licencias, credenciales y organizaciones profesionales del candidato.

Declaración de propósitos Identifica el propósito de la empresa u organización.

Dermatología Estudio de la piel y sus estructuras.

Dermatólogo Especialista de la piel y sus estructuras.

Descripción del Trabajo Explicación por escrito de las responsabilidades del empleado.

Detallado Nivel de historia y examen que requiere más información, pero no es comprensivo.

Determinación de cobertura nacional (NCD) Política unificada de Medicare para determinar si un servicio o procedimiento será cubierto bajo el CMS.

Deudas incobrables Deudas que no pueden ser pagadas, como en el caso de un paciente fallecido con ninguna finca. Cuando un equilibrio debe ser eliminado de la cuenta de un paciente permanentemente.

Deudas incobrables Pacientes que no han pagado sus facturas e no pueden pagar mismo con el uso de una agencia de cobros.

Directiva avanzada Una manera de generar información sobre el centro de salud con el fin de promover negocios futuros.

Elementos de diseño Artículos incluidos en el anuncio para atraer a los pacientes o clientes deseados.

Encuesta de análisis del mercado Lista de preguntas que pertenecen a los servicios y cuidado a pacientes ofrecido actualmente para el centro de salud, o que se puede ofrecer en el futuro.

Encuesta de paciente Encuesta enviado para averiguar lo que les gusta y no les gusta acerca del centro de salud, con el fin de mejorar el servicio.

Enfermedad Pulmonar Obstructiva Crónica (EPOC) Enfermedad progresivo de los pulmones, en que hay dificultad a respirar a causa de bloqueo de las vías respiratorias.

Enfermera anestesista titulada certificada (CRNA) Enfermera que se especializa en la administración de la medicación para la reducción de dolor.

Equipo de protección personal (PPE) Protege al empleado durante el tratamiento de los pacientes e incluye guantes, batas, mascarillas y gafas. Cuando fluidos corporales están involucradas en el cuidado del paciente, lo mejor cobertura que tiene empleado, la menor posibilidad de exposición.

Especialidad Tipo de tratamiento médico que se ocupa de las enfermedades y trastornos de un sistema corporal determinado.

Especialista Médico que tiene la educación adicional en un área específica.

Estación de lavaojos Equipo conectado directamente a un grifo existente, fácilmente visible y accesible, en caso de que hay accidente. Es diseñado para tratar agua en ambos ojos en el caso de una sustancia peligrosa que se obtiene en los ojos. Los ojos deben ser vaciados para 15-20 minutos o hasta que el empleado puede obtener más ayuda.

Evaluación comparativa Herramienta estándar en el sector para evaluar la eficacia de las prácticas del centro de salud.

Evaluación y manejo (E & M) Servicios incluyendo exámenes de oficina, visitas de hospital, visitas de consulta, gestión de caso y códigos de observación.

Evento centinela Un error o una acción que puede causar daños graves o la muerte a un paciente.

Examen Una revisión del área de cuerpo u órgano afectada así como otros sistemas de cuerpo afectados por el problema actual.

Explicación de beneficios (EOB) Declaración con información sobre el servicio, fecha del servicio, código CPT, deducibles, coaseguros, copagos y pagos de seguros. También puede incluir información sobre los pagos reducidos o denegado si algo no estaba cubierto o pagado adecuadamente.

Fecha de nacimiento (DOB) Fecha de nacimiento del paciente.

Fichas de datos de seguridad (MSDS) Formularios de empresas y proveedores médicos sobre materiales que podrían ser peligros si no se usan correctamente, incluso el alcohol, y incluyendo pruebas de los materiales.

Folleto Un aviso que proporciona información sobre una empresa, incluyendo la información de contacto y los servicios prestados.

Fuera del mercado Audiencia externa e individuos que no son pacientes actuales.

Gastroenterología Especialidad tratando con el estómago, intestino grueso y delgado, y boca al ano.

Gastroenterólogo Especialista en la medicina interna con formación adicional en el campo del estómago, intestino grueso y delgado, y boca al ano

Gerontología Especialidad tratando con la salud de mayores y condiciones normales y anormales del envejecimiento.

Gerontólogo Especialista con formación adicional en los procesos normales y anormales del envejecimiento.

Historia y física (H & P) Documento médico en que la paciente enumera toda la información necesaria a su llegada al departamento de ingresos o antes de un procedimiento. Esto incluye su información de salud anterior que se relaciona o puede afectar a la visita actual.

Historia Queja principal, una descripción del problema actual, una revisión de la historia propia de los pacientes, así como sus antecedentes sociales y familiares.

Hoja de día Papel en la cual los gastos y pagos del paciente fueron recordados.

Horas de Trabajo Requisito del personal para trabajar en la publicidad, usando métodos o internos o externos.

I-9 Una forma documentando información sobre la identidad y ciudadanía.

Identificador de proveedores nacional (NPI) Número de proveedores junto a cada código de procedimiento para identificar al proveedor médico. Los proveedores pueden los usar para identificarse con todas las aseguradoras, en lugar de números diferentes para cada aseguradora.

Intercambio electrónico de datos (EDI) Transmisión de documentación médica por medio electrónico.

Ley de acceso libre al información (FOIA) Permite el acceso a la información del Gobierno Estadounidense anteriormente prohibido.

Ley de mejora de laboratorios clínicos (CLIA) Aprobado para el Congreso en 1988, esta ley estableció las normas para todas las pruebas realizadas para laboratorios, incluso los de consultorios médicos, para asegurar la precisión, exactitud y puntualidad.

Ley de portabilidad y accesibilidad de seguro médico (HIPAA) Reglamento devolviendo al paciente el derecho de indicar cómo el centro de salud puede comunicarse con el paciente u otras personas.

Ley de Seguridad Social Asistencia federal dando un ingreso constante a los ancianos, pobres y desempleados.

Ley de tratamiento de emergencias medicas y trabajo de parto (EMTALA) Previene salas de emergencia o departamentos que participan en la asistencia médica de rechazar a pacientes pobres o no asegurados, o de transferir a pacientes antes de que ellos hayan sido evaluados para condiciones de emergencia y estabilizados.

Ley para Estadounidenses con discapacidades (ADA) Ley que prohíbe estrictamente todo discriminación en la contratación basado en invalidez, estado mental, niños, preferencia sexual, sexo, edad y raza.

Licencia Permiso de realizar responsabilidades de trabajo que demuestra la prueba de calificaciones y el seguimiento del proceso apropiado.

Listas de correo electrónico Direcciones electrónicas de los clientes y pacientes que se utiliza para transmitir información publicitaria.

Lugar de Servicio (POS) Ubicación donde se realizaron procedimientos.

Mantenimiento de archivos Documentación detallada de los empleados, incluidos de capacitación, e informes de lesiones como el registro de lesiones penetrantes. Es el método por el que OSHA justifica el cumplimiento y el centro de salud puede demostrar el cumplimiento durante una investigación.

Manual en Línea de Internet (IOM) Cambios recientes en el sistema de codificación HCPCS que puede encontrarse en Internet.

Médicamente necesario Diagnóstico que justifica los servicios y el procedimiento: el paciente solo será responsable para un monto de copago, deducible o coaseguro.

Medicare como política secundaria (MSP) Cuando un paciente tiene dos aseguradoras incluso Medicare, y el otro aseguradora es el primero a pagar.

Médico de Atención Primaria (PCP) Especialista que se ocupa de los trastornos comunes que afectan a todos los miembros de una familia, de los niños a través de los ancianos.

Mercadeable La publicidad cumple con las necesidades del público objetivo y tiene una respuesta exitosa.

Mercadotecnia Determinación si el centro de salud tendrá éxito en aquella área y como se puede hacer publicidad para promover sus servicios.

Metas nacionales para la seguridad de los pacientes (NPSG) Estándares diseñados para promover el mejor cuidado del paciente.

Modificador Código de 2 caracteres agregado al código de procedimiento para cambiar el significado.

Naturaleza del problema presentado Tipo de enfermedad, dolencia o condición con que el paciente ha presentado al centro de salud, y el nivel de intensidad necesaria en el tratamiento de la enfermedad, dolencia o condición.

Negaciones Reclamaciones de seguros rechazadas por un motivo concreto. Pueden ser cancelados o transferidos al paciente.

Neumología Estudio de las enfermedades y los trastornos de los pulmones.

Neumólogo Especialista en medicina interna y que tiene capacitación adicional en el área de los pulmones y sus trastornos.

Niveles de E&M Opciones de código de visita, en cual se determina la historia, el examen y la decisión médica y se elija el código apropiado según el trabajo implicado por el proveedor.

No participantes Un médico que no ha firmado un acuerdo con una aseguradora para aceptar un reembolso fijo.

Noticia de beneficiario avanzada (ABN) Manera de generar información sobre el centro de salud.

Objetivo Como parte del curriculum vitae, declaro el objetivo del individuo durante su empleo.

Oficina del Inspector General (OIG) Agencia federal que desarrolla proyectos en el área de auditorías y inspecciones de programa, investigaciones de fraude o mala conducta y resolución de fraude y casos de abuso. Cada año el OIG publica su plan propuesto en el registro federal.

Organizaciones profesionales Grupos sin fines de lucro de las personas con los mismos antecedentes educacionales, que hacen conexiones de redes para promover el ámbito de sus competencias y tener reuniones de educación continúa.

Orientación Reunión en que se dan normas y reglamentos al nuevo empleado.

Paciente externo Paciente que no está admitido, pero consigue tratamiento y deje el mismo día.

Paciente hospitalizado Paciente que es admitido al hospital.

Pacientes internos Personas que ya presentan al centro de salud para tratamientos.

Participando Médico que ha firmado un acuerdo con una compañía de seguros para aceptar una cuota de reembolso establecido.

Pediatra Médico que ha capacitado en esta especialidad. Debe ser consciente de todos los tipos de condiciones médicas y quirúrgicas para niños.

Pediatría Estudio y la práctica del crecimiento y trastornos de los niños, generalmente entre los recién nacidos y los adolescentes.

Plan de acción Una resolución del problema cuando ocurra, para asegurar que no volverá a suceder.

Plan de exposición Plan escrito que defina como el lugar de trabajo protege a sus empleados contra la exposición a patógenos transmitidos por la sangre. El plan expone en detalle que tipos del equipo son usados, y es mantenido al corriente cada año para reflejar métodos nuevos y más seguros.

Plan de Trabajo Plan escrito para proteger a los empleados de la exposición a materiales peligros.

Post operativa Período de tiempo después de un procedimiento en el que el proveedor tiene que cuidar al paciente como parte del procedimiento original.

Pre operativa Período de tiempo antes de que el procedimiento en el que el médico debe evaluar al paciente y asegurarse de que esta listo para el procedimiento.

Preguntas cerradas Proveen una respuesta de "sí" o "no" para obtener la información apropiada.

Presentación oportuna Período de tiempo en el que el centro de salud debe presentar una reclamación de procesamiento a la compañía de seguros.

Problema centrado (PF) Nivel de la historia y el examen únicamente enfocado a la condición o enfermedad de la visita.

Procedimientos de microscopía realizadas para proveedores (PPMP) Autorización de CLIA para realizar pruebas de laboratorio con un nivel de dificultad mediana y que requieren el uso de un microscopio por un proveedor autorizado.

Proceso en capas Pasos para la creación del formulario de reclamación. El primer paso es el registro de paciente, luego la visita y finalmente la presentación de la reclamación con procedimiento apropiado y códigos diagnósticos.

Proveedor Centros de salud que están bajo contrato con Medicare y están obligados a seguir sus reglamentos, así como aceptar la asignación de los reclamaciones.

Publicidad en los medios Utilizando los periódicos, la radio o la televisión para demostrar lo que ofreces y conseguir clientes o pacientes interesados.

Publicidad Una manera de generar información sobre el centro de salud a fin de promover negocios futuros.

Público objetivo Grupo de individuos que ven el anuncio.

Queja principal, Historia, Examen, Detalles, Medicinas, Evaluación & Vuelta (CHEDDAR) Documento médico con un formato especifico describiendo el problema del paciente, un informe breve, examen, y expectativas después de la visita.

Recepcionista Empleado quien saluda a los pacientes y les registran para sus citas.

Reclamación limpio Un reclamación de gastos médicos que se envía a la compañía de seguros sin errores y esta pagada a la primera presentación.

Redes sociales en línea Grupos que se crean en internet y permitan el intercambio de mensajes o blogs entre sí.

Registro Federal Publicación oficial diaria del gobierno que incluye el plan de trabajo OIG.

Registro Formulario con secciones múltiples que debe completarse la primera vez que un paciente acude a un centro de salud, incluyendo los datos personales y del seguro.

Remisión Proceso de notificación al aseguradora de procedimientos previstos, los servicios y la cirugía y obtener autorización para esos.

Rentable Publicidad económico para el centro de salud que contribuye al crecimiento de ingresos.

Renunciado Abstenerse de imponer restricciones sobre una prueba de laboratorio.

Resumen de alta Documento médico enumerando la información completa relacionado con el alta del paciente hospitalizado o externo, incluida la condición actual y planes para el futuro.

Seguimiento posterior a la exposición Dado a cualquier empleado que ha estado expuesta a materiales peligrosos, tales agentes patógenos de la sangre o cualquier otro tipo de líquidos. Después de dicha exposición, el empleado esta instado a buscar atención médica en función del tipo de exposición, que se debe controlar.

Seguridad Reglamentos que forman parte de la regulación HIPAA para mantener confidencial la información del paciente.

Sin Límite Preguntas de una encuesta que se permita explicar la respuesta.

Sistema de codificación de procedimiento común para cuidados a la salud (HCPCS) Código con 5 caracteres alfanuméricos que representa los procedimientos o servicios prestados a la paciente.

Sistema de pago prospectivo para pacientes ambulatorias (OPPS) Pago inclusivo al hospital para servicios de reembolso CMS.

Solicitud de empleo Una lista de información personal que les pidió al solicitantes para una puesta, durante o después de la entrevista.

Subjetivo, objetivo, evaluación y plan (SOAP) Documento médico que contiene información sobre la visita del paciente en un formato especifico, con las quejas, exámenes, resultados y expectativas futuras del paciente.

Suscriptor Persona asegurada.

Tecnólogo de información de salud (HIT) Profesionales involucrados con datos, comunicación electrónica, y documentación y codificación. Tienen formación a nivel técnico o universitario y conocimiento tan diverso como el informático, registros médicos y codificación.

Tecnólogos médicos americanos (AMT) Organización que certifica al profesionales de la salud aliadas y mantiene su afiliación y educación continua.

Terceros pagadores Tipo de seguro y la compañía con la que un individuo puede tener un plan de seguro. Procesará reclamaciones por servicios presentados.

Terminología procesal corriente (CPT) Código numérico o alfanumérico con 5 dígitos para identificar el procedimiento o servicio proveído al paciente.

Tiempo Contacto de cara a cara en el que el médico realiza una historia clínica, examen y aconseja al paciente y/o a su familia en cuanto a la problema presentado y el tratamiento.

Toma de decisiones médicas (MDM) Resultado final que implica el número de diagnósticos, la cantidad de pruebas e información para ser examinada, y el riesgo de morbosidad o mortalidad.

Triage Evaluación para dar prioridad a la urgencia de llamadas de teléfono y hacer decisiones apropiadas.

Unidades de educación continua (CEU) Horas de capacitación completadas después de certificación para mantener información y habilidades actuales.

Urología Estudio del sistema urinario y sus partes incluyendo la vejiga y los riñones.

Urólogo Especialista en enfermedades y trastornos del sistema urinario.

Vacuna contra la hepatitis B Vacuna para prevenir la Hepatitis B que debe ser disponible a todos los empleados dentro de un período de tiempo dado, por lo general aproximadamente 10 días.

Vinculación Mostrando la relación y la coherencia de los procedimientos, servicios y POS en el formulario de reclamación y justificándoles como médicamente necesario con un diagnóstico apropiado.

W-4 Formulario necesario por el empleador para que el impuesto federal correcto puede ser retenido del sueldo.

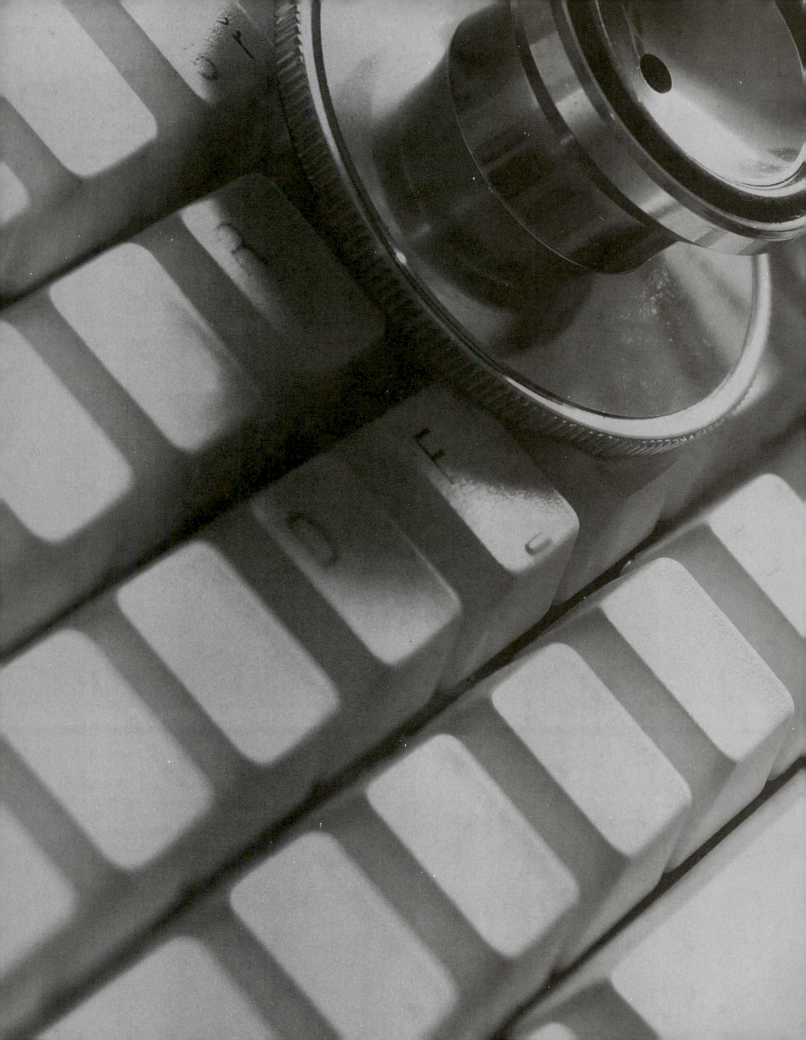

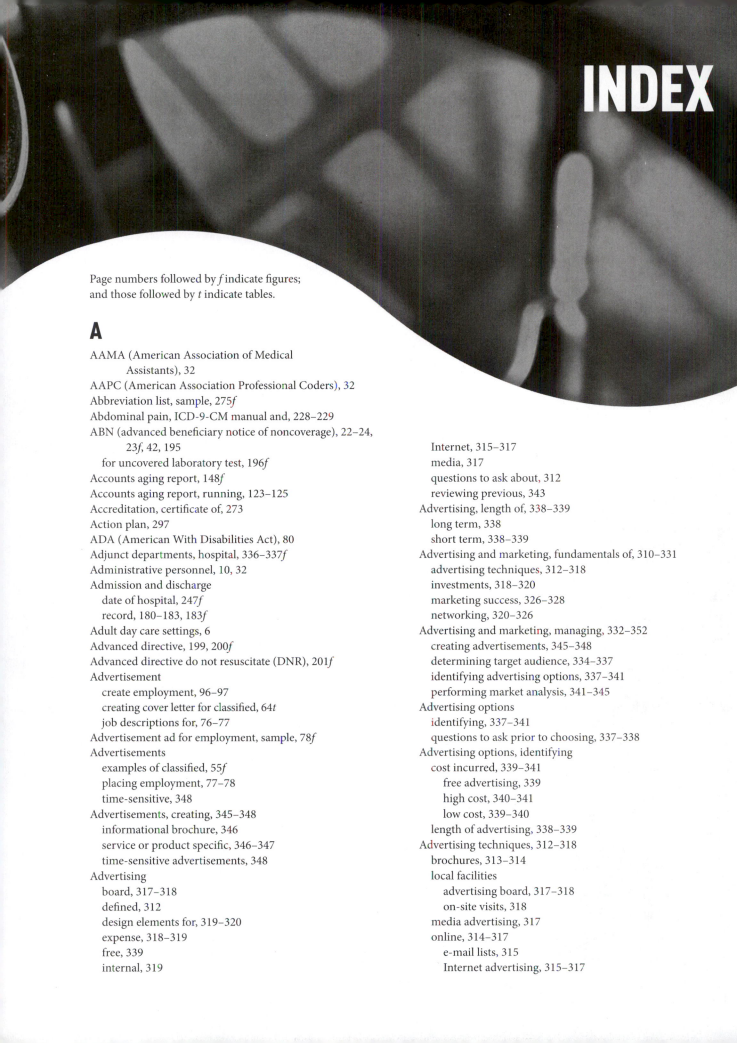

INDEX

Page numbers followed by *f* indicate figures; and those followed by *t* indicate tables.